Perceptual and Motor Development in Infants and Children

Third Edition

Bryant J. Cratty

University of California, *Los Angeles*

Prentice-Hall, Englewood Cliffs, New Jersey 07632

Library of Congress Cataloging-in-Publication Data

CRATTY, BRYANT J.
   Perceptual and motor development in infants and
children.

   Includes bibliography and index.
   1. Child development.   2. Developmental
psychobiology.   3. Motor ability in children.
4. Perception in children.   I. Title.
RJ131.C7 1985   612′65   85-25763
ISBN   0-13-657164-6

Editorial/production supervision: Mary Bardoni
Cover design: Lundgren Graphics, Ltd.
Manufacturing buyer: Harry P. Baisley

ISBN   0-13-657164-6   01

PRENTICE-HALL INTERNATIONAL (UK) LIMITED, *London*
PRENTICE-HALL OF AUSTRALIA PTY. LIMITED, *Sydney*
PRENTICE-HALL CANADA INC., *Toronto*
PRENTICE-HALL HISPANOAMERICANA, S.A., *Mexico*
PRENTICE-HALL OF INDIA PRIVATE LIMITED, *New Delhi*
PRENTICE-HALL OF JAPAN, INC., *Tokyo*
PRENTICE-HALL OF SOUTHEAST ASIA PTE. LTD., *Singapore*
EDITORA PRENTICE-HALL DO BRASIL, LTDA., *Rio de Janeiro*
WHITEHALL BOOKS LIMITED, *Wellington, New Zealand*

CONTENTS

PREFACE

An effort was made in this third edition to accomplish two goals. First, the book was updated to include current research information dealing with how children's movement behaviors change with maturation. The second, and most important goal, was to introduce several new and useful threads into the material and the thinking about motor development. It was with this second objective in mind that several content areas new to books on motor development were added to this edition. These include: (a) an overview of early neural changes, and how these influence the acquisition of movement capacities; (b) a chapter on motor learning—how learning and learning strategies are modified in younger and older children; (c) a section dealing with the way in which physiological capacities evolve throughout childhood and early adolescence; (d) a chapter dealing with various qualitative changes in movement development, including overflow, motor planning, reaction time, and rhythm; and (e) a discussion of the variables that negatively and positively influence early motor development. The book concludes with an overview of currently available evaluative tools.

In addition to the new material, several threads of thought are woven into the text. For example, the emphasis is on individual differences. Instead of becoming preoccupied with spurious assumptions about how "all" children must certainly throw a ball at the age of 6, data are presented that illustrate the wide range of qualities seen in children's movement behaviors at various ages. Contemporary directions in research have also provided useful new ways of looking at motor development. Examples of these new directions include modern views of how infants see, look, and perceive; the fascinating study of movement stereotypies; as well as the new research dealing with early social behaviors. Finally I have attempted to "operationalize" ideas and concepts by describing how they are measured, rather than simply employing ill-defined words and vaguely descriptive phrases. This focus on evaluation has permeated most of the text, as well as the final chapter.

Motor Development has been considered by many during the past decade or two as a rather sterile field, one in which new developments are not plentiful. However, I found the writing of this edition fascinating, as I explored the dimensions of movement reflected in the new material, as well as the interactions of other variables as they impinge upon the emerging actions patterns of youngsters.

Among the other fields of knowledge that have important relevance to the study of motor development are those of social psychology (studying play), cultural anthropology (exploring intercultural differences in childrearing), biochemistry (studying the effects of environmental stimulation on brain growth), ethnology (looking at rhythmic behaviors of animals and children), and linguistics (exploring how language and actions at play intermesh).

I am indebted to several people who helped with the content and production of the text. Larry Hawley, a professional photographer from Hollywood, California, produced many of the strobe pictures found in several of the chapters. Dr. Glen Glaesser helped in the review of the chapter dealing with physiological changes. The parents of 14 infants and children permitted me to photograph their offspring. I would like to thank these parents and their patient children. Esther Thelen and Jana Parizkova pemitted me to use data from their scholarly work. I hope they will be pleased with how I interpreted their findings.

This book is intended as a textbook for upper-division students in physical education, physical therapy, kinesiology, and elementary education. It may be used as a resource for courses in or students of child development, developmental psychology, dance therapy, nursing, and related disciplines. I hope that some of the hypotheses, substantiated and unsubstantiated, that are presented throughout the text will encourage energetic researchers to pursue some of the ideas that are only barely traced in the dirt at present.

B.J.C.

CHAPTER ONE
SENSORY–MOTOR BEHAVIOR AND DEVELOPMENT THEORIES, MODELS, AND SPECULATIONS

Since the early part of the present century, scholars have been speculating concerning the meanings of the movements appearing during the first days and weeks of human life. These observations have been backed up by increasingly sophisticated instrumentation. The earlier writings of Piaget, based upon penetrating observations derived from watching his own daughters as they developed, are being replaced by the more recent and equally creative work of T. G. R. Bower, Jerome Bruner, and others. They have used sophisticated measuring instruments that reflect such subtle behaviors as breathing patterns and eye blink rates, as well as other physiological and neurological evidences of changes in the infant's emotional and/or intellectual state.

Most writers have not concentrated solely on the manner in which beginning patterns of movement are generated in and of themselves, but rather have attempted to explore the antecedents of intelligence through the use of the most measurable behaviors available, voluntary action patterns. Some have also concentrated on the reasons for the movements shortly after birth. In this chapter two contrasting models dealing with the development of motor behaviors will be briefly explored.

The first is the traditional ideas of Jean Piaget, reflected in his formulation of the sensory-motor period and its six phases. The second model covered is a contemporary framework formulated by the author.

PIAGET

Perhaps no other man in the twentieth century has sparked more interest in the early acquisition of human abilities than the Swiss scholar Jean Piaget. The scope of his writings is immense, as is the library of books and monographs he has produced. His work encompasses the genesis of numerous facets of children's grasp of both the concrete and abstract concepts of their world.[1] If important criteria with which to judge the worth of theoretical speculations are the amount and quality of research they produce, Piaget's work readily meets the test. Hundreds of studies, monographs, and books have been stimulated by Piaget's penetrating discussions about the unfolding of the child's mind.

The Background to Piaget's Ideas

Piaget grew up in a family of scholars. He spent his early years in intellectual debate with his father, a history professor at the University of Neuchatel in Switzerland. Even during his formative years, he displayed a talent for carefully observing the processes of nature. His first published work, at the age of 11, was a brief article dealing with the behavior of an albino sparrow in a park near his home. This article attracted the attention of the curator of the museum of natural history in his town, Paul Godet. Piaget's friendship with Godet led to joint observations in the countryside near Piaget's home, and he continued to observe and record nature. His next publication, at the age of 16, dealt with the development of shellfish that inhabited some nearby lakes. His first books, written as a young man observing the horrors of the First World War, dealt with philosophical as well as natural issues. He argued the question as to whether the aggression he saw around him was an inherent and "natural" part of human behavior, or whether love was the more basic human trait. Piaget turned from philosophy and biology to psychology through a series of accidents. After writing a thesis on mollusks, he traveled to Paris, then the center for psychiatry. This exposure led Piaget to what he called "the clinical method," which involved the careful questioning of patients to discover the deep-seated sources of their confusions.

While he was in Paris, Piaget became acquainted with Theodore Simon, who had been a co-worker of Alfred Binet. Binet had died in 1911, and Simon had continued his work on standardized intelligence tests. Piaget accepted a position on this project. For the next several years he not only did work on test standardization, but more important, during the testing of children from 5 to 6 years of age, became interested in the deeper question of how intelligence unfolds. Piaget became intrigued by the nature of the "wrong" answers the children gave to questions on the tests. Using the clinical methods he had learned from psychiatrists, he probed immature psyches in an attempt to discover not only quantitative, but qualitative dif-

---

[1] A manageable survey for undergraduates has been produced by Ginsbury and Opper, *Piaget's Theory of Intellectual Development* (Englewood Cliffs, N.J.: Prentice-Hall, 1969). The review and critique by Cohen (1983) may also prove helpful.

ferences between the thinking processes of children and of adults. The titles of the articles he wrote during this period reflect his interest in the use of clinical methods, together with his awakening concern about the intelligence of children. These included "Psychoanalysis and Its Relationship to the Psychology of the Child," and "On Studying the Explanations of Children." He continued to be concerned about moral values, however, as articles such as "Psychology and Religious Values" attest.

Piaget quickly gained prominence as a young man. Recognition brought him an appointment to the University of Geneva, where he was later named director of the Jean-Jacques Rousseau Institute. In 1925 he married one of his students, Valentine Chatney. Together they began detailed observations of the development of two daughters and a son born to them during the latter part of the 1920s.

One of the conclusions Piaget drew from watching his children grow was the conviction that thought sprang from actions, and not from other sources such as language. Perhaps frustrated by his work with abnormal children, during which he attempted to assess them via verbal behaviors, he came to look upon the concrete manipulations of objects via the child's motor abilities as important clues to the quality of emerging intelligent behavior.

Several concepts proposed by Piaget at this time are reflected in his writings on the relationship between movement and intellectual development. A primary concept was his feeling about the term *intelligence* itself. In general, he held to a rather broad definition: He suggested that intelligent behavior was both a type of biological adaptation to an environment,[2] as well as evidence of attempts to bring about what he termed a "harmonious equilibrium" between environmental problems and objects and the child's "mental actions." He did not believe that intelligence was totally inherent, but that within the first days of life the child began to modify even simple reflex actions, evidencing the beginnings of mechanisms he termed "psychological structures." These structures were examined in some detail within the six components of what he called the early sensory-motor period.

Piaget employed several other words in an effort to illuminate how knowledge is acquired, and how the infant and the child adjust to the environment. He used the terms *correspondence* and *transformation* to explain intellectual unfolding. First, the infant and child may merely copy a tree when drawing it, for example. This is a case of simple *correspondence,* with no modifications by the child. With experience, however, the child may begin to draw trees of all types, with or without the presence of a model to copy. The latter, a more sophisticated level of functioning, is what Piaget termed *transformation.*

The terms *accommodation* and *assimilation* were used to denote stages through which a child passes as confrontations with new environmental events (objects, people) take place. The first stage is called *assimilation.* For example, on seeing a rattle for the first time, the infant grasps it in a manner previously learned for

---

[2]The phrase "biological adaptation" springs from his early background as a biologist; "equilibrium" was probably formulated from his interest in and study of physics.

getting hold of something. Later, however, the infant will begin to *accommodate* to the rattle and learn to shake it, first with effort and concentration, and then with apparently little effort or attention. Moreover, the infant and child often engage in both accommodation and assimilation at the same time. One object may be grasped, and even used, while another is being visually inspected, or assimilated. Accommodation (using the first object) occurs as a second object or event is being assimilated.

Through these complementary processes, the maturing human organism seeks to bring about a balance, or equilibrium, between itself and an environment composed of events and problems of increasing complexity, Piaget believed.

The Six Phases

The "action base" to the formation of intelligence Piaget divided into six primary phases, marked by behavior that at first includes simple "experimentations," primarily sucking, on the part of the neonate and progresses to more complex two-handed coordinations that signal the onset of more sophisticated intellectual behaviors. These six phases will be considered in the following paragraphs: the age ranges indicated are approximate.

Phase I.   Struck by the variations in sucking behavior in his own newborn children, Piaget characterized this phase (from birth to one month) as a time during which the infant shows both generalized assimilation of sucking to the nipple, and also differentiated responses involving sucking. That is, he noted that the so-called reflexlike sucking reaction, even during these early days of life, manifests itself in a variety of ways. At times the sucking seems to be motivated simply by the ability to suck! He suggests that this first phase is characterized by the infant's need to seek stimulation, to exercise variations in what simple capacities he or she possesses, and at the same time to manifest various kinds of accommodation as he or she learns to seek the nipple in a variety of ways. Thus, both "seeking responses" as well as sucking responses themselves assume a variety of forms during the first 30 days of existence. In recent experiments, contemporary researchers, whose work will be covered later, have further exploited the ability of the infant to suck in a variety of ways.

This first phase, like Phase II which follows, involves reactions to and about the body itself; it does not involve actions directed toward external people or things. These initial behaviors suggested to Piaget that a kind of self-actualization is beginning to occur, through the exercise and expansion of primitive psychological-behavioral "structures."

Phase II.   This second stage within the sensory-motor period, lasting from 1 to 4 months of age, is characterized by what Piaget terms "primary circular reactions." These behaviors, still centered about the child's body, involve attempts by the infant to discover how to repeat actions that initially (and often by accident) lead to satisfactory conclusions.

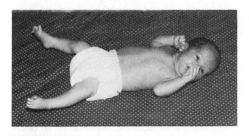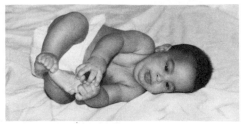

FIGURE 1.1 Primary circular reactions involve the infants own body. Sometimes the thumb, while at other times the feet may prove fascinating.

An expansion of response patterns also occurs during this second period. A child, for example, will tend to expand the sucking response to include thumb sucking, sucking nearby objects as the head is turned, and so on, rather than confining sucking efforts to the nipple. Bruner has noted further that during this period an infant may behave like a child evidencing athetoid tendencies.[3] Piaget, on the other hand, assumes that these are the child's awkward attempts to repeat a satisfactory action. The ability, first an accident, to bring the hand to the mouth, is another example of a primary circular reaction (see Figure 1.1).

Another behavior that appears during this second phase is a kind of perceptual readiness Piaget calls "primitive anticipations." A primitive anticipation would include a sucking response occurring well before the bottle or nipple is brought to the child's mouth.

Two types of behavioral characteristics also make their appearance during this period. These are (a) *curiosity,* a motivational point of great importance, evidenced primarily by visual searching behaviors of nearby objects (see Figure 1.2); and (b) *imitation.* The behaviors imitated during this period are necessarily primitive, and include the echoing of simple vocalizations, as well as of an adult figure's mouth movements with no accompanying sounds.

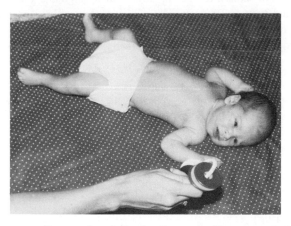

FIGURE 1.2 During this second period, curiosity makes an appearance, as the infant visually searches the nature of nearby objects.

[3]A type of cerebral palsy characterized by constant and relatively uncontrollable movements.

Phase III.   From the fourth to the tenth month, the infant continues to engage in circular reactions, but they begin to include objects external to his or her body. The infant starts to crawl and to manipulate objects of a variety of types; and to attempt to repeat enjoyable manipulative experiences with increasing precision (accommodation). It is interesting to note that Piaget views a chain of events (both actions and causal events in space) as operative and beginning at either end. Thus, he does not rule out the possibility that the child moves because previous movements have caused a dangling object to sway and make a noise, instead of in order to cause the object to make noise and sway. This kind of secondary circular reaction may be depicted as shown in Figure 1.3 and Figure 1.4.

Also apparent during this third phase, according to Piaget, is the presence of "partial reactions"; these are abbreviated movements involving the apparent awareness by the child that classifications of things exist which may not be fully exploited at all times. Piaget cites as examples of these signifiers the tendency to kick partially at a toy that has been previously dealt with in other ways, while not responding at all to unfamiliar toys. Most important, during this third sensory-motor stage, the child manifests the ability to differentiate between strong and weaker movement patterns. Cited as an example was the first chance striking of a chain by Piaget's son Laurent, followed by first a gentle tug and then by increasingly stronger and stronger attempts to swing the chain while grasping it.

A final kind of behavior seen during this period is what Piaget called "deferred circular reactions." These are signified by the termination of a reaching movement, with the later resumption of the movement, after a time delay. Thus, partial or incomplete movement schemas seem capable of being stored, at least for a short period of time, by the child.

Phase IV.   The final two months of the first year, according to Piaget, is a time for "coordination of secondary schemes." Unlike the previous stages, in which actions began as accidental behaviors, during this fourth stage the child seems to manifest intention, and then to try a variety of ways of reaching some goal—for example, grasping a matchbox held just out of reach. This child may evidence originality in attempts to reach some goal via the efforts of his or her own

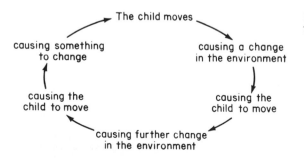

FIGURE 1.3 Secondary circular reaction.

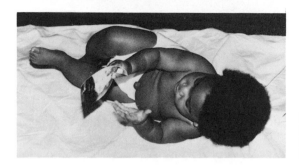

FIGURE 1.4 Circular reactions after the fourth month include the examination of objects external to the body as is happening here.

body; these original actions may not have had any direct or similar antecedents. Formation of original schemes is the hallmark of this fourth period and an extremely important type of event in the life of a child. It would seem to indicate that intention and thought become initiators of action, rather than an accidental movement and its result being instigators. Imitations of movements and tasks improve and refine themselves during this period. The simple anticipatory actions, seen initially in stage III, also assume more distinctive forms and manifest increasing precision.

Phase V. This fifth state (15 to 18 months) is also marked by an increasing variety of behaviors, actions which suggest the child is attempting to learn about the properties of objects he or she is manipulating. Thus the child learns that dropping a bar of soap produces results different from those achieved when a block is similarly released. These explorations in turn lead to a less conservative use of action patterns. Movements are increasingly productive in an exploratory sense, as most children are walking quite well by the beginning of this period.

New means are employed to attain a goal. The imitation of models is expanded to include movements that may not resemble closely those the child has been using previously. In addition, according to Piaget, at times the child's exploratory tendencies are so marked that accommodation takes precedence over assimilation. In other words, the child may evidence more pleasure in relatively brief and crude movement encounters with environmental objects for novelty's sake.

Phase VI. This final period is seen by Piaget as the bridge between sensory-motor behavior and intellectual endeavor. He suggests that children are fully aware and make that awareness known as they actively attempt to search for hidden objects, evidencing the importance of the emergence of thought independent of the sensory stimuli present. Moreover, actions are increasingly delayed, or postponed altogether, unlike the other periods, in which thought and direct and immediate action were often close companions. For example, a child, frustrated and/or confronted with a problem, manifests anger at a later time. It is this final period, lasting from about 18 months to 2 years, that Piaget suggests signals the end of the sensory-motor period and the beginning of cognitive behaviors.

Overview and Contemporary Evaluation

From 1920 to 1980, Piaget broadened his work, and its impact on American psychology was profound. The entire subfield of developmental psychology in the United States may be traced to the interest in Piaget's work which was translated in the 1950s and later. Piaget set about to formulate a system to explain problems that had plagued philosophy and philosophers for centuries. Many Americans of his generation studied only minute portions of human behavior within tightly controlled laboratory settings that usually included a maze and a near-by cage of rats. Piaget, like Europeans before and since, painted theories and models in broad, philosophically rich strokes.

At the same time, Piaget was not the deity that some of his contemporary biographers would have us believe. His insights, while profound, were like those of all of us, at times constricted by the limitations of time and energy, and by the society within which he studied infants and children. Moreover, some have suggested that his ideas were not always subjected to the critical scrutiny of those surrounding him in the institute, where he was known as *le patron,* the boss.

During the past three decades scholars have begun to scrutinize closely some of the ideas in the writings of the prolific Swiss philosopher-psychologist. Some of these questions have been focused on the methods used by Piaget and on the restricted cultural environment in which he formulated his theories about intellectual development.

Other critical reviews have contrasted basic assumptions made by Piaget with research data from the laboratories of others who began to study infants more closely in the 1960s and 1970s. Some of these writers have examined some of the primary ideas Piaget held about the orderliness of the stages through which infants purportedly pass from egocentric infancy to cognitive adolescence. During recent years, useful questions have been arising about various hypotheses found within Piagetian thought and theory.[4] Some of these contemporary insights are useful for those interested in the "movement component" within the unfolding personalities of infants and children. Among some of these recent elaborations upon, and contradictions of, Piagetian theory are the following.

The Infant: A Social Isolate?   Piaget painted a picture of early infancy that excluded social influences. Developmental substages within the sensory-motor period were believed to take place during what Piaget termed an egocentric phase of development.[5] Social influences were ignored both in early sensory-motor development and in later intellectual phases. Evidence from carefully arranged experimental studies of infants' responses conducted since the 1960s, however, more than

---

[4]These critical reviews range from the questions posed by Flavell in the 1960s (Flavel, 1962), to more penetrating efforts at Piagetian analysis carried out by Donaldson in the 1970s (Donaldson, 1978) and Cohen in the 1980s (Cohen, 1983) and include useful experimental tests of Piaget's notions about stages in object acquisition and exploration (Willatts, 1984).

[5]Actually, Piaget believed the infant to be "solipsistic," the most extreme form of egocentricity.

suggest that the child almost from birth is not only socially responsive, but initiates and stimulates the social behaviors of others (see Chapter 13).

Fantz, for example, finding that infants spend a great deal of preferential visual behaviors scanning the details of the human face, suggested that there may be innate structures within the brain of the neonate that are somehow "wired" to respond to the appearance of others (Fantz, 1961). Infants and their mothers rather early in life begin what Cohen has described as a "ballet of interaction" (Cohen, 1983). For example, when Trevarthen (1972) brought infants into the laboratory and separated them by glass from their mothers, 3-month-olds were found to use smiles, noises, and looks to engage in nonverbal social conversations with their mothers. The common game of peek-a-boo is found in all cultures in which it has been searched for. Although initiated at first by adults, by the twelfth month of age infants will begin the game without any prompting (Bruner, 1977).

Piaget, as a result of his observations, claimed that children did not play together at all before the age of 4½, nor could they engage in conversations with others before 5½ years. But Rosenthal (1982) found that babies of only 3 *days* of age made different vocalizations when their mothers were present than when they were absent.

Piaget thus paints a picture of early learning which suggests that infants and young children acquire knowledge as the result of rather solitary interactions with and interpretations of various aspects of the environment. The role of social stimulation and learning seems to be ignored. Even as late as 1975, in his dialogue with the linguist Noam Chomsky, Piaget declared that a child learns not by imitating a person, but by using gestures that reflect the nature of an object. He explained that if a child is presented with an object containing a hole, he may imitate the hole. Piaget thus seemed to reject the possibility that even speech may be acquired through social imitation (Cohen, 1983).

Not only were the social and cultural influences impinging upon individuals not considered within Piaget's speculations, but possible differences in the manner in which children and infants from various cultures may learn were also neglected. Piaget somehow believed that the orderly stages of development he identified within his own children within the culture of Switzerland in the 1920s was somehow reflective of the levels through which infants the world over inevitably must pass.

The Nature of Experience, Interaction, and Manipulation. Critical to the central thrust of this model is Piaget's view of what he terms the genesis of intellectual development: action. In the vast majority of phrases that are used in his writings to describe action, it is clear that motor manipulation of the environment is what is meant. Several writers have said that one of the primary weaknesses of Piaget's theory is that he leaves the concept of experience vague (Cohen, 1983; Brown & Desforges, 1979).

Piaget believed that action, or specifically manipulative efforts, during the sensory motor period are important precursors to even primate cognitive operations. One of the most important milestones in intellectual development was believed by

Piaget to consist of the infant's ability to form mental representations of objects not directly seen (or touched, or heard). Evidence of this quality of what he termed *object permanence* must, according to Piaget's experiments, be confirmed through actions taken by the infant. The infant must be cognitively aware of the presence of a hidden object, and must then reach, grasp, and remove its covering in order to confirm this knowledge.

Piaget's naturalistic research, conducted in the nursery of his home, required his own children to make ever more intricate movements, graspings, and manipulations involving the precise movements of the arm and hand. It was only through these action-based behaviors that he believed evidence of the unfolding intelligence was demonstrated. However, more thorough explorations of the abilities of infants since the early 1970s have brought to light the fact that infants, even before they acquire precise manipulative behaviors, can indeed behave as if they know previously seen objects continue to exist even when screened from view. That is, object permanence can be demonstrated even if the infant does not actually engage in physical interactions with the environment. Tom Bower, for example, found that infants of 4 months would visually follow the pathway of a ball once it had disappeared behind a screen (Bower, 1973).

Throughout the 1970s, Bower and others employed physiological responses made by infants in order to determine whether or not they were surprised when objects were made capriciously to appear and disappear under and in back of coverings. These measures consisted of fluctuations of heart rate, respiration, and the like that purportedly accompanied surprise reactions by infants a few weeks of age and older. Generally the results of these studies indicate that infants are indeed aware of hidden objects, and of the pathways moving objects took, even when parts of their trajectories were hidden from view. This awareness of objects, and the expectation that hidden objects would reappear, indicate that infants, well prior to gaining the ability to remove obstacles themselves through their own efforts, were well aware of the continued and sustained existence of things, even without continually keeping those things in view.

The heart rates of babies in these studies predictably reflected surprise when objects were made capriciously to appear and disappear, independent of the infants' direct physical contact. These results suggested that (a) cognitive qualities could exist and be measured independent of intentional actions engaged in or possessed by infants, and (b) that many of the cognitive qualities believed critical by Piaget occurred far earlier in life than his theorizing suggested.

Other data continued to point out rather vividly that thought, even in infancy, can exist independent of action, or even of direct sensory experience. Bower and Wishart (1972), after permitting babies to interact manually with various toys, plunged their laboratory into darkness. Using an infrared camera, it was found that even at 2 to 4 months of age, infants continued to engage in searching behaviors independent of the presence of vivid sensory cues given off by the desired objects.

The rigidity of the position that only through action can one learn would seem to fly in the face of the evidence of the adequate to superior mental abilities possessed by many children who may lack adequate movement capabilities. At the same time Piaget's position about the centrality of human action in the learning process undoubtedly has pleased several generations of movement educators. It is not hard to locate self-congratulatory passages in the books written by physical educators and others who, like Piaget, believe that movement is the basis of intelligence.

There are glimmerings, however, even in the writings of *le patron* himself, which suggest that what Piaget termed *action* is a broader concept than the simple muscular contractions that move bone on bone. For example, he seems to insist that meaningless actions will not lead to learning in a passage in which he states: "Action . . . is only constructive when it involves the spontaneous participation by the child . . . it is necessary that they [children] form their own hypotheses and verify them through their own active manipulations" (Piaget, 1973). What Piaget has sometimes referred to as "messing about," according to one critical review, actually requires mental representations of the actions taking place in order for true learning to take place (Murray, 1979). Furthermore, co-workers of Piaget seem also to be intent upon clarifying what is meant by action as the term is used by Piaget. Inhelder, Sinclair, and Bovet write that "being cognitively active does not mean that the child merely manipulates a given type of material. He can be mentally active without physical manipulation, just as he can be mentally passive while actually manipulating objects" (Inhelder et al., 1974). Murray (1979) also alludes to the notion of "mental actions" as he reviews Piaget's ideas (Murray, 1979, p. 174).

In the main, however, Piaget leaves no doubt in the vast majority of his writings that he never changed the beliefs he adopted in the 1920s about the imperative nature of movement in learning. His belief that thinking starts with action perhaps contributed to the appeal his theorizing has had. For after all, what Piaget talked about could be seen and thus verified by the senses of the teacher, researcher, and parent. But that same rigid insistence that thought starts with movement, instead of with thought itself, may well be a major weakness of the Piagetian model of intelligence.

Other shortcomings have been pointed out by contemporary critics. Piaget's serious children seem to be continually engaged in deep and logical thought. However, careful analyses of the components of human thought by Czimenthalyi (1982) reveal that little more than 10 percent of a child's time is taken up with cognition and problem solving. Children become angry, they laugh, and they use their imaginations in ever quickening ways as they mature. And yet Piaget's archetype seems to be rather emotionless, having little time or energy for the arts, for feeling, or for random daydreaming.

Piaget was careful not to assign his various stages and substages to exact chronological ages. He was inflexible, however, in that he clearly believed children must pass through each stage, in precise order, before successive levels could be reached. Cohen (1983) and others have reviewed a great deal of experimental evidence that infants and children often seem to ignore the need to pass through "lower" stages before exhibiting relatively sophisticated signs of intellectual competence. Gelman (1982), for example, writes about "pockets of competence" that reflect instances of mature thought processes in infants and children at ages far younger than Piaget declares such competencies will occur. Zajonc (1979) has proposed the concept of *hot cognitions,* or thoughts that are highly influenced by intense emotion. It is difficult to reconcile the notions of both Gelman and Zajonc with the carefully plotted stage theory of Piaget. Indeed, some have expressed wonder at how a Piagetian child is able to pass so quickly from intellectual neophyte to full-blown theoretical physicist between the ages of 6 to 14, as Piagetian theory suggests is possible (Cohen, 1983).

Thus the feelings of many contemporary observers about Piagetian theory, including those of this writer, are ambivalent. *Le patron* is viewed by most as a great stimulator, the impetus for a whole generation of experimenters and model builders in developmental psychology. He was a teacher of careful observational methods. He asked simple questions, while providing answers that were filled with philosophical insight. Historically, he provided a refreshing new breeze through the whole of psychology, which seemed stalled between Freudian vagueness and the sterility of American behaviorism during the first half of this century.

At the same time, many of Piaget's notions today seem constrained, if not quaint. Cognitive theory is perhaps not quite ready to produce a formula for a cognitive theory of development, but when it comes, its tenets may be difficult to reconcile with the simple notion that action breeds thought. The idea that action begets thought may be an attractive one to some movement specialists, but they need to look at the cognitive approach taken by many developmental linguists. Rather than insisting that language begets thought, they believe that thought is a stimulator of language. I believe a more rational idea than that action produces thought is that thought, action, verbal behaviors, and perceptual activities stimulate and interact in intricate ways. This more expansive concept is portrayed in the second model in this chapter.

THE DIFFERENTIATION AND INTEGRATION OF BEHAVIOR:
A PICTORIAL MODEL

This second model was formulated in an attempt to depict the manner in which the abilities of the human infant seem to mature. It presents a "picture" of just how specific abilities may diffuse, collect together, and otherwise interact in the maturing infant, child, and adolescent. The model suffers from the fact that it is presented in only two dimensions, whereas motor behaviors and the other behaviors alluded to are multidimensional in nature. Further shortcomings of the model include the exclusion of extensive reference to motivation and/or emotion as possible instigators and/or blunders of performance, as well as the omission of discussion of *how* the behaviors present unfold as maturation takes place.

This model is in some ways similar to the theorizing of Piaget. Both models describe the simultaneous processes of integration and differentiation, while both indicate how complicated skills may be builtup from subskills.

There are major differences, however, in the two theoretical approaches to the emergence of human behaviors. Piaget emphasizes the imperative action-base to the formation of intelligence; whereas in this second model it is proposed that perceptual, intellectual, verbal, and motor abilities appear early and simultaneously in the personality of the infant. Piaget's model is a fully developed theory, whereas this second model presents simply a picture of the emergence of abilities as a function of age. Piaget deals carefully and in depth with learning, while this second model does not. Piaget outlines a "stage" theory, whereas this second model outlines mutually interdependent stages of abilities. This second model is based upon research using correlational and factor analytic techniques, whereas Piaget's ideas are based upon naturalistic observations. And finally, Piaget's model does not account well for how atypical populations may develop, particularly those lacking adequate movement attributes; whereas this final model, through the use of the concept of "selective blunting," is more applicable to a variety of atypical groups of children and youth.

Many theories of child development contain stage models that consist of a number of reasonably discrete horizontal layers. The model presented here is more like a lattice. It encompasses several concepts. The idea of bonds formed horizontally between various channels of development interacts with the idea that the evolution of various vertical classification abilities is at times uneven in nature. An attempt has been made to explain the way in which both the normal and the atypical child mature, as well as the way in which educational programs may modify unfolding attribute patterns.

A theory has been defined as an attempt to explain and thus to predict. A theory of human behavioral development, then, is an attempt to explain and to predict the ways in which the infant and the child change as a function of age. A model, on the other hand, may be viewed as an outline or skeleton of a theory. The extent to which this attempt to construct a viable "skeleton" for the study of processes of human maturation is successful may be judged by reference to the research literature, as well as by the sensitive observation of children engaged in both thought and action.

Upon consulting the research, it appears that the child's behavioral patterns evidence both diffusion and integration.[6] The processes of diffusion and integration occur simultaneously at times. To explain these processes, several terms have been employed. An *attribute* may be defined as a cluster of scores in similar tasks denoting a relatively specific ability trait. The phrase *classification of ability traits* has also been used to refer to a group of ability traits that are relatively similar. Four general classifications are dealt with in the pages that follow: the motor, the percep-

---

[6]The theory is based on various measures of behavior to be found in the literature, with particular emphasis on factor analyses. Additional research studies have been consulted in an attempt to evaluate the manner in which experience modifies behavior.

tual, the intellectual, and the verbal. As the model unfolds, it will become apparent that these four "simple" classifications become increasingly fragmented as a child ages.

Because of the focus of the text, the emphasis is on explanations dealing with the interrelationships between the motor and perceptual classifications. However, since cognitive processes are important when trying to gain a comprehensive understanding of the growing child, references to cognition and verbal behavior are made at several points in the discussion.

The second important term in the model is *bond*. It is suggested that, owing to a number of variables, bonds are formed between various facets of the child's behavioral attributes. These bonds are conceived of as functional connections between attributes that in the child's life have previously been operating independent of one another. The formation of a bond may often signal the emergence of a new ability trait within a larger classification of attributes.

Another term in the discussion that follows describes the manner in which attributes may be retarded, terminated, or otherwise reduced in efficiency or in the incidence with which they occur. It will thus frequently be stated that certain conditions may *blunt* some attribute or classification of attributes.

The term attribute is used often in the conceptual schema that follows. In this context, an *attribute* is taken to mean an ability trait reflected in a score obtained from a test of motor, perceptual, verbal, or cognitive functioning. Separation of motor, perceptual, or verbal from cognitive attributes is of course difficult, and indeed the theory has as one of its primary tenets the bonding of various different ability traits in the performance of a new type of task, reflecting an emerging attribute. At the same time, it is possible to determine whether a score derived from a given task is *more* indicative of an individual's verbal ability, movement competence, ability to organize and to interpret sensory information, or ability to think. Most of the time some kind of verbal and/or motor response is required when testing subjects in various kinds of batteries, but the motor response (checking a yes or no answer) is often incidental to the validity of the score obtained.

The outline that follows is presented in the form of axioms and the postulates derived from these axioms. After each of these generalizations is drawn, examples taken from the research literature, as well as from observations of the behavior of children, will be presented.

AXIOM 1   Attributes emerge and mature at various rates, and at the same time overlap in time. These attribute "families" may be classified as cognitive, verbal, motor, and perceptual (Figure 1.5).

In general, it appears that efficient visual behaviors precede the acquisition of motor accuracy, and that these two classifications in turn are followed by the acquisition of verbal competence coupled with cognitive abilities. A child first becomes able to track moving objects using both eyes together for short periods of time during the first weeks of life. Not until several months later, however, can a child be

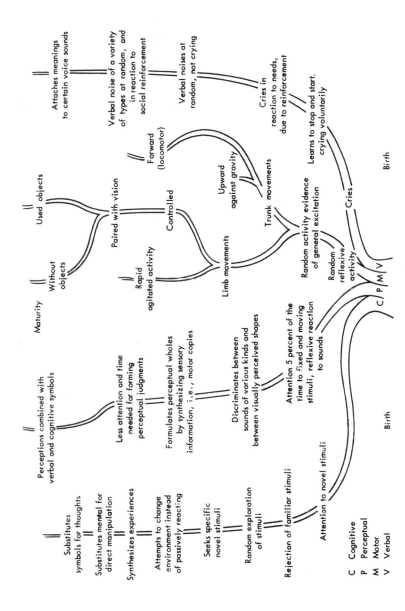

FIGURE 1.5 Four attribute channels illustrating examples of behaviors each contains, as well as the manner in which each tends to branch as a function of age.

15

expected to evidence motor behavior accurate enough to enable him or her to intercept a toy swinging on a string by using a crude swiping motion of the hand. The
child will probably not call the object thrown to him or her a ''ball'' until about 2
years of age, and an understanding of the laws of motion governing the trajectory of
a thrown missile may not be evidenced until adolescence.

> *POSTULATE 1 . The rate of change shown by a given classification of attributes
> varies at different times in the life of the infant and child.*

The greatest change in visual perceptual abilities and in perceptual abilities
coupled with motor attributes occurs early in the life of the child, from birth to the
seventh year. On the other hand, verbal behavior, reflected in vocabulary increase,
shows marked acceleration from the second to the eighth year of life.

> *POSTULATE 2   The change in a given classification of attributes, which may be ex-
> pected through the efforts of others such as teachers and parents, will be most pro-
> nounced at the time of the child's life during which those attributes are in the greatest
> state of flux because of normal maturational processes.*

The causes for this proliferation and differentiation are partly programmed by
the genetic make-up of the child.

Learning experiences also play a role; while as Bower has pointed out, both
the physiochemical environment as well as their psychological environment may
exert marked influences in what and how the infant and child learns and performs
(Bower, 1979). It is thus becoming increasingly apparent that gene expression and
learning, as well as what is termed *epigenesis,* contribute in interacting ways to the
development of the child. Untangling the relative contribution of each of these
groups of causes remains a formidable undertaking.

> *POSTULATE 3   Exercise of one's capacities may be motivating for its own sake, in-
> dependent of any apparent material reward for performance.*

Children acting as subjects in innumerable experimental studies and taking
part in a variety of educational programs have been observed to continue to perform
tasks in the absence of any obvious reinforcers other than mastery of interesting
tasks that test their capacities.

> *POSTULATE 4   Success perceived by the child elicits exercise of groups of attributes
> and thus is likely to result in marked changes in levels of performances within a given
> classification. Lack of success leads to less participation in tasks, which in turn is
> likely to blunt the performance levels of tasks requiring those abilities.*

In a study carried out several years ago, we found that groups of atypical children, who evidenced mild coordination problems and who were likely to be aware
of the degrees of ineptitude they evidenced, demonstrated performance in late childhood that represented their best efforts. After the ages of 12 and 13 years they were

performing as a group at levels similar to the proficiency evidenced in early childhood. It was apparent that a syndrome of failure was reflected in our data: There was withdrawal of exercise of abilities and a resultant lack of proficiency in perceptual-motor tasks (Cratty, 1966).

AXIOM 2   As the child matures, the number of individual and relatively independent attributes evidenced within a given classification of abilities will tend to proliferate.

At birth, the child cannot move his or her hands with precision. The neonate generally shows birth reflexes in the hands, as well as rapid and inaccurate "thrashing movements" of the arms and hands reflecting general excitation. Later, ability to deal with objects "branches," and the child evidences two important abilities: the manipulation of objects, and the making of marks with objects, such as scribbling with crayons.

By either the end of the second year or the beginning of the third, this scribbling again branches into two subattributes: relatively free movements of the arms, and the growing tendency to draw accurately. Geometrical figures appear in drawings. Again, in the fourth year the ability to draw geometric figures subdivides: The child begins to draw letters and numbers, and continues to draw geometric shapes.

Later in childhood, geometrical figure drawing continues and becomes more complex, while at the same time the simple circles and squares come to represent faces and houses. The child's effort to print continues, but he or she will also evidence another branch, that of cursive writing. In late childhood the inclination to translate cognitive symbols into the written word may take the form of typing.

Big muscle activity undergoes this same process of division as a function of maturation. At birth the child is generally either active or inactive. Upper limb movements soon become observably different from leg and trunk movements. The latter subclassification of movements begins to separate into those showing that the upright is being sought and those involving some kind of movement forward in a horizontal place. Following the acquisition of walking behavior, the child begins to devise innumerable ways of moving forward.

Evidence of this kind of differentiation of abilities can be found in literature as early as 1946, in a study which analyzed intellectual test scores (Garrett, 1946). Other research, notably that by Dye and Very in 1968, as well as by Kalm in 1970, also alludes to this differentiation of mental abilities. The tendency of motor abilities to become more specific as a function of age has been apparent in the literature for the past decade (Rarick and Dobbins, 1975). Broadhead et al. (1985) have recently summarized this work and confirmed the tendency for motor abilities to become more discrete and differentiated as a function of age.

This process of division of attributes as a function of maturation, using two subclassifications of motor abilities, is depicted in Figures 1.6 and 1.7.

POSTULATE 1   Severe and/or moderate intellectual deficits are likely to impede the proliferation of attributes and to render the total attribute structure less specific and complex.

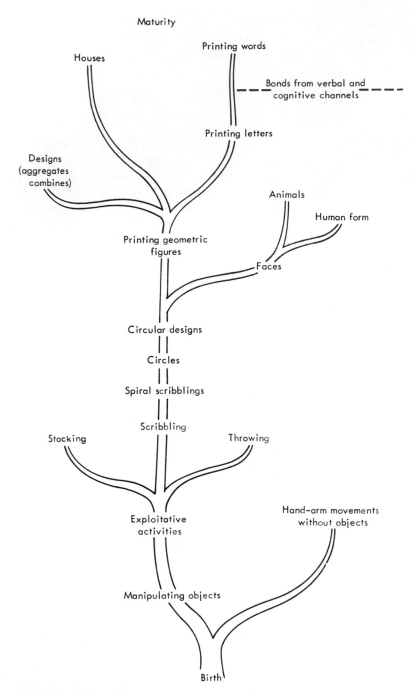

FIGURE 1.6   A detailed examination of the manner in which the attribute channel containing arm, manipulative, and drawing abilities tends to diffuse.

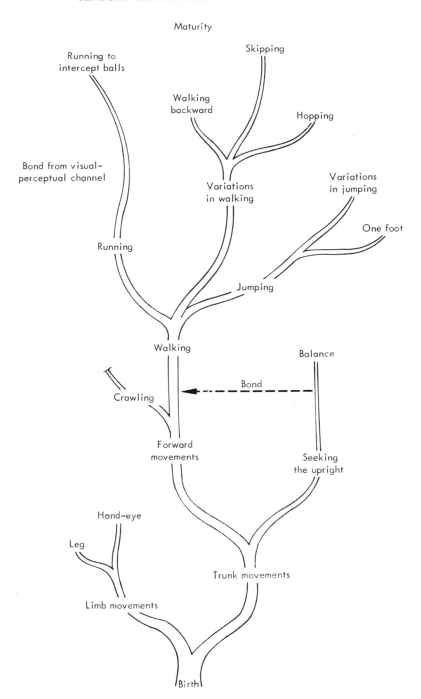

FIGURE 1.7 The differentiation, diffusion, and bonding that occur within the attribute branch containing locomotor and trunk behaviors.

Studies of retarded children indicate that the lower on the intellectual scale performances are sampled, the more likely are high correlations between performance traits. It has been hypothesized by more than one researcher that retarded children's ability trait structures stop becoming diffuse by the age of 10. On the other hand, as normal children continue to mature, they evidence an attribute structure indicative of increased specificity and complexity (Cratty, 1966).

AXIOM 3   A "blunting" either of a total classification of attributes or of individual attributes may occur for a variety of reasons.

POSTULATE 1   If some subattributes within a classification are found to be relatively ineffectual in coping with the environment, they may tend to disappear or to be evidenced very seldom as the child matures.

Simple arm waving due to excitation by the presence of an object is likely to disappear from an infant's motor ability repertoire as more effective uses of the hands and arms can be found. Crawling gives way to effective means of locomotion as the child acquires the upright and learns to walk.

POSTULATE 2   Moderate and severe sensory, motor, and intellectual deficits may tend to blunt or accelerate another classification of attributes, depending on the type and the severity of the defect.

The child with moderate motor problems may tend to compensate by seeking scholarly outlets for his efforts. However, if the motor problem is serious enough, efforts to coordinate the hands when writing may be so constrained as to make much classroom work either difficult or impossible.

The child who is born blind, in the absence of cognitive deficits, will tend to learn about space in other ways. Results of studies of the blind show that there are close relationships between measures of kinesthesis, manual competencies, and scores gained from tasks involving spatial orientation of the total body (Juurmaa, 1967).

POSTULATE 3   Not only does there seem to be an optimum time for the insertion of educational experiences to elicit the most improvement in an attribute or group of attributes, but the reverse also seems to be true.

The extent to which some kind of environmental or nutritional deprivation is likely to affect an attribute or classification of attributes negatively is dependent on the time in the child's life during which this deprivation occurs. When the negative factor is inserted, the greatest blunting of ability is likely to occur during that time of life in which that attribute or classification of attributes evidences the greatest amount of change caused by normal maturation processes (see Chapter 2, "Brain Growth Spurt").

Thus, cortical cell proliferation is likely to be more negatively affected during the early months of life by dietary deficiencies. If the child experiences a similar deprivation of nutritional intake later in life when the growth of the central nervous system has stabilized, little or no nervous system damage may occur.

The early deprivation of normal visual experiences is likely to produce more marked changes in the infant's visual-motor behaviors than if this occurs later in life. If the infant is permitted to move when capacities for action mature, any early deprivation of movement experiences will not exert a marked effect on motor development (Dennis, 1938).

POSTULATE 4   An overexercise of a group of attributes may tend to blunt the emergence of ability traits within another classification or to delay their appearance to some degree.

The hyperactive child is likely to have learning problems because an overzealous exercise of movement capacities may block intellectual growth to some extent. Early enriched visual environments may tend to delay slightly the beginnings of hand-eye coordinations. The contemplative infant may appear relatively immobile in the play yard.

AXIOM 4   Many attributes within several channels, particularly those involving an observable response, may be "taken over" via mental functions as a child matures. A child may become able to "mentally manipulate" the environment without the need for direct experience after he or she has stored a number of types and classifications of experiences.

Contemplative babies between the ages of 15 and 18 months have been found to evidence better intelligence later in life. One important criterion of intelligence may be the appearance of this more efficient type of coping behavior (Bayley, 1968).

Kilpatrick, Judd, French, and others have identified the ability of individuals to formulate perceptual judgments via analytical processes (thought) without the need for direct action. Even animals (cats) have been found to be able to learn escape problems through observation, rather than through physical practice (French, 1965; Judd, 1908; Kilpatrick, 1946).

AXIOM 5   As maturation proceeds, innumerable bonds are formed between previously independent attributes residing within the same or within separate classifications. At times, this pairing signals the emergence of a new attribute within a classification of attributes (Figure 1.7).

As visual regard becomes bonded to crude voluntary hand movements, visually monitored manipulative and rudimentary drawing behaviors are triggered. Later, as the maturing child is increasingly confronted with the necessity of catching balls, previously formed abilities to track moving objects and to run become welded together, and he or she is able to anticipate and to intercept the missiles.

As the child becomes able to draw more precisely in later childhood and early adolescence, previously acquired and little used abilities to scribble may again be "called up" and employed to depict shadows and shadings in landscape drawings.

POSTULATE 1   At times a bond may be formed between three or more attributes in different classifications. This bond may not become established between all three attributes at the same time in the life of a child (Figure 1.8).

POSTULATE 2   Some bonds formed early in life may become less distinct with disuse as the child matures or disappear entirely when their continuance may tend to impede efficient functioning.

Several of the important bonds pairing movements with vision formed early in the life of the child will become less distinct. Visually directed walking is important to the child of 1 and 2 years, but is of little use to the child of 4 and 5.

POSTULATE 3   At times, the problem of the educator is to aid the child to form useful bonds between previously unassociated attributes and at other times to aid in terminating useless bonds.

The child, when beginning to draw and to write, may need aid in pairing movement with vision. On the other hand, when learning to walk, he or she may need to be aided to watch the goal ahead rather than to watch the alternative placement of the feet.

As a child first learns to read, lip movements representing vocalizations of the words are paired with attempts to decipher the printed page. However, in the normal child, these will usually "drop out" when it is found that reading speed will be impaired and/or that the reading speed tends to exceed the ability to match the slower lip movements with each word.

The young child, and later the older individual, may need to watch the hand as it approaches, contacts, picks up, and returns the water glass to the mouth. This type of commonly performed task is seldom accompanied by the same degree of visual monitoring when performed by the older child, adolescent, and adult in the middle years of life.

The child of 5 or 6 similarly needs to observe every constant hand movement when learning to write, whereas adolescents and adults pay considerably less attention to each movement of the pen when doing the same kind of task.

POSTULATE 4   The educator at times must aid in the formation of bonds that would not normally be formed in order to enhance the emergence of a given set of attributes.

The author has formulated a program of total body movements that have been found to aid a number of cognitive operations and classroom skills (Cratty, 1969). Montessori and others have utilized a variety of sensory experiences to aid children in acquiring concepts of weight, size, texture, and the like (Montessori, 1914). These types of programs may prove inefficient with the normal child who may be quickly and easily forming subtle cognitive bonds between various classifications of

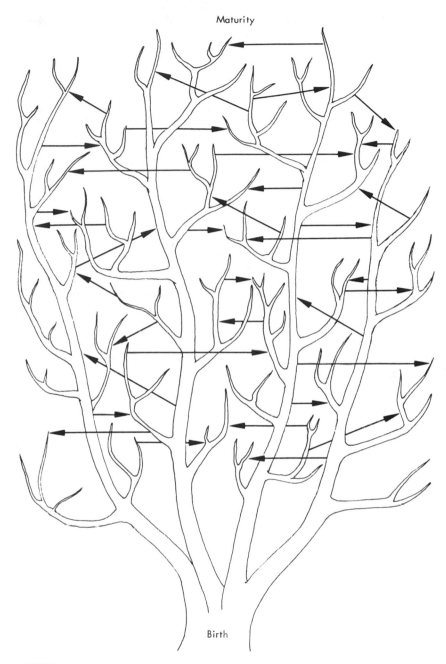

FIGURE 1.8 A schematic representation of the attribute channels and the bonds that tie appropriate abilities together.

stimuli and may not need this kind of ''artificial'' bond building. The atypical child, on the other hand, is often in need of programs that lead toward the enrichment of associations between cognitive, perceptual, motor, and verbal activities by using ''new routes.''

> POSTULATE 5   The formation of one bond leads to the formation of other bonds. The formation of bonds between facets of behavior proceeds in a reasonably orderly manner in normal children.

A child usually crawls before he or she walks, and on walking will engage in a variety of modifications of locomotor activity. A child must see his or her hand prior to using it, but once the child begins to use it in primitive ways, he or she soon discovers innumerable variations of manipulative behavior in which he or she may engage.

> POSTULATE 6   Failure to form a bond may be due to a lack of appropriate prolifer- ation within classifications of attributes between which the bond must be formed, to a lack of cognitive ability to perceive relationships, to a lack of experience at observing others, to a lack of motivation, and/or to a lack of appropriate educational experi- ences.

If a helpful bond is not being formed in a child, it should be determined whether perceptual, cognitive, motor, or attitudinal deficits or some combination of these is present. The 3- and 4-year-old child may not evidence efficient drawing behavior forming a visual-manual bond because he or she (1) may not feel that it is important (attitude); (2) may not have observed other individuals drawing or may lack drawing implements at home (cultural deprivation); (3) may not realize that it can be done with crayons and pencils (cognitive), or (4) may lack the ability to guide the hand visually on a reasonably accurate course.

> POSTULATE 7   The bonds formed by a child may be basic, necessary for survival and for efficient performance for all children within a culture. On the other hand, a bond may be unique to an individual. Both types of bonds are formed in children under most circumstances.

As a normal child matures, more unique bonds are formed as experience be- comes more specific. It must be determined in atypical children which bonds are important to form—that is, which bonds are basic and which bonds are less impor- tant. Early in life, a child forms bonds between classification of attributes that ena- ble him or her to walk; to think through basic processes, such as to remember items in a series; to write, and to form verbal connections to common objects, move- ments, and situations in the environment. Unique bonds would be connections formed, for example, as the son of a naturalist learns the names of various water- fowl.

POSTULATE 8   The effectiveness of educators, of curriculum developers, and of parents when attempting to deal with children lies in the facility with which they can identify those bonds that are dependent on other bonds. In the life of a normal child, various types of bonds and the manner in which various subattributes may be expected to appear within a given classification of attributes should emerge.

POSTULATE 9   At times educators must aid a child to strengthen bonds between facets of behavior that may be indistinct because of some kind of maturational delay or sensory-motor or cognitive deficits or because of lack of practice.

AXIOM 6   With maturation and the evolution of intelligent behavior, the child will quickly become able to select from the several clusters of attributes at his or her command those that will enable him or her to deal effectively with situations. The facility with which the child "calls up" attributes may be an important index of intelligence and emotional stability.

There is less time delay between the presentation of stimuli and the appropriate reactions by older people than there is by younger people. Learned response patterns are more quickly reacted to than are new response patterns. Several authors have cited the development of efficient work methods as important to efficient motor and perceptual-motor performance, as are basic movement and perceptual capacities.

POSTULATE 1   With maturation, the "calling up" of appropriate attributes is carried out with less and less conscious effort. Exercise of capacities and learned experience results in efficient selection of appropriate work methods from a storehouse of attributes.

The theory outlined could be elaborated on by reference to the expanding literature in neurology, and in particular by texts such as those by Konorski (1967) and by others who have attempted to relate neurological function to behavior. Konorski utilizes the concept of bonds formed between various components of the human personality; however, his theoretical assumptions are more static and at the same time are more global than the assumptions contained in our model. Hebb's concept of cell linkages, written years ago, as well as John's exposition of contemporary molecular trends in biochemistry of neural functioning, also offer physiological and anatomical support for the statements made here (Hebb, 1949; John, 1967).

It is believed, however, that a model of the type sketched here may rest simply on supports formed by data collected from various studies of *behavior,* and that it need not be made more "respectable" by allusions to neurological "models," which in themselves are to a great extent speculative in nature. Rather, the attempt has been to formulate a series of statements that weld themselves into a cogent and rational raft of thought. It has been said that the worth of a theoretical tenet may be assessed by consulting the evidence that has inspired it, as well as by inspecting the quality of the research that, in turn, has seemed to provide the impetus. My purposes will be served if the reader, after reviewing the previous paragraphs, is encouraged to engage in either endeavor.

The model outlined in this last part of the chapter differs in several ways from the stage theory postulated by Piaget. The evidence upon which it is based involves more than the observational data obtained by Piaget. Most important, however, is the assumption within this lattice-work theory that sensory-motor performance is not an imperative base from which perceptual, cognitive, and linguistic qualities must arise. This latter model does not assume motor primacy, but rather that one must consider the fluctuations, consistencies, and inconsistencies of all kinds of abilities from birth onward if one is to truly understand the developmental process. Development involves both consistencies and inconsistencies, as Clarke has recently pointed out (Clarke and Clarke, 1983).

Moreover, an action-based notion of the developing intellect fails to account for the presence of intact cognitive operations within populations of children who may display less than adequate movement qualities, including cerebral palsied children (Holman and Friedman, 1959), congenital amputees (Robinson and Tatnall, 1968), and thalidomide children (Decarie, 1969).

SUMMARY

The lattice-work model described here is based upon the supposition that maturation is a parallel interaction between various aspects of the unfolding personality, rather than a stratified appearance of horizontal stages. Generally the model rests upon data obtained in contemporary work dealing with early cognitive qualities in infants, as well as upon information emanating from factorial studies of human abilities (Clausen, 1966; Cumbee, 1954; Fleishman, 1964; Kalm, 1970; Rarick and Dobbins, 1975; Smith and Smith, 1966; Broadhead et al., 1985).

Further research should attempt to determine the manner in which unique attributes emerge in the several classifications as the child matures. There are few factorial studies employing children under the age of 5 as subjects, and I am not aware of an extensive and detailed research program in which the emergence of various factors of either perceptual or motor ability traits have been studied as a function of sex and of age.

The manner in which bonds are formed between various attributes in children is a topic that has been studied by educators for years. The concept of bond formation utilized within the previous paragraphs is similar to the concept of learning used by many behavioral scientists.

The clinician may also gain some guidance from a careful consideration of the theoretical pronouncements within this final section. It is believed that, to successfully modify the behavior of both normal and atypical children, those wishing to bring about change should be aware of the complexities of human development and the numerous variables that modify this development. Grasping at naive theoretical guidelines may result in the formulation of simple-minded and ineffective curricula.

QUESTIONS FOR DISCUSSION

1. Discuss Piaget's concepts of assimilation and accommodation. Differentiate between the two concepts, and give concrete examples for each term.
2. Contrast Piagetian theory with regard to the sensory-motor period of life with the model of human attributes. What would each approach imply when formulating a motor development program for normal and/or atypical children?
3. What does Piaget mean by secondary circular reactions? Give several examples of this kind of chain of events.
4. Discuss the concept of diffisuion of attributes, as outlined in the model.
5. Discuss and give examples of the concept of "bonding" found in the model of attributes.
6. What implications might the model of attribute change have for the education of the child who is somehow different from his peers?

STUDENT PROJECTS

1. Observe an infant within the first four months of life, and attempt to identify some of the behavior referred to by Piaget as occurring during the sensory-motor period of life. Within what specific stage does the infant you observe seem to be?
2. Throw a ball, from some distance, to some 5-year-olds. Observe the manner in which they coordinate watching the ball, moving their body to its arrival point, and/or placing their hands in proper position for the catch. What implications can you draw from your observations relative to the concept of bonding?
3. Using a child from 6 to 10 months of age, study his or her reactions to objects first shown, and then hidden. Discuss the reactions in relation to Piaget's concepts regarding object permanence. Observe the same reactions in the family dog to objects first shown and then hidden. What conclusions can you draw from contrasting these two types of observations?
4. Observe a young infant watch and swipe at a stabile hanging over the crib. What conclusions can you draw in relation to Piaget's concepts of primary and secondary circular reactions?
5. Discuss with parents of the child about a year old the manner in which he or she attempted to learn to walk.

CHAPTER TWO
NEUROLOGICAL
BEGINNINGS
OF MOVEMENT
CAPACITIES

The complex movement capabilities discussed in this book stem from a variety of neural processes having their genesis before birth. At from two to three weeks after conception, specialized cells that will form the nervous system are seen to differentiate from those cells that will make up the skeletal-muscular systems and the other organ groups of the body. These cells migrate together, forming a neural plate, a structure that soon folds, making a groove. This folding continues until the edges meet, making a cylinder. The early migration of cells is called *gastrulation;* the formation of the cylinder is called *neurulation* (Figures 2.1 and 2.2).

The formation of the structures in the central nervous system are dependent upon and reflected in three major types of processes. At the cellular level, the constitution, size, and location of cells change. With time, the cells migrate, finally coming together to form functional neural pathways and structures. Second, the overall appearance and bulk of the nervous system undergoes change. The appearance of the brain itself changes from a smooth organ to a complex one as surface convolutions appear. Its size and weight increase due to the addition of neural cells and of supportive or *glial cells*. Third, in a healthy fetus, neonate, and infant, the muscular and bony systems develop their capacities to move as nerve structures and pathways join them in intricate ways.

Neural development and the acquisition of these neuromotor connections and integrations represent a process that is continuous from conception to death. The

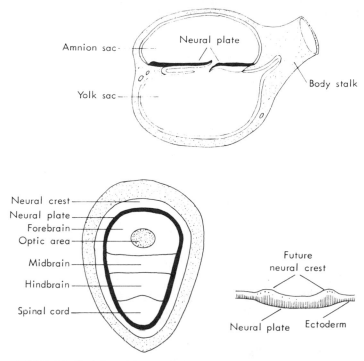

FIGURE 2.1   Depiction of the neural plate and its early subdivisions prior to the formation of the neural groove and channel. From W. M. Cowan, "The Development of the Brain," *Scientific American, 241* (1979), p. 114. With the kind permission of W. H. Freeman Publishers.

entry of the human into the world at birth represents only a shift of environments, rather than a radical change in the developmental patterns of the nervous system. Processes that accompany changes in the constitution and location of the cellular makeup of the nervous system are closely interwoven with the more observable changes in the brain size and action capacities of the developing fetus.

It is the purpose of this chapter to survey some of these interrelated dimensions of early maturation that, if thwarted, are likely to impose either subtle or profound limitations on the child's later abilities to move with precision, speed, and force.

EARLY BEGINNINGS

The formation of the neural plate undergoes a folding during the third and fourth weeks after conception (Figure 2.1). The upper end of the tube widens to form the ventricles (cavities) of the brain. The peripheral nervous system comes largely from the cells of the neural crest and from the nerve fibers that will leave the lower part of the brain at each section of the spinal cord. By the fourth week, the neural tube is

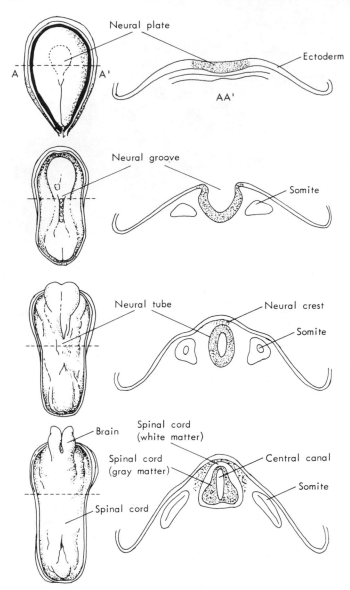

FIGURE 2.2 The closing of the neural groove. The nervous system's beginnings, about 18 days after fertilization. The future spinal cord is seen in the bottom cross-section. The early formation and changes in somites are also shown. From W. M. Cowan, "The Development of the Brain," *Scientific American, 241* (1979), p. 116. Reproduced with the permission of W. H. Freeman Publishers.

completely closed and covered with a skinlike ectoderm. At this time it also becomes separated from the amniotic space. During the fourth week, as the canal is formed, cube-shaped somites are seen (Figure 2.3). These somites later contribute tissue to bony portions of the skull and to the musculature and bones of the spinal

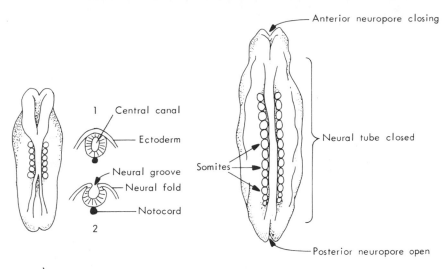

FIGURE 2.3 (a) Neurulation, a back view of a 24-day embryo's canal during the initial closing of the neural folds. (b) The neural tube largely closed, with the exception of the anterior neuropore, depicted as open in this drawing. The posterior neuropore at the bottom of the drawing will close slightly later. With permission from R. E. Lemire, et al., *Normal and Abnormal Development of the Human Nervous System,* New York: Harper and Row, 1975.

cord itself. By the thirtieth day of gestation, thirty-eight pairs of somites appear, and six more pairs are added later. Failure of the neural tube to form during these early weeks will result in an aborted fetus, or abnormal conditions seen after birth, such as spina bifida.

The three main parts of the brain, the forebrain, midbrain, and hindbrain, originate from prominent swellings at the end of this neural tube. In the human infant, the cerebral hemisphere will later overgrow the hindbrain and midbrain and partly obscure the cerebellum at the time of birth (Figure 2.4).

Also during the fourth week, the beginnings of the arms and legs are apparent. From the fourth to the eighth weeks these rudimentary arm and leg "buds" evolve into more recognizable appendages, which begin to separate into fingers and toes (Figure 2.5).

The fourth week also marks the beginnings of movement by the fetus as the heart begins to beat. Movements of other muscle groups do not begin until the fourth month, when the nervous system begins to acquire myelin sheaths. During these early weeks and months of life, individual rudimentary masses of muscles may react to specific and localized stimulation. This type of twitching to stimulation applied directly to a muscle is termed *myogenic movement.* It is not, however, until the nervous system is more mature, at about the fourth and fifth months, that the fetus will respond to stimulation from "messages" carried by the nervous system. This mature type of action is called *neurogenic movement,* meaning that it has been generated from a source other than the muscle itself and has been transmitted by the nervous system in some manner.

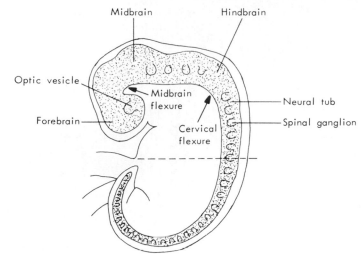

FIGURE 2.4 A side view of the embryo at about 28 days after conception, showing the initial bendings or flexures that are beginning to become subdivided into the primary divisions of the brain. Also seen are somites that later become portions of the spinal cord and cranium. From K. L. Moore, *The Developing Human*, 3rd ed. Philadelphia: Saunders, 1982. Reproduced by permission.

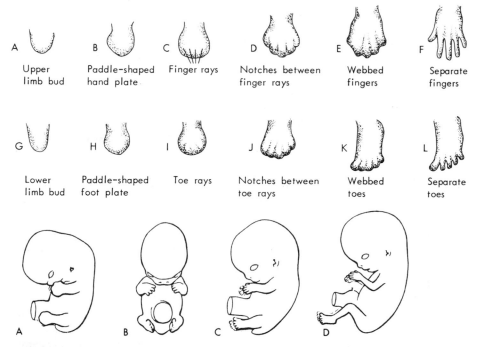

FIGURE 2.5 (a) The beginnings of the development of the hands, feet, and limbs, 28 to 32 days after conception. The formation of the hands slightly precedes that of the formation of the feet and toes. (b) Limb formation and their positions relative to the trunk from A, at about 40 days after conception, to D, at about 56 days after conception. From K. L. Moore, *The Developing Human*, 3rd ed. Philadelphia: Saunders, 1982. Reproduced by permission.

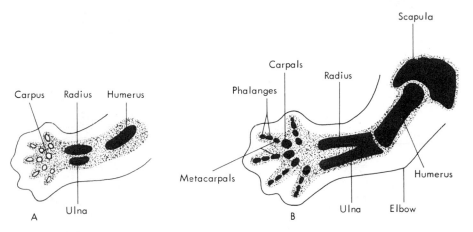

FIGURE 2.6 (a) The embryo at about 28 days, showing the early appearance of the limb buds, and the beginnings of cartilage models of the bones that will later appear. (b) Arm formation at about 40 days, showing more completed models of the various bones of the upper arm. From K. L. Moore, *The Developing Human,* 3rd ed. Philadelphia: Saunders, 1982. Reproduced with permission.

By the eighth week the rudimentary beginnings of all essential neuromotor structures and organs are present, and the *embryonic period* ends. The *fetal period* then extends from the ninth week to birth, and is characterized by the growth and elaboration of neuromotor connections, structures, and pathways. The overall appearance of the infant changes in the ways shown in Figures 2.8 and 2.9.

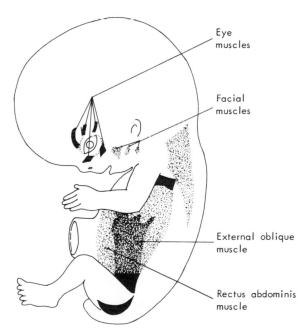

FIGURE 2.7 The appearance of the first, dissociated, musculature of the trunk at about eight weeks after conception. From K. L. Moore, *The Developing Human,* 3rd ed. Philadelphia: Saunders, 1982. Reproduced by permission.

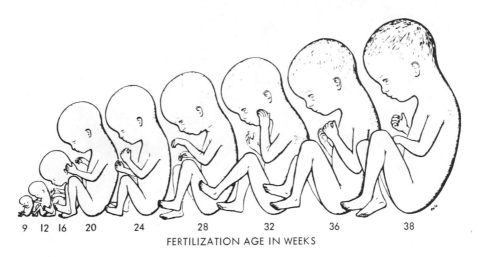

9 12 16 20 24 28 32 36 38

FERTILIZATION AGE IN WEEKS

FIGURE 2.8 Changes in the appearance of the fetus from the end of the embryonic period at 8 weeks until the end of the fetal period and birth, which normally occurs at the 38th week. From K. L. Moore, *The Developing Human,* 3rd ed. Philadelphia: Saunders, 1982. Reproduced by permission.

During the next weeks and months, three important types of changes take place. These include the enlargement of and increasing functional sophistication of the brain itself. Marked changes also occur in the cellular makeup of the nervous system. These changes are accompanied by the functional maturation of the bones

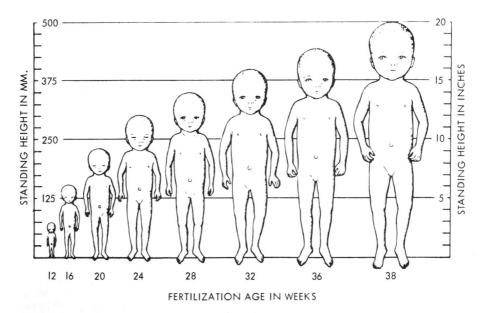

FERTILIZATION AGE IN WEEKS

FIGURE 2.9 Proportional changes in the segments of the fetus's body, head, and limbs from the 12th to the 38th weeks. From K. L. Moore, *The Developing Human,* 3rd ed. Philadelphia: Saunders, 1982. Reproduced by permission.

and muscles needed to engage in movement. The neurological bases of these changes are surveyed in the sections which follow.

THE DEVELOPING BRAIN

The three main parts of the brain are seen forming as early as the second and third month (Figure 2.4). However, after that time the size and appearance of the brain changes rapidly (Figure 2.10). Convolutions do not appear on the surface of the

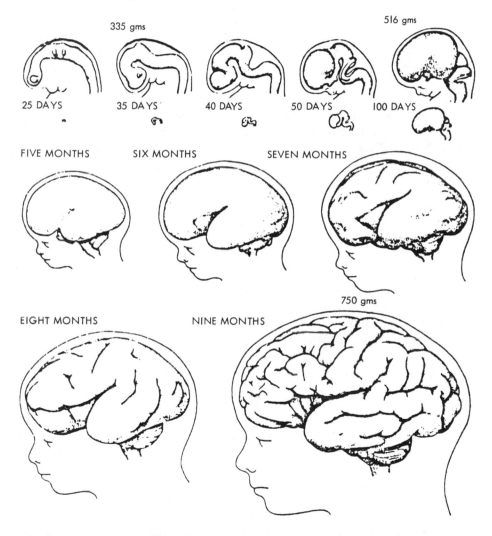

FIGURE 2.10 Changes in size and appearance of the brain from 25 days to birth. From W. M. Cowan, "The Development of the Brain," *Scientific American, 241* (1979). Reproduced with the permission of W. H. Freeman Publishers.

cortex until about the middle of the fourth month, and increase rapidly after that time. These convolutions result in the unseen portion of the brain's surface becoming approximately twice as great as the area that can be viewed at the time the child is born.

During the latter months of gestation, the weight of the brain changes rapidly due to several kinds of simultaneously occurring processes. (a) There is an increased growth of the spines of the dendrites. (b) There is an increase of blood vessels within the brain. (c) There is a rapid increase of the cells which support the nervous system, the *glial* cells. (d) There is an increased amount of myelin coverings around the various structures.

Neurons are generated by the developing brain at the rate of about 250,000 a minute! It has been estimated that at adulthood the total number of brain cells present numbers about 100 billion. The size of the brain continues to increase after birth, weighing about 1,000 grams at the age of two years. During this time, the area of the cortex devoted to movement, the *motor cortex,* continues to increase in size. Other parts related to movement also expand, including areas devoted to the regulation, formulation, and storage of motor programs.

Portions of the brain devoted to the storage of motor programs, the *basal ganglia,* become distinguishable deep within the cortex at about the 36th week after conception. However, these and other structures undergo maturation well after birth.

At the age of 5 years, the various cellular layers of the motor cortex are well differentiated. The brain's weight at about 6 years of age is often that of the average adult (1,350 grams). However, numerous important milestones of the maturation of the brain continue into early and even middle adulthood.

All portions of the brain, however, do not mature at the same rate. Nerve pathways that tie brain function to movement also do not mature on an even and similar schedule. For example, pathways that interact with the motor system mature before some pathways carrying sensory information to the brain. It seems as though nature is preparing the organism to move before equipping it to obtain accurate information from movement receptors and from other sensory end organs.

This principle of motor primacy before birth does not mean that the sensory systems are nonfunctional during prenatal development. Different parts of the sensory system mature before and after birth. In general, reflex capacities come before sensory development, while structures needed to control voluntary movements mature later.

This uneven development of the various systems, both motor and sensory, is evidenced in the various ways portions of the cerebral cortex mature, usually measured by their thickness. The overall thickness of the motor cortex, for example, reaches adult levels at about 2½ years of age. However, its mature functioning also depends upon the maturation of pathways that both enter and leave this part of the brain. This final process continues until about the sixth year of life.

As would be expected, the parts of the cerebral cortex that receive and process information from the environment mature and thicken after the child is born into the external world. Parts of the *temporal lobes,* on the sides of the brain, which contain portions devoted to the processing of sound and memory, do not show much maturation prior to birth. After birth, however, until about six months, they evidence rapid maturation. The visual center in the rear of the brain, in the *occipital lobe,* similarly evidences rapid maturation just after birth through the sixth month of life, after which its rate of maturation tends to slow down, until it assumes adult maturation (thickness) at about the first year of age.

Several sections of the brain evidence more than one period of rapid maturation, separated by periods during which maturation proceeds at a less rapid rate. For example, the *parietal lobe,* which processes information about the body's positions and parts, undergoes a period of rapid maturation and growth one and two months prior to birth, and then again a second period of maturation (thickening), at from 4 to 6 years of age. This same pattern of irregular change is noted when the growth of portions of the front of the cerebral cortex is studied (the frontal lobe). This part of the brain, controlling hand movements, evidences a first period of rapid growth just prior to birth, and a second period of rapid maturation after the age of 6.

In contrast, the frontal associational areas increase in thickness rapidly from the prenatal period to the age of 2 years, after which the increase is slow although steady throughout most of adulthood. There thus seems to be neurological evidence, in the form of structural changes, which suggests that while first there is formation of basic structures for so-called high-level thinking, the acquisition, storage, and use of information at a relatively sophisticated level proceeds throughout the major part of the individual's life span. That is, structure formation precedes exploitation of the structure mediating higher thought processes.

BRAIN GROWTH SPURT

Lasting from the third month of gestation into the third and fourth year of life is a period of rapid acceleration of brain growth. This period is called the *brain growth spurt.* During this time of rapid growth, the brain is particularly vulnerable to various kinds of trauma, nutritional deficiencies, and other types of "insults." The first part of this period is marked by the multiplication of cells that support the maturation of and changes in the nerve cells, or neurons. The second and longer part of this period of rapid growth occurs because of maturation of the coverings of the nerves and nerve pathways. This development of the nerve sheath, or myelination, is discussed in the section that follows.

Various nutritional deficiencies, as well as trauma occurring during this period, will result in functional and structural problems, some of which are difficult to modify later through education and remediation. Among the problems seen in children who have somehow been "damaged" during this critical period of brain growth are those which are reflected in physical awkwardness. The structural problems seen as a result of the disruption of normal development during this period of fast brain growth include: (a) an overall and permanent reduction in brain size; (b) a reduction in the total number of brain cells; (c) effects on the presence and/or quality of the myelin sheaths; (d) deficits in the amount and quality of branches from the neurons, which in turn reduce the number of joining of neurons into functional groups; (e) negative effects on important enzyme functions that regulate nerve cell transmission and migration. The results of these kinds of neural deficiencies may include not only motor clumsiness, but an inability to handle stress, learning difficulties in school, and problems with retention.

Studies of children who have suffered nutritional deprivation during this critical period of rapid brain growth are often seen to evidence poor motor function into middle and late childhood, despite the fact that the nutritional problems were later rectified. Of particular importance seems to be the amount of protein available to the infant and child during this important period of neural maturation (see Chapter 4).

CELLULAR-LEVEL CHANGES AND MATURATION

More important from a functional standpoint than a survey of how the brain looks or how much it weighs during early development is the integrity of the cellular-level processes occurring during the first weeks, months, and years of life. Four major cellular processes are important:

These include: (1) Cell *proliferation,* a period of time marked by the generation of immature neurons. This period is also marked by a separation of these neurons into specialized functions. (2) *Cell migration,* which begins to occur during the time neurons and other support cells are being generated. The precision of this migration is critical, and the precise mechanisms that cause various similar cells to collect together is just being unraveled by neuroscientists. (c) An *elaboration phase,* which begins once the cells reach their final destinations and hookups (synapses) within the nervous system. Increasing numbers of branches (dendrites) appear, branches that are able to accept synaptic output from other cells that are similarly branching and elaborating. If this elaboration phase does not proceed well because of faulty help from "location" blood chemicals (enzymes), various forms of mental retardation, perhaps accompanied by motor ineptitude, may occur. (d) Last there occurs a *myelination phase.* This stage is marked by the formation of sheaths over neurons and nerve pathways, a process that marks the maturation of various portions of the nervous system, and a readiness of various parts to receive and send precise and rapid "messages" to each other.

These complicated processes of cell proliferation, migration, elaboration, and myelination are interdependent, and consist of numerous substages. Moreover, during this time millions of cells that appear to support some of these mechanisms are removed. Apparently more support cells and neurons are needed during the formation of the nervous system than are required as mature functions are begun. These redundant cells are then passed off and disappear. This cell death has been estimated to involve from 40 to 75 percent of the cells originally generated. It has been postulated that since most cells die at about the time neurons are establishing synaptic

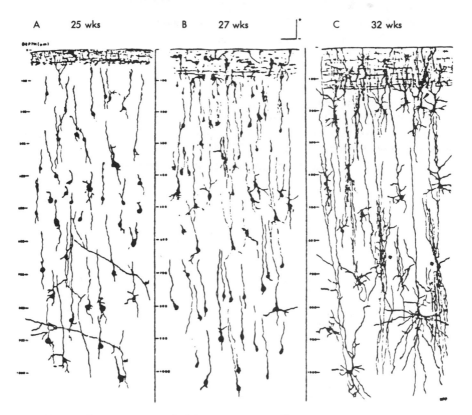

FIGURE 2.11 Cell production and death in the visual cortex. The initial proliferation and overproduction of cells as well as of dendritical spines and cellular contacts is first seen in (a) and (b) at weeks 25 and 27, respectively. Cell death, which may signal specificity of function, is seen in (c) at about 32 weeks after conception. From R. Katzman (ed.), *Congenital and Acquired Cognitive Disorders,* New York: Ravens Press, 1979. Reproduced with permission.

connections with each other, cells not successfully competing for the limited number of connections available disappear. The death of the nonessential cells suggests that toward the final periods of neural maturation a kind of stabilization of the nervous system takes place. An example of how cells proliferate and then die within the visual cortex is shown in Figure 2.11.

Proliferation and Migration

The processes of migration and proliferation often overlap in time. The manner in which these two processes are biochemically controlled is still not well understood. Groups of cells seemingly have a chemical affinity for each other and thus somehow find each other, forming neural pathways and structures that have common functions. The increases seen in both RNA and DNA within the formative periods for brain maturation are probably linked to these processes. For example, the amount of DNA increases over 20 times during the period from 4 weeks to the end of gestation. RNA seems more important to postnatal maturation of the nervous system, since it increases more after birth than before. Deficits in nutrition are likely to disrupt these controller nucleic acids (RNA and DNA), which in turn will disrupt the migration of cells to their final proper locations.

The migration of neural cells to their final locations involves processes whose complexities boggle the mind. In general, the first cells formed reside within the center of the nervous system, while those forming later come to occupy the periphery. Some have suggested that neurons may be divided into two classes relative to their migrational tendencies. Type I, it is suggested, is composed of larger neurons with long axons having pathways and target locations that are genetically determined. Type II appear later and are less limited and "strict" in their formation of connections and groups. The final location of these latter cells, it is postulated, may be determined by both the functional demands placed on the organism as well as the kinds of stimulation imposed on the young human. Slight but consistent differences seen in the cellular-level makeup of the nervous systems of animals that have been exposed to various kinds of enrichment and stimulation would seem to support the assumptions about type II neurons. Differences seen in neuromotor as well as perceptual and intellectual functioning in children subjected to various kinds of demands and stimulation might also be due to the differences in the two types of migrating cells. Developmental psychologists have referred to the apparent cellular-level changes occurring as the result of the psychological environment in which the child emerges as "epigenesis" in contrast to those modifications induced by learning and due to inherited genetic make-up.

In summary, the control of the complex processes of proliferation and migration, as well as of cell elaboration, stems from genetic plans contained in the chromosomes. Migrating cells must not only somehow communicate and chemically "recognize" similar migratory cells when seeking their final destinations, but also somehow "communicate" with dissimilar cells and act upon information received from them. The final location of neurons, or nerve cells, is dependent upon two other qualities contained in substances that somehow "tell them" to group together. One additional type of locator information that is important is the physical location of the intended destinations of cells. A final variable influencing the proper collection of "correct" neurons into groups during these periods of migration involves timing. The biochemical receptors that group neurons seem to be active and operable for relatively brief periods of time, after which they are not helpful in the formation of proper connections.

These elaborate plans in turn are carried out by what are termed *inducers,* or tissues that seem to influence the development of adjacent tissues. Once a primary embryonic plan has been established by primary inducers, a group of *secondary* inducers is activated to further elaborate neural pathways and structures. Science is still exploring the exact ways in which compatible neural cells locate each other and form unifying structures and pathways that terminate in muscle, brain, and organs.

Axon Development and Elaboration of Dendrites

The single type of mechanism that results in the assumption of increasingly complex sensory-motor behaviors involves the ways in which the nerve cells branch and connect, or synapse, with each other during early stages of neural maturation. As the neurons grow axons and dendrites during and after the period of cell migration, support cells are also formed and become differentiated as to function. These support cells later become important for their ability to form myelin sheaths around neurons and groups of neurons.

Nerve fiber formation occurs as tissues are formed in the developing fetus. New sensory neurons send out axons that often travel long distances to synapse with other neurons with which they will function. The axons of sensory neurons have a biochemical affinity for the specific kinds of tissues with which they will later function. The terminal targets of the axons of motor neurons do not seem to be as specific. However, they too have ultimate goals, guided by the time they mature as well as by their biochemical make-up. When a motor neuron and the muscle it innervates match up biochemically, it is probable that the neuron somehow induces some of its biochemical properties into the muscle. In this way a completed functional hookup is formed between the central nervous system and peripheral muscles.

As neurons connect, or synapse, with other neurons, a series of stages has been identified. First, cells before the synapse develop cells that contain *neurotransmitters,* substances that enhance nerve impulse transmission. Next seen is a thickening of the membranes of the two cells that will form the synapse. Finally, the connection is formed.

Beginning as early as the eighth week after conception, there is an increase in the density of the synapses in the nervous system. The number further increases until synapses are formed in the cortex itself at about the 23rd week. Nutritional problems resulting in a deficit of biochemical transmitter substances may detract both from the formation of an adequate number of synapses and their later functions. These structural deficiencies at the cellular level in the nervous system in turn may cause various behavioral problems, including mental retardation, coupled with motor and perceptual delays.

Dendritic maturation. The branches forming on the neurons, which in turn offer an increasing number of possible synaptic relationships, undergo observable changes as normal neural maturation takes place. With maturation more branches or dendrites appear, and with this increase more possible connections or synapses are possible with other neurons and neuronal networks. The vast amount of information transmitted through the nervous system occurs because of the elaboration of the dendrite system within the cortex. It thus follows that lack of healthy dendritic growth and maturation will cause moderate to profound problems in cortical functions, including perceptual, motor, and intellectual deficits.

The first dendrites appear on axons in the cortex as early as the sixth month of gestation. By the eighth month, thick dendrites with obvious spines are present on many cells. There are, however, differences in the speed with which dendrites appear in various portions of the cerebral cortex. Most advanced in dendritic growth are cells deep within the cerebral hemispheres and cells within the motor cortex, which controls movement. Later, dendritic maturation is seen in the visual cortex.

Dendrites appear within predictable and qualitatively different stages as maturation occurs. Their shapes change, and various types are seen at various stages. For example, during the second and third week of gestation, only a few thick dendritic processes are present anywhere in the cortex. By the fourth and fifth weeks after conception, long, thick spines proliferate, and a number of shorter stubby spines may appear. After birth, fewer long spines remain, and instead there are more of the thick, broad spines (Figure 2.12).

Infants suffering from oxygen deprivation at birth and/or other pre- or parinatal birth insults, including malnutrition, are likely to evidence abnormal dendritic characteristics. These include spine loss and spines of unusual shapes. The development of healthy and normal dendritic configurations seems to occur most rapidly from the latter stages of gestation to the sixth month of life. Noxious events to which the infant may be subjected during this same time period may thus lead to inalterable patterns of dendritic growth that are abnormal, and that in turn result in behavioral characteristics which may mark the individual as developmentally delayed (see Chapter 4).

Myelination.   One of the major signposts of neural maturation most cited involves the changes seen in the development of the sheath or covering that spreads

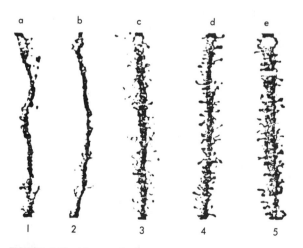

FIGURE 2.12 Microscopic characteristics of normal dendritic changes during maturation. *Dentritic spine and shaft changes.* Moving from growth cones and thin spines, (a), to an increase in number of long, thin spines by 22 weeks of fetal life, (b). By the 33rd week of fetal life, (c), the dentrite pattern shows long, thin spines, as well as a few more mature mushroom-shaped spines. By six months after birth, and by the seventh year (d and e), the pattern is more stubby spines, which are almost identical during these postnatal months and years. From R. Katzman (ed.), *Congenital and Acquired Cognitive Disorders,* New York: Ravens Press, 1979. Reproduced with permission.

over most of the fast-conducting pathways of the central nervous system. The growth of these sheaths seems to help the overall precision and speed with which nerve impulses pass over groups of neurons that may be functionally interdependent. The myelination may help groups of pathways and neurons removed from each other in the nervous system to become highly integrated units. The functions of myelination thus involve maintaining and permitting high-velocity transmission of "messages," as well as aiding in the maintenance of the overall functional integrity of the sensory and motor pathways. Again, nutritional deficiencies may detract from the myelination process. For example, protein-bound lipids facilitate normal myelination, and thus dietary problems detract from adequate and normal myelination of the nervous system.

Structurally, myelin sheath formation is seen in two ways. (1) A maturational component is observable, and is reflected in a gradual thickening of the sheath along its length (Figure 2.13). (2) A growth component is also apparent. This refers to the overall increase of the length of the sheath along a given nerve fiber(s). Overall neural maturation and growth and the function this maturation infers may be estimated by measures of how far these two processes have progressed in a given infant, child, or adult. A number of motor behavioral "milestones" are able to be paired with the myelination of various pathways, including the appearance of primitive pre- and postnatal reflexes, discussed in Chapter 5.

Like other indications of neural maturation discussed in this chapter, myelination does not proceed in a uniform manner in all portions of the nervous system at the same time. In general, the myelination of pathways depends partly on their relative importance to the maintenance of life. The pathways controlling the sucking responses, for example, mature quite early. The auditory-acoustic track is myelinated at birth so that the child may become aware of the environment, and to provide the bases for language and speech. In general, functional myelination occurs both in response to survival demands and in response to stresses the environment is likely to place on the human infant and child.

Myelination generally proceeds upward within the nervous system. Portions

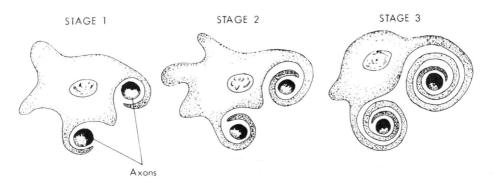

FIGURE 2.13   A cross-sectional look at successive stages of myelination by the glial cells around an axon. From H. Lou, *Developmental Neurology*. New York: Ravens Press, 1982. Reproduced with permission.

of the spinal cord are myelinated first, beginning during the fourth and fifth month after conception. Also during this fourth fetal month, the motor roots within the spinal cord undergo myelination. Sensory roots in the spinal cord receive myelin coverings about one month later. Motor mechanisms within the spinal cord are almost completely myelinated by about the first month after conception, while sensory mechanisms take longer to mature and are not completely covered with a myelin sheath until about six months after birth.

Based on this kind of evidence, the newborn infant appears to be more mature sensorially than motorically. That is, while simple motor spinal reflexes are functionally ready at birth, myelination of functional motor pathways from the periphery of the body to the cortex are not as mature as sensory pathways. The newborn, for example, is quite sensitive to and dependent upon tactile stimulation, as most mothers know. The second of the major sensory systems to develop is the visual system. Myelination takes place on the visual pathways from birth to 6 months of age. Last to mature are the auditory pathways, reflected in myelination that is not completed until about the fourth year of life.

The major pathways carrying motor functions from the cortex undergo rapid myelination during the last month of gestation and the process is complete at about the age of 2 years. The last areas and pathways to evidence myelination are those involved in the storing and integration of information. The frontal associational areas, as well as the large stalks connecting the two hemispheres (cerebral commissures) are the last to mature. Their maturation continues into the third decade of life, even though they have undergone more rapid myelination near birth (see Figure 2.14).

It is also probable that attentional qualities undergo positive change during the first decades of life. A relatively prolonged period of time is devoted to the maturation and myelination of the reticular formation, a structure in the brain stem purportedly devoted to attention and self-control.

In summary, therefore, first to mature, as evidenced by the progress of the myelin sheath, are pathways and areas devoted to simple prebirth reflexes. Next to mature are those involving sensation. Next to mature are pathways mediating voluntary movements, and integration of the peripheral neuromotor system to the central nervous system and motor cortex. Last to mature are pathways and structures that control attention, self-control, memory, and learning (see Table 2.1).

SUMMARY

Neurological maturation is a process that begins shortly after conception and continues throughout life. The first signs of the emergence of the nervous system involve the formation of the neural tube. It then folds and begins to evidence various parts of the brain within the first month after conception. The first movements of the fetus involve localized reactions to stimulation, termed *myogenic* movement. Later,

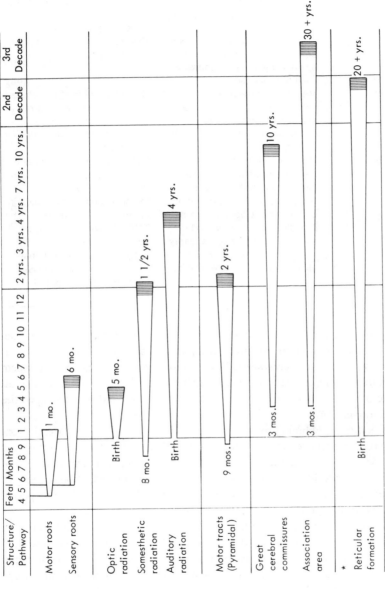

FIGURE 2.14 The rate of myelination of selected structures and pathways. From A. Minkowsky (ed.), *Regional Development of the Brain in Early Life*, Oxford, Eng.: Blackwell Scientific Publications, 1965. Reproduced with permission.

*Width and length of bars indicate increasing density of myelination; blacked-in areas at end of bars indicate approximate age range of completion of myelination process.

TABLE 2.1   Selected Milestones of Myelination and Behavior During the Prenatal Period

AGE	MYELINATION	BEHAVIOR(S)
4th fetal month	First appearance of myelin, confined to spinal cord.	Change from *myogenic* contractions to first *neurogenic* contractions; motor neuron is functional.
6th fetal month	Tracts involving head and body coordinations myelinated; spinal-cortical motor pathways still unmyelinated.	First reflex behaviors appear, including grasp.
7th fetal month	Medulla and midbrain myelinated; also reflex arcs of spinal cord and pathways controlling vital functions such as respiration.	Stimulation of medulla results in respiratory and sucking responses; mass muscular reflexes appear—Moro, righting, tonic-neck.
8th fetal month	Motor tracks in spinal cord well myelinated; some evidence of motor tracts to higher centers.	Reflexes appear in legs and lower extremities.
Birth	Motor pathways myelinated to cortex; most advanced in cortex, including motor areas and somatosensory areas; auditory areas less mature, while association areas show little myelin.	Motor responses are reflex in nature; now include swimming, TNR, righting, stepping; good tactile responses to any part of body; early visual responses present; auditory responses only gross reactions to loud noises.

by the third and fourth month after conception, *neurogenic* movement occurs, actions in parts of the fetus removed from the point of actual stimulation.

Generally, many structures needed to monitor and modify movement appear by the fourth to fifth month after conception, including the basal ganglia. In general, sensory systems and pathways mature earlier than the fetus's and infant's capacities for accurate movement.

The period of rapid brain growth, termed the brain growth spurt, extends from the third trimester to between the third and fourth years of life. It is during this time that various kinds of biochemical, nutritional, and mechanical insults to neural structures and cells are likely to result in the most significant reduction of sensory and motor capacities. This is particularly true if the insult has occurred over a period of time; for example, protein deficiencies lasting throughout infancy.

Cellular-level modifications of the nervous system include (a) proliferation of cells, neurons, and support cells; (b) the migration of these cells, and the clustering of cells into groups, to form structures and functional pathways; (c) the elaboration of cells reflected in dendritic branching; and (d) the myelination of neurons and nerve pathways, reflected in the growth of sheaths that expand longitudinally as well as in thickness. This latter process results in faster nerve impulse transmission, as well as in more discrete "messages" carried by nerve pathways.

A number of fluctuations and variations are seen when studying neural maturation. For example, the rate and timing of myelination differs from structure to structure, and from pathway to pathway. Fluctuations occur in the rate of maturation of various parts of the cerebral cortex. Additionally, fluctuations in the rate of development of individual parts of the cortex occur. These individual differences and variations have significance when planning programs of motor development and of infant stimulation.

QUESTIONS FOR DISCUSSION

1. Discuss the significance of the period identified as the brain growth spurt, with reference to variables discussed in Chapter 4.
2. What is the possible behavioral significance of the myelination process?
3. Discuss the concept of neurological maturation as a continuous process, from conception to death.
4. What may be the behavioral significance of the uneven development of parts of the cerebral cortex?
5. How might the fact that cell deaths occur as the nervous system seems to somehow stabilize itself relate to the concept of behavioral bonds outlined in Chapter 1?
6. How might incomplete myelination of the higher centers result in the continued appearance of less useful reflexes, as discussed in Chapter 3?
7. Why might "useless" dendrites break off and disappear? What behavioral significance might this have?
8. What kinds of deficiencies might the nervous system evidence if the fetus and infant fails to obtain sufficient protein to nourish "locator" enzymes?
9. Discuss the significance of type II neurons with regard to programs of infant stimulation.
10. What seems to mature first in infants, the ability to take in and process information, or the ability to move with accuracy? What significance does the uneven development of the sensory and motor systems have when planning programs of early infant stimulation?
11. What possible educational significance does the relative late maturation of myelin sheaths within associational and attentional areas of the brain have upon programs of motor skill acquisition for young adults and the aged?

CHAPTER THREE
PHYSICAL GROWTH AND THE CHANGING BODY IMAGE

Those who have studied the maturation of the child's body have taken two avenues. The most frequently traveled road contains rather well-defined measures of stature, muscle, and fat tissue, as well as body shape. The second road has relied upon psychological rather than physical measures. Studies in this latter category have focused on children's feelings about their bodies, their perceptions of its shape, size, movement capacities, and spatial dimensions.

Both sets of variables, one composed of physical measures, the other of less precise signposts, usually interact to determine and influence how, why, when, and with what effort the maturing youngster engages in physical activities. The effort expended, and the frequency and types of actions exhibited by the child, in turn influence the acquisition of movement capacities. Finally, children's satisfaction or dissatisfaction with their bodies is likely to exert important influences on their self-concept.

Commonsense observations suggest the close interaction of mind and body as the maturing youngster plays and interacts with his or her peers. The thin, shy, withdrawn child is a stereotype familiar to everyone; so is the muscular, supremely self-confident bully. Generally it has been found that children's satisfactions with their bodies and themselves depend upon how close their feelings about their bodily conformation coincide with their, or society's, ideal. The literature has often documented how important athletic prowess is to achieving social recognition in both childhood and adolescence.

The close association between the psychological and physical selves prompted the discussion in this chapter. Children's changing bodies, and their continual adjustments in how they feel about those bodies interact to determine modifications that form an inseparable duo. It was for this reason that information about the nature of physical as well as psychological modifications is found here.

PHYSICAL SIZE, MATURATIONAL SIGNPOSTS, AND BODY BUILD

Humans have long been interested in variations in physical size and in the proportions and shapes of their bodies. Writings from ancient Rome, Greece, Arabia, and China reflect this interest, as do the sketches of early artists. With the dawn of the scientific age many centuries later, assessments of the body's dimensions became more exact. One mathematician affiliated with the armies of Napoleon found, upon measuring the heights of thousands of soldiers, that the measures obtained produced what satisticians now describe as a normal bell-shaped curve. The discovery of X-rays in the early 1900s permitted a look at the maturing skeleton as an additional measure of maturation. In the 1940s exact measures of body build appeared in the work of the anthropologist Sheldon, assessments that more exactly delineated the concepts of fatness, thinness, and muscularity than had been possible in the past (Sheldon and Stevens, 1942).

The evaluation of the physical size and body types of children and youth has been stimulated by several factors. Medically marked deviations in growth rates are cause for concern, and may lead to interventions intended to accelerate or slow down unusual rates of change in the young child.[1] Physical educators as well as developmental psychologists have been interested in variations in physique among the young because of the possible relationships between exercise tolerance, power, and strength, as well as personality and the manner in which the child's body develops. Coaches and scientists interested in high-level athletic performance regularly descend upon Olympic Games competitions to explore just what highly specialized body builds seem best prepared to exhibit prowess in some of the more exotic events. It has been discovered, for example, that about half the body types evaluated among Olympic athletes are not found within the general population.

As a result of scientific work, as well as speculation about physique-temperament relationships, it is unlikely that a child will grow up without hearing references to fat-lazy, thin-nervous, or perhaps strong-silent people. At times, particularly if the child's body build differs markedly from the average, these often

---

[1]Medical interest was also spurred because of the possible relationship between body types and susceptibility to disease.

derisive pairings are applied in direct ways to him or to her. If negative judgments of the child's body build are confirmed when that same child confronts a mirror, the youngster's self-concept may be undermined at an early age. Conversely, if positive comments about body build are received from others and the child's first experiments are successful when confronting physical tasks, an early and positive charge is put into the battery representing the youngster's total feelings about himself or herself. It is for this reason that consideration of body build, rate of physical maturation, and changes in bodily proportions and size are important from the standpoint of both physical performance and psychological and social-emotional growth and development.

Assessment Procedures

Evaluation procedures can reflect several kinds of scientific orientations when used to measure physical maturation. Moreover, historically we can trace a gradual but steady rise in the validity and sophistication of the measures applied to physical changes in children. For example, the first assessments of children's growth and development often included norms based on height, weight, or combinations and ratios derived from these measures. However, these often did not provide the precision necessary to deal accurately with maturational status and variations within such general notions as stockiness or thinness. For example, it was more useful to know whether or not a "stocky" child (whose height was minimal, but whose weight was high) was fat or muscular. At the same time, a tall, thin child's ratio of trunk length to leg length was not included when only height and weight were measured. Additionally, it is important not simply to trace height changes in children as a function of age, but also to inspect how height may tend to accelerate and decelerate at various ages, thus displaying normal growth spurts during the development of the maturing child.

Growth Changes

For the most part, the growth rate of the average infant is extremely rapid during the first year and a half of life, as shown in Figure 3.1, which graphs changes in body length. The growth rate tends to level off by the ages of 2, 4, and 6. Additionally, if data from large numbers of children are inspected, we see that the growth rate remains relatively stable from the fifth to about the twelfth to thirteenth years, followed by a period marked by the adolescent growth spurt. Some have suggested that this is why the child in these middle years is able to acquire a great number of skills so rapidly; somehow such children do not have to worry about sudden changes in stature and can concentrate on using their relatively unchanging bodies to full advantage.

We obtain a very different picture of physical growth when we look at an *individual* child. The individual child is a product of the genes of the parents and of *their* parents, and of subtle genetic programming which is just now beginning to be studied. Various other factors, including the opportunity to play and encouragement

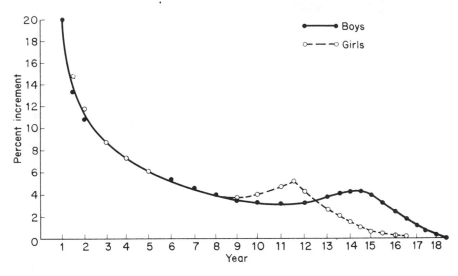

FIGURE 3.1 Relative growth rate. From Leona M. Bayer and Nancy Bayley, *Growth Diagnosis,* Chicago: The University of Chicago Press, 1959. By permission of the publisher.

by parents in physical efforts, add further complexity to the picture of growth. A single child may, for example, evidence the relatively steady growth rate typical of the charts emanating from group studies. He or she may evidence relatively rapid early growth in childhood and a later leveling off; still another pattern of growth may include a slow start, followed by a marked change in late childhood. An even more complicated pattern may include changes in size that show stops and starts during the period of time from the fifth year to puberty.

Researchers of the 1960s and 1970s began to look at human growth in a number of ways. For example, they separated the plottings of yearly increments from what is called the *velocity* curve. Figure 3.2 shows two charts for the same boy. One shows simple change from year to year; the second shows the velocity curve, illustrating annual increments to inches. The former is thus a relatively smooth, regular curve, whereas the latter indicates just how irregular changes were from the second to the twentieth years. Figure 3.3 shows average velocity curves of both males and females from birth to adolescence. As can be seen, the growth spurt occurs much earlier in females than in males. As late childhood and early adolescence are reached, marked individual differences are likely in the onset of growth spurts on the part of both males and females. Differences in the timing of these accelerations in growth are shown in Figure 3.4, which gives the growth velocities of three boys.

Indexes and Factor Analyses

In the search for more precise measures of physical stature, maturation, and body build, various index numbers have been employed. Some of these combined

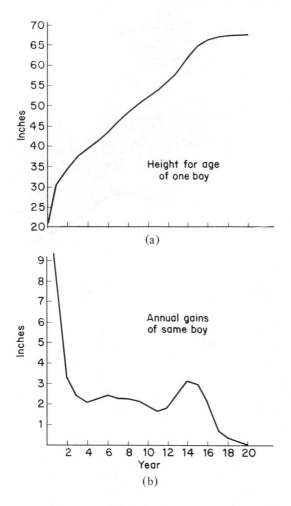

FIGURE 3.2
(a) A "distance" curve showing the height of a boy at various ages. (b) A "velocity" curve showing annual gains, plotted from first curve. From F. Falkner, "The Physical Development of Children. A Guide to Interpretation of Growth- Charts and Development Assessments: And a Commentary on Contemporary and Future Problems," *Pediatrics, 29* (1962), pp. 448-66. Copyright, American Academy of Pediatrics, with permission of the author and publishers.

height and weight, as represented by the Ponderal Index, which is the height divided by the cube root of the weight. Others began to incorporate such measures as chest circumference (Seagraves, 1970). Based on the assumption that growth may be placed into several distinct channels represented by common variations in children's body builds, Pryor formulated width-weight tables (Pryor, 1966) suggesting that body weight is an index of nutritional status. She employed measures of chest circumference and shoulder width in addition to height, age, and weight.

Longitudinal measures of height, and weight changes in and of themselves, even in combination with indexes, did not always reflect modifications and variations in body build that are commonly seen among both children and adults. So large numbers of measures of the body were intercorrelated to determine what measures seemed to cluster together, and to identify "basic" or general physique factors in children.

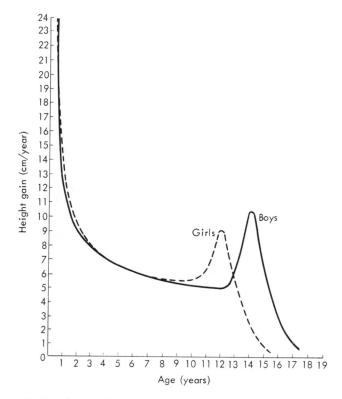

FIGURE 3.3 Typical individual velocity curves for supine length or height in boys and girls. These curves represent velocity of typical boy and girl at any given instant. From J. Tanner, *Archives of Diseases in Childhood*, 1966, *41*, pp. 454-71; p. 613-35.

For decades factor analyses have been conducted, using various kinds of data emanating from the measurement of body build. Generally studies (Barry and Cureton, 1961; Hammon, 1957) have brought to light three factors. These include one associated with the development of subcutaneous fat, usually obtained from skinfold measures. A second factor reflects linearity, as reflected in limb and trunk length. A third factor reflects thickness of the body, and consists of measures of the diameters of body parts.

Measures of Body Composition

During the past several decades, more and more studies have delineated the nature of various components of the body, including the presence of fat, muscle, and bone. The first approaches tried to identify the quantity of lean versus fatty tissue in the total body, but as measurement procedures became more sophisticated, fat versus muscular and bony components were studied in various limbs. Changes in percent of fat tissue present were studied as a function of age and sex. In other stud-

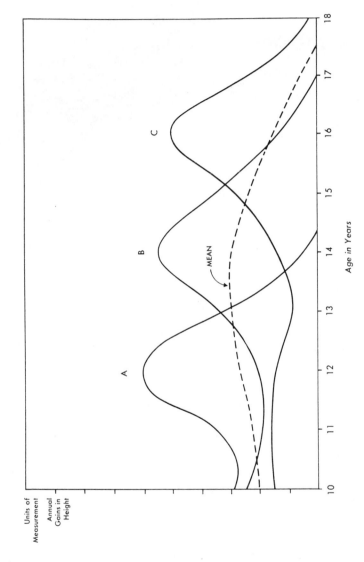

FIGURE 3.4 Curves of annual gains in height of three individual boys (A, B, and C). The dotted line shows the mean annual gain of the three boys. From F. Falkner, "The Physical Development of Children. A Guide to Interpretation of Growth-Charts and Development Assessments: And a Commentary on Contemporary and Future Problems," *Pediatrics*, 29 (1962), pp. 448–66. Copyright, American Academy of Pediatrics, with permission of the author and publishers.

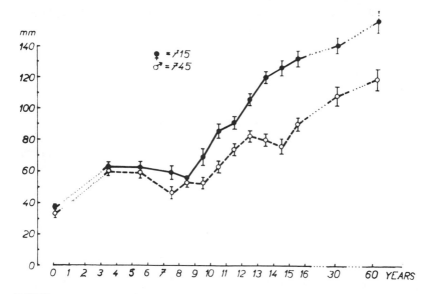

FIGURE 3.5 Development of subcutaneous fat, expressed as the sum of skinfolds measured at ten sites. From J. Pařiźková, 1963. *Impact of Age, Diet, and Exercise on Man's Body Composition*, Ann. N.Y. Acad. Sci. 110:661-675. With the kind permission of the editors.

ies, modifications in the percent of fat present were depicted as influenced by exercise programs of various intensities (Parizkova, 1960); see also Chapter 12.

Early in the lives of children, sex differences in body composition have been identified (Garn, 1956, 1965; Parizkova, 1963). Newborn infants of both sexes were evaluated, and based on a measure called a fat-weight-ratio,[2] it was found that females were significantly more obese than were males. Moreover, skinfold thicknesses have been found to be significantly thicker over the hips of newborn girls than at corresponding sites in boys. Maresh (1961) also found that during the first year of life, girls evidence more adipose tissue, while boys evidence more thickness of muscle.

These sex differences in subcutaneous fat (or more properly skinfold plus fat measures) continue to be slight, but measurable, during childhood, and tend to diverge, as shown in Figure 3.5, during late childhood and early adolescence, with girls as a group evidencing a greater percent of fat tissue than boys. This same pattern of skinfold differences in boys and girls is apparent when skinfolds from various parts of the body are compared, as has been done by Tanner and Whitehouse (1962) in the area below the scapula and in the triceps area.

In general, the growth of fat in all children increases quite rapidly during the first 9 months of life, and then a plateau is reached reflecting little or no fat increases

---

[2]The thickness of the skin plus adipose tissue in millimeters divided by body weight in kilograms.

recorded when taking skinfold measurements. At the same time, the bone-muscle core of a limb around which the fat is arranged increases, and thus skinfold measures taken during childhood may seem to decrease when actually the fat is merely being stretched thinner because of the larger limb core that it covers. Thus both the measurement of fat through skinfold measures and the interpretation of these measures in growing children must be carried out with care.

As children mature, relatively high correlations are found in measures of fatness reflected in skinfold measures taken at various parts of the body. However, there appear to be only low to moderate relationships between measures of bone and muscle widths in various locations, and even these relationships are higher in younger than in older children (Malina, 1969). In contrast, the percent of lean body mass, when viewed in relationship to height, is not different in males and females during childhood, and only becomes different as adolescence is reached. Figure 3.6 illustrates these two trends. When corrected for height, measures of lean body mass do not differ greatly prior to adolescence when the sexes are contrasted. It is only as adolescence is reached that marked differences in both the percent of body fat and its locations become apparent. Some males may experience what is known as a puppy-fat phase during the preadolescent period. The female, on the other hand, does not lose as much baby fat as the male, and finishes as an adult with a good deal more total fat than the average male.

Maturity and Skeletal Age

Around the turn of the century, scientists became interested in the maturation of the long bones of the body, as reflected in skeletal maturation. Not only could bone density be ascertained, but also the degree to which the growth centers at the end of the long bones (epipythesis) had become "wedded" to the entire shaft. The remainder of the shaft was first ascertained on cadavers, and then later through the

FIGURE 3.6 Ratio of the fat-free mass ("LBM") to height for both sexes as a function of age. From G. B. Forbes and J. B. Hursh, 1963. Age and Sex Trends in Body Mass. Ann N.Y. Academy of Science, with kind permission of the editors.

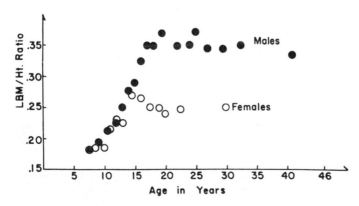

use of X rays. Pioneers in this work, such as J. W. Pryor, T. M. Rotch, Wingate Todd, and others, began to differentiate between what might be termed *growth,* the simple elongation of the bones of the body, and *development,* the metamorphosis of the chemical nature of bony tissues. These early scholars identified principles that are generally accepted today, even though the methods used to assess skeletal maturation have gone through several modifications. These principles include the following:

1. The bones of the female ossify in advance of the male; initially this difference may be measured in days, later in weeks, and at puberty in years. In females bone maturation is completed from 19 to 20 years after conception, whereas in males the process takes about three years longer. These 20-year periods are divisible into three phases. Though they overlap, they are relatively distinct. The first involves the ossification of the diaphyses of both the long and short bones, and is completed prior to birth. The second phase, starting just before birth, involves osteogenesis in the epiphyses of both the shafted and the round bones. This second phase is completed by puberty, and in girls takes about 12 years. The final phase, starting at puberty or later, is not completed until the seventeenth to twentieth year. This involves the invasion of the growth cartilage places that lead to the functional destruction, and the bony fusion of the epiphysis and the diaphysis. These differing rates of skeletal maturation are depicted in Figure 3.7, based upon skeletal maturation of the hip and pelvis in both females and males.

2. Independent of normal variations in maturity, the two sides of the body tend to ossify in a symmetrical fashion.

3. The various bones of the body tend to ossify at different rates. Furthermore, differences in the rate of maturation of various bones seems to be an inheritable trait. For example, as Figure 3.8 shows, the various bones of the hand, a portion of the body most often used to ascertain a single skeletal age, actually ossify at different times. The numbers on the chart indicate the order in which they ossify. Thus the evenly maturing skeleton is a myth. Each child must be considered as an individual in terms of the differences in maturational rates of bones in various parts of the body.

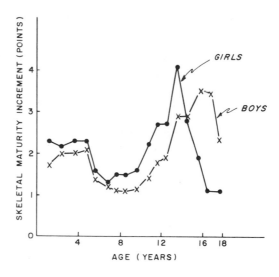

FIGURE 3.7
Velocity curves (B) for skeletal maturation of the hip and pelvis, computed by Oxford Method for the Bruxh Foundation (Cleveland) children together with others from a longitudinal study in Oxford, England. This method permits the differing rates of skeletal maturation to be demonstrated graphically and also shows that there is a pubertal spurt in skeletal maturation. Hewitt and Acheson, 1961. "Some aspects of skeletal development through adolescence, Part I, variations in the rate and pattern of skeletal maturation at puberty," *American Journal of Physical Anthropology, 19,* pp. 333-34. With permission of the publishers, Alan R. Liss, Inc., New York.

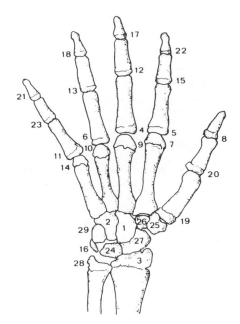

FIGURE 3.8

The individual centers of ossification (separate bones) numbered approximately in the order in which their ossification begins. Based on a photograph from *Radiographic Atlas of Skeletal Development of the Hand and Wrist* by W. W. Greulich and S. I. Pyle, Stanford, Calif.: Stanford University Press, 1959, p. 187.

4.   At the same time, however, individuals may be classified as fast or slow or early or late maturers, based upon skeletal age.

Falkner (1962), for example, has proposed that six different patterns of maturation may be identified. These include:

1.   An average child who will closely approximate the mean curve for height and weight at stated ages.
2.   Early maturing children who are tall in childhood only because they are more mature than the average; they will not become unusually tall adults.
3.   Early maturing children who are also genetically taller than average from early childhood. They mature rapidly and remain taller than average throughout their lives.
4.   Late maturing children who are short in childhood, but who later evidence reasonable growth. They will not remain unusually small in adulthood.
5.   Late maturing children who are genetically short and who remain short adults.
6.   An ''indefinite group'' whose members must often be exposed to medical evaluation; they may be children whose adolescent growth ''spurt'' starts unusually early, by the eighth or ninth year, or their growth may evidence unusual delay and be the cause for parental and medical concern.

Thus, just as is true with simple measures of height and/or weight, indexes of skeletal maturity reveal marked individual differences within relatively ''normal'' ranges.

For example, in Figure 3.9, the skeletal ages for three hypothetical children have been plotted. Child C evidences consistently below average maturity and is

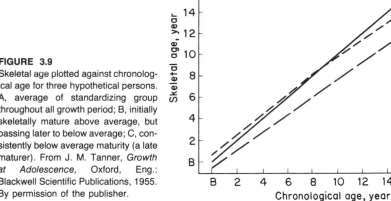

FIGURE 3.9

Skeletal age plotted against chronological age for three hypothetical persons. A, average of standardizing group throughout all growth period; B, initially skeletally mature above average, but passing later to below average; C, consistently below average maturity (a late maturer). From J. M. Tanner, *Growth at Adolescence,* Oxford, Eng.: Blackwell Scientific Publications, 1955. By permission of the publisher.

thus a late maturer. Child B, on the other hand, while evidencing an early advance (better than the mean indicated by the solid line A), later shows a deceleration in growth, passing below the average (A).

Despite the possible limitations of X-ray techniques for ascertaining skeletal maturity, this method has several practical uses. It may be used in conjunction with other measures of physical maturity (strength, height, weight) to classify children and youth for equal competition in athletics. Skeletal maturity may be used to assess present maturity and possible problems.

Assessing the Body's Form

The historical roots of attempts to evaluate and classify the various shapes the human body assumes go back centuries. Hippocrates proposed a two-way classification system composed of linear types (*habitus phthisicus*) and lateral types (*habitus apoplecticus*). In the last century the German psychiatrist Kretschmer developed a three-part typology: fat, muscular, and lean. This same three-way classification is to be found in the system of somatotyping[3] formulated by the anthropologist Sheldon in the 1940s and 1950s. Modifications of Sheldon's system are those most used today.

Sheldon suggested that, instead of the placement of an individual's body build into rigid categories, it was more valid to rate a human physique according to the *degree* to which fat, thin, and muscular qualities were present. These components, now found in the common vernacular, were named endomorphy (fatness), ectomorphy (thinness), and mesomorphy (muscularity). Each component in a physique was rated individually from standardized photographs, and a rating for each of

---

[3]Literally, the typing of the soma or body.

the three qualities was made on a 1 to 7 scale; with 1 representing the least expression of a quality and 7 the fullest expression of a given component. The resultant three-number scale represented the person's somatotype. The method also made use of the Ponderal Index, anthropometric measures of bodily girth, and measurements and estimates taken from photographs. Thus an individual with a 1-3-7 somatotype would be an ectomorph with slight mesomorphic tendencies, while a 2-5-1 would be a mesomorph with slight endomorphic qualities.[4]

Sheldon expanded his research and formulated other physique categories. He also explored possible relationships between character, physique, and personality. Overall, however, Sheldon believed that physique type was inherited, and underwent relatively little change during childhood and adolescence. This notion of the inflexible somatotype (or morphogenotype) was not accepted by all. Sheldon's notion that personality and body type were closely linked also attracted numerous critics. However, the other physique qualities he assessed continue to be of interest today, as are his general measurement techniques.[5]

More flexible systems have evolved from Sheldon's rather tedious and expensive methods of photography analysis. For example, Parnell (1958) has modified Sheldon's methods in order to derive what he terms a phenotype, using fewer measurements. *Phenotype* is defined as how the body appears at a given moment, and thus takes into consideration changes from the more rigid notion of an unchanging inherited physique. The concept of phenotype superimposed upon morphogenotype allows for expected deviations of body build elicited by nutrition, living conditions, exercise, and the like. (An example of the alteration of physique in children through exercise is described in Chapter 12.)

In the 1960s Petersen extended Sheldon's methods to evaluate the body builds of children. Heath in this same decade modified Sheldon's somatotyping methods by eliminating adjustments for age and by extending the component rating scales in order to accommodate a greater range of variations in physiques. In 1966, Heath and Carter formulated an approach using easily obtained measures of skinfold thickness, bodily girth, and the ponderal index. The latter method is now most commonly used. Petersen generally agrees with Sheldon's assumption that the basic physique is relatively fixed. However, he also suggests that physique changes during adolescence present special problems for those assessing physique and body build developmentally.

A number of researchers have studied the nature and the consistency of body builds in childhood and adolescence. These have ranged from studies of nursery school children, reflecting efforts to contrast physique type to personality, to longitudinal studies of youth during their adolescent years (Walker, 1952; Hunt and

---

[4]All the permutations of 1 to 7, in all three places, do not occur in life, nor in Sheldon's system. An individual cannot, for example, be both fat and thin, and have a somatotype of 6-1-7.

[5]Among the other physique qualities he assessed are dysplasia, or the unevenness of the physique qualities in various components of the body (literally bad shape or form); gynandromorphy, the adherence or deviation of the physique type from the biological sex of the individual; and coarseness, or angularity, of the body and its parts.

Barton, 1959). Studies contrasting the body builds of children to those of their parents have provided interesting information (Parnell, 1958). More recently, somatotypes have been used in various social-psychological studies relating a youngster's perceptions of his or her body type to such measures as their ideal body type and their actual somatotype (Tucker, 1983; Collins and Proper, 1983). Somatotype ratings have also been contrasted to children's performances on tasks requiring power, strength, and/or endurance (Malina, 1973; Barry and Cureton, 1961).

In younger children, linearity has been associated with slightly more precocious walking and other locomotor behaviors (Bayley, 1935; Shirley, 1939). In an unpublished study recently completed in my laboratory, children midway in the second year of life whose ponderal indexes reflected linearity were able to move significantly more rapidly when encouraged to run than were the more stockily built youngsters in the study. At a relatively early age, it is also possible that physique and tendencies to exhibit movement begin to interact in ways that persist throughout childhood. Walker (1952), for example, found, upon obtaining the somatotypes of 125 nursery school children from 2 to 4 years, that (a) mesomorphic children tended to exhibit more energy than those possessing other somatotypes, and (b) that the directions of these energies differed between boys and girls, with the mesomorphic girls expressing themselves more in social activities, while the boys engaged more in vigorous gross motor actions. Using teacher's assessments of the personalities of these youngsters, the data strongly suggested that even at this early age, cultural expectations concerning stereotyped relationships between physique and behavior are already exerting influences upon people's perceptions of children with various body builds.

Parizkova (1984) has also identified body-build differences in pre-schoolers that correlate significantly with performance measures, and conceivably with the children's social acceptance, and with that part of their self-concepts that impels them to move vigorously.

Studies of individual differences in body build of youngsters within middle childhood generally have focused upon intra-individual consistency as well as the prediction of body build from other information about the child, notably the body builds of parents. Thus, from a strictly anthropometric standpoint, body-build measures in children have been used as predictors of (a) their own later body builds, and (b) parent-child relationships in physique.

It seems clear from the available evidence that during growth and even into adolescence, a child's basic somatotype undergoes little alteration. The genetic regulation of both ultimate size and rate of growth is well documented, and adult height may be predicted from about 2 to 3 years of age. Indeed, the old wives' tales which say that adult height is approximately twice that of the child at 2 years are confirmed by contemporary scientific evidence (Garn, 1966; Tanner, 1978). At the same time, the child's physical constitution may be altered, particularly the fat component, through diet, exercise, and extreme food deprivation (Parizkova, 1984). Thus it may be generalized that while somatotype seems rather fixed, phenotype is alterable. Hammond, for example, noted (1953, 1957) that changes in size and proportions during childhood do not fundamentally alter somatotype. In children of 5 through adolescents of 18, for example, correlations between somatotype measurements ranged from + .65 to + .92 for both males and females. Several researchers, however, including Hammond and Peterson, have noted that consistency in physique tends to be lower during puberty. Hammond found, for example, that 18 percent of the males in his investigation changed somatotype after 14 years of age, whereas 22 percent of the females from 10 to 13 years of age in his longitudinal study changed somatotype. In general it seems that measures of linearity, perhaps because they are generally of bony girths, tend to be more consistent in children, while measures of muscularity and fatness are less consistent across ages. Generally, the percent of body fat decreases from birth to the 5th year (Parizkova, 1984; Parnell, 1958). Muscularity and fat are most modifiable by exercise, diet, and other components of a child's life style. This same lack of consistency in muscularity and fatness was observed in a longitudinal study of adolescents by Barton (1959).

Even the casual observer is aware of the tendency for children, in at least general ways, to acquire body builds that resemble those of their parents. Research in general confirms this observation. For example, there is a strong tendency for large-chested parents to have large-chested children (Garn, 1966), and conversely for small parents to beget offspring whose breadth of chest is equally limited. Relative to overall physique, the parental line principle has been noted by several experts (Parnell, 1958). It has been found that from 70 to 75 percent of physique ratings of children fall roughly on a line connecting their parents' physiques on a somatochart. This leaves, however, over 20 percent of children whose physiques do not closely resemble some kind of average of their parents' bodily shapes.

PHYSIQUE AND PERFORMANCE

At extremely high levels of athletic competition, there are desirable body types in many sporting activities. These demands are not as high in some events and sports as in others. For example, sprinting competitions seem amenable to a wider variety of body builds than do distance running and gymnastics. Body types found in various outstanding female and male athletes are shown in Figures 3.10 and 3.11. However, in a recent and extensive study of various measures of body build and performance among children of nursery-school age, there were definite relationships between throwing, running and jumping tasks, and the body builds of the children evaluated (Parizkova, 1984). In this investigation obesity was negatively correlated to many measures including running; while muscular children, as would be expected, performed most motor tasks better. Of additional interest in this investigation was that nursery school children who had received the most and best physical education not only performed better in many tasks, but also displayed superior postural alignments.

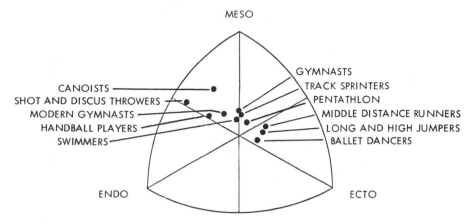

FIGURE 3.10 Mean somatoplots of selected groups of outstanding female athletes. From J. E. L. Carter, "The Prediction of Outstanding Atfhletic Ability: The Structural Perspective," in F. Landry and W. A. R. Orban (eds.) *Exercise Physiology,* v. 4, Miami: Symposia Specialists, 1978, pp. 29-42. With permission of the publishers.

Early walkers are those who have large muscular legs, and whose bones are not overly large (Shirley, 1931; Norval, 1947). Throughout childhood, as numerous researchers have found, early skeletal maturation is associated with superior motor performance (Seils, 1951) and with memberships on teams as adolescence is reached (Clarke, 1971). At the same time, it is important to differentiate between what kinds of physique components and qualities are contrasted to just what kinds

FIGURE 3.11 Mean somatoplots of selected groups of outstanding male athletes. From J. E. L. Carter, "The Prediction of Outstanding Athletic Ability: The Structural Perspective," in F. Landry and W. A. R. Orban (eds.) *Exercise Physiology,* v. 4, Miami: Symposia Specialists, 1978, pp. 29-42. With permission of the publishers.

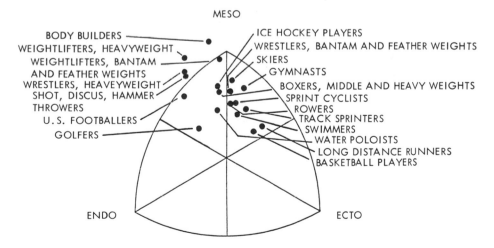

of motor tasks before sweeping generalizations are formulated about relationships (or the lack of relationships) between physical tasks and physique qualities during both childhood and adolescence.

In the early school years, data relating physique variables to physical performance are not plentiful. More work has been done using children in later childhood and adolescence. For the most part, there are usually low to moderate correlations between physical performance and mesomorphy, or muscularity, as would be expected. Agility tasks are generally performed better by children with linear and muscular builds than by children who are obese. The same is true when ectomorphic children are contrasted to those with muscular physiques in strength tasks; the mesomorphs are superior. However, it is usually easier to find slight correlations between children evidencing extremes in ectomorphy and endomorphy and physical performance than when trying to derive predictable relationships between mesomorphic physique qualities and physical performance measures. Children within the mid-ranges of physique qualities are less predictable when exposed to both strength and endurance tasks than youngsters evidencing extremes in physiques, either extreme to moderate fatness or thinness (Wear and Miller, 1962; Bookwalter, 1952).

In adolescence, the best-performing boys are generally those within the medium physique categories (mesomorphs) who have relatively short legs and narrow hips, in contrast to poorer performing boys with stocky builds, wide hips, and relatively long legs (Espenschade, 1940). Girls in adolescence who perform best are usually characterized by a slender, muscular physique, as would be expected (Espenschade, 1940).

However, when data from more recent studies of body build using the somatotyping methods devised by Sheldon are inspected, the expected relationships between adolescents' body builds and performance are slight. In a 1967 study, for example (Espenschade and Eckert, 1967), it was found that high-performing boys were only slightly higher in mesomorphy and considerably lower in endomorphy, with little difference in ectomorphy, than more poorly performing male adolescents. Similar trends were noted when the body builds of high- versus low-performing girls were compared in the same study. The mesomorphic girls were only slightly superior to girls with other somatotypes. Generally, however, endomorphy correlates negatively with endurance tasks; ectomorphy combined with mesomorphy predicts good endurance efforts in adolescents (Cullumbine et al., 1950).

The presumption that body build is a clear-cut indicator of superior performance in a variety of tasks is perhaps a myth engendered by inspection of Olympic athletes, rather than a solid scientific fact based on surveys of large populations of youngsters and adolescents. Scientists in the countries of Eastern Europe, always eager to learn the correlates of athletic excellence, have coined the word "anthropomotorics" to reflect the search for an ideal body build for each and every athletic feat. However, in the real world populated by the large mass of children and adults, variables other than simply the shape of the body contribute to or detract from motor performance and athletic prowess. It seems particularly difficult to predict how the "average looking" child will perform physical skills without having more information about the youngster than simply physique conformations. Motor performance in childhood is formed and enhanced by many subtle factors, such as the quality of the motor programs inherited from the family, as well as the nature of the fiber types and capacities for endurance work acquired from these same relatives. Access to coaching and facilities, as well as the child's unique motivational make-up, are further contributing factors.

In the 1980s anthropometric research reflecting an interest in measuring body build has lost some degree of popularity. Perhaps it has become tiresome to determine that indeed Olympic weight lifters are muscular, or that gymnasts are small-boned and short. Perhaps those measuring body build have simply become overwhelmed by the task of classifying and norming body builds within the many ethnic and racial groups represented both in the world and in the United States. For without ethnic-racial specifics, so-called norms for body build, as well as for weight-height ratios at various ages, are difficult to interpret.

One of the most promising new uses for body-build data apparent in contemporary research is to contrast it to various psychological measures. For example, the child's feelings about his or her body are often correlated with the child's actual body build. Differences are obtained contrasting measures of the youngster's perceptions of an ideal body build and the child's somatotype. These psychological measures of the child's body concept are used to ascertain how total self-concept is reflected in youngsters' perceptions of their physiques. Psychological measures of this type are also explored as possible predictors of efforts children make when performing physical skills, and the tendency to participate in competitive sports.

BODY PSYCHOLOGY AND THE CHILD

The body is something to be looked out from. It is several months, and even years, before infant and child begin to form even general impressions of bodily conformations, capacities, and size. Still later, the child begins to become able to compare his or her body to those of others, and to begin to make "liking" decisions about the platform from which movement arises.

It is understandable that various discrepancies occur between how children perceive their bodies and how they are viewed by others. Social psychologists interested in the formation of what are termed the social cognitions that form "other" schematas as well as "self" schematas tell us that the way we form self-perceptions is generally based upon verbal data coming to us in the form of self-talk about how we are, what we can do, and how we appear. On the other hand, these behavioral scientists contend, the formation of ideas and perceptions about others is based upon data taken in visually—information about behavior and about body size and shape.

As children mature, they form two large classifications of ideas about their bodies. On one hand are easily researched ideas about the names of body parts, what movements these parts can make, and about their left and right body parts. A second classification is more difficult to objectify and involves feelings about the body, its acceptability to the child, its movement capacities in a variety of situations, as well as what the child feels about how others view the shape and movement potentials of his or her physique. The child's body, when viewed both physically and psychologically, is a multifaceted vehicle moving at times hestitatingly through infancy, childhood, and adolescence. It consists of a firm genotype (or morphogenotype), as well as a more modifiable phenotype. From a social-emotional-psychological perspective, children's bodies also consist of how they believe themselves to be, as well as how they think they are viewed by others. Action capacities may also be viewed operationally and physically as well as psychologically. That is, the child has the objective capacities to perform various tasks and at the same time holds less concrete ideas as to what might be accomplished, colored by what the child believes is expected by others viewing the body and the apparent capacities it possesses.

If a child is within some elusive norm deemed acceptable or average by parents and friends, little social-emotional trauma may occur. However, if the youngster is "too" something (fat, thin, wide, tall), marked distortions may occur. These problems and distortions may be reflected in the child's self-perceptions, as well as in the expectations of both parents and peers. Moreover, marked variations in maturational rate or size and shape of the child are likely to have rather direct impacts upon the child's ability and willingness to participate in physical skills. To cite some examples, during evaluations of several thousand youngsters in our laboratory at UCLA over the years, we have been struck by what has been called an "age-size" illusion. This refers to the fact that some children do not appear in line with their chronological age. They may be bigger and thus appear older than the number of birthdays they have experienced. Conversely, they may be smaller and immature-looking compared to children of a similar chronological age. In either case, there are predictable social-emotional as well as physical outcomes. The child who seems mature and/or large for his or her age elicits expectations from others in the areas of physical skill and emotional control that may be difficult to satisfy. The immature, small youngster may be expected to react in ways that are immature and physically inept, and these expectations in turn may begin to mold the actual abilities acquired by the undersized youngster.

The youngster in late childhood who may be maturing earlier becomes a valued member of sports teams and the subsequent recipient of adults' coaching efforts. This early start, in turn, is likely to heighten both self-esteem as well as the willingness to train hard, both requisites to later sustained athletic performance of a high quality. Late maturing youngsters may receive little or no early support for their physical efforts, but in fact may face derision when physical acts are attempted in early and middle childhood. These youngsters are far less likely to persist in sports and games, and may instead turn toward more sedentary endeavors likely to elicit recognition, including music, scientific efforts, computers, and other forms of academics. Less acceptable social compensations than these are also often acted out by the youngster who is immature and inept physically.

Within the past two decades, more and more attention has been paid to the interaction of the child's and adolescent's self-concepts with feelings they have about their changing bodies. These studies have also concentrated on how the child who somehow feels different in body build functions socially and emotionally, as well as how the youngster whose physique is deviant feels about himself or herself (Hendry and Gillis, 1978; Stager and Burk, 1982; Tucker, 1983; Collins and Propert, 1983).

Liking and Disliking Bodily Conformations

One critical factor in the formation of at least part of maturing children's self-concepts is whether or not youngsters accept and like or reject and dislike the shape and size of their bodies. A second important variable involves children's perceptions of how they believe one with their bodily conformation is expected to act both in general ways and when confronted with opportunities to move. Still another important aspect of this problem is how acceptable the child is to himself or herself relative to various areas of functioning, including physical and athletic competence. Since the late 1970s and 1980s, more and more researchers have begun to deal with these and related concepts. Moreover, how a child may preceive his or her bodily conformations may be situationally specific, rather than a generalized perception (Stager & Burke 1982).

Essentially this work revolves around the assumption that simply evaluating body build with the anthropometric tools described in the previous section reveals only a rather superficial aspect of the body and body image. What is of more importance are judgments society as a whole makes about people with various body types. Almost a half-century ago, Sheldon suggested that human behavior is influenced by the body build and the genetic and physiological qualities that may influence the physique. More recently, a number of researchers have modified that assumption after finding few relationships between personality and body types. A more enlightened contemporary view is one revolving around principles of social learning. This viewpoint, first proposed by McCandless (1961), is that any relationship between body build and behavior is caused by social expectations that people with various body builds will behave in stereotypic ways. This expectation theory linking body build and behavior has been validated in several studies, some of which have involved children (Lerner, 1969; Staffieri, 1967). For the most part, like findings among adults, children tend to rate the mesomorphic physique most desirable and also attach more favorable social evaluations to those with muscular and trim body builds.

An important research program has been conducted at the University of Denver by Susan Harter and her associates (1981). This research has involved the use of a self-perception scale for children involving the degree to which children accept in a positive way their competencies in three areas: social competence, athletic and physical competence, and cognitive or scholastic competence. Although at times these researchers have attempted to divide the assessment of these purportedly separate domains, some of their data reveal that in young children the separation of how a child feels about social versus physical self is difficult. So ingrained are the abilities to *do* things physically with the younger child's total self-concept that these two qualities are not always perceived as separate when younger children are evaluated. The evaluative instrument recently formulated by Harter includes six separate subscales, several of which have relevance for further research on children and physical activity. These subscales include scholastic competence, social acceptance, athletic competence, physical appearance, behavior/conduct, and self-worth.

Furthermore, in both adolescents and children there are important relationships between a positive self-concept and how far a youngster feels his or her own body build deviates from a hypothesized ideal, usually a mesomorphic build (Tucker, 1983; Guggenheim, Poznanski, and Kaufmann, 1977). These associations between self-concept and idealized mesomorphic body build can produce negative social-emotional outcomes in children and adolescents who may deviate from the ideal average (Hendry and Gillies, 1978). It is a consistent finding that especially among older children and adolescents, obesity or undue thinness can have negative influences upon the maturing youngster's self-concept (Guggenheim et al., 1977; Hendry and Gillies, 1978).

Body Image in Late Childhood

It is probable that as a child matures from early to middle and then to late childhood and finally adolescence, concern about bodily conformation increases. This heightened concern is probably brought about by the fact that the youngster becomes increasingly aware of both negative and positive social evaluations from sexually desired others, as well as youngsters' more mature perception of life in general as they grow older. However, it seems apparent that even at relatively young ages, children attach both negative and positive connotations to individuals simply because of the appearance of their physiques. Staffieri (1967) studied the reactions of 90 boys from 6 to 10 years of age when presented with silhouettes that represented extreme endomorphy, mesomorphy, and ectomorphy. All the adjectives the children attached to the mesomorphy physique were positive and included such descriptions as "strong," "best friend," "clean," "lots of friends," and "healthy." The words and qualities associated with the endomorphy were for the most part unfavorable and socially aggressive. The fat silhouette was characterized as "fights," "nervous," "gets teased," "lies," "naughty," "stupid," and "dirty." The thin silhouette was described by these children in terms that reflect a passive and submissive nature. A thin body type drew such descriptions as "quiet," "worries," "lonely," "afraid,' and "sad."

Further, the data in this investigation indicated a gradual evolution from the sixth to the tenth year in preference for a mesomorphic physique as a personal ideal, with this preference starting to be seen by the age of 7 or 8. Moreover, by the eighth and ninth years the children's perceptions of their own body builds tended to match with some accuracy their actual physical conformations. It thus appears that during middle childhood, youngsters begin to evidence reasonably accurate judgments about the shapes of their bodies. At the same time they become increasingly likely to evidence concern about whether or not their bodies match some hypothesized ideal. Williams (1983), for example, reported the results of two unpublished studies which indicated that children at 5 are not very accurate when attempting to describe the shapes of their bodies. In a 1967 study by Staffieri, it was found that children 8 years of age and older were able to report self-perceptions of body build that were quite accurate. Support for the contention that children at about this same time begin to register unhappiness if they feel their bodies are not somehow ideal are found in the data from Dibiase and Hjelle (1968). They found that children at 8 years not only began to assign favorable and unfavorable social attributes to various physique types, but also began to evidence some signs of social retardation if they believed their own body build was not pleasingly mesomorphic.

Before middle childhood, children are able to make various simple judgments about the height and widths of their physiques. However, formation of the body concept probably begins to assume new and important dimensions during middle childhood (Stiles, 1975).

The Body Image in Adolescence

As adolescence is reached, feelings about their bodies heighten in both female and males. In a 1973 study by Wiggins, for example, both male and female adolescents, while having an overall positive self-concept, indicated that they were dissatisfied with both their heights and weights. As might be expected, deviations in body build are also reflected in more deviant social-emotional behaviors, and in distortions of self-concept during late childhood and early adolescence. Hendry and Gillies (1978), for example, studied the interplay of social forces revolving around 1,000 youngsters 15 to 16, classified into three groups labeled overweight, underweight, or average. It was found, as expected, that the overweight youngsters were the most unfit of the groups, but additionally they also possessed lower body esteem than the other youngsters. The underweight adolescents, on the other hand, appeared more socially isolated than their more robust peers, while evidencing a higher self-concept. These findings are reflected in numerous other studies evaluating body build and social-emotional variables among teenagers of average and atypical physiques, body weights, and height-weight ratios (Guggenheim et al., 1977). It is usually found that overweight girls seem to suffer more than their male counterparts. Dwyer and Mayer (1967) have suggested that the cause for this is that females appear more dependent upon social success and positive feedback from others, whereas males are more anchored in personal achievement. However, this kind of assumption needs further clarification in the light of changing social pressures for success in females. Indeed, teenagers of the 1980s perceive all slim people as possessing innumerable positive traits, whereas fat people are viewed negatively (Worsley, 1981).

Obesity in children is often a function of social class, with lower-class young-sters often tending toward obesity more than is true among those more favored eco-nomically. Concern about their figures among females in their early teens, and the subsequent stringent diets that may be instituted, may lead to a condition receiving more and more publicity in the popular press during the 1980s, *anorexia nervosa* (Crisp, 1977). Often pubertal females wish to minimize their changing shapes and thus characterize themselves as fat when in truth they are not obese (Guggenheim et al., 1977). This forced dieting may result in extreme weight loss and in actual termi-nation of a main signpost of puberty, the menarche. If the dieting continues, severe weight loss can lead to profound psychophysical consequences. The condition, which involves an extreme psychotic distortion of the body image, is correctable only through psychotherapy and medical intervention. Its course is depicted in Fig-ure 3.12.

Marked concern with physique is not a sole concern of females, however. In studies we have carried out with young adolescents and boys in late childhood, they have been asked to "draw a picture of yourself." Often the outcome is a stylized muscular depiction of Conan the Barbarian, often suspended in an iron cross from the gymnastic rings. Likewise, the overall self-concept of young males seems closely linked to the physique type they are perhaps fortunate enough to pos-sess.

Tucker (1983) recently studied 284 young males, presenting each with seven drawn somatotypes ranging from extreme ectomorphy, through mesomorphy, to the obese endomorph. He, like other researchers over the years, was interested not only in the self-concept scores of the males in various categories but also in how far their perceptions of an ideal physique varied from their actual physiques. Positive per-ceptions of the physical self were higher in the mesomorphic males than in the thin or obese young men. The overall self-concept scores obtained from the subjects de-clined in individuals who were thin or fat. Although the majority of the males be-lieved the mesomorphic physique to be ideal, 35 percent believed a build that was slightly obese or thinner was better. Most important in this investigation was the finding that the young men who perceived the ideal physique as quite different from their own scored significantly lower on the self-concept scale administered. It ap-peared that there was a critical point in the score reflecting discrepancy between the ideal physical self and the actual physical self at which the young men's feelings about themselves tended to diminish.

Evidence from various cultures indicates that satisfaction with one's size and weight may be influenced by self-imposed racial-ethnic stereotypes. For example, Mizuno and his colleagues (Mizuno et al., 1968) found that Japanese children and youth tended to view ideal body builds as similar to larger youngsters in English and American cultures. In several studies, this group of researchers found: (1) Boys in all cultures studied wished themselves taller and heavier than their national aver-ages; (2) girls studied in the various countries wished to be slimmer than national means; and (3) Japanese youth wished both their stature and weight to be near the national averages in England and America (Mizuno, 1967, 1968).

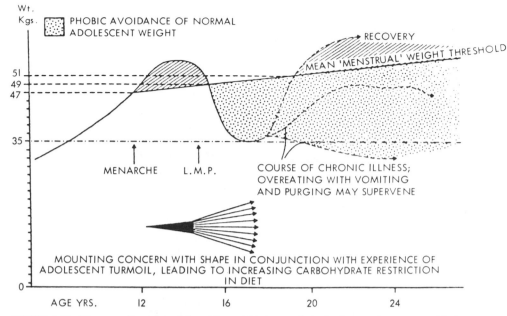

FIGURE 3.12 Diagrammatic representation of the weight changes that arise in anorexia nervosa and their relationship to mounting concern about shape once the "menstrual" weight threshold has been exceeded. The stippled area is the range within which the syndrome operates (actual thresholds will vary from person to person but will be of this order). L.M.P. = last menstrual period. From Crisp. 1977.

THE VERBAL IDENTIFICATION OF BODY PARTS

Numerous attempts have been made during the past fifty years to obtain verbal responses from children indicating their awareness of the names of body parts, their left-right dimensions, as well as other judgments about the planes of the body. These investigations have at times contrasted these judgments in normal and in atypical youngsters. Other studies of this nature have been employed to ascertain how general judgments about the body's space reflect accurate awareness of components of more distant elements of space. Left-right responses are often obtained to ascertain whether so-called assessments of laterality have anything to do with the child's attempts to organize the up-down and left-right of words, letters, and sentences.

Correct reactions to verbalizations of body parts is seen in normal children by the end of the first year and the beginning of the second year of life. Even though at this period the infant does not possess expressive language, and thus cannot both point to and name body parts, he or she is able to indicate correctly many body parts when their names are spoken by an older child or an adult. Thus the infant at from 10 months to 16 months enjoys playing games involving "Where is your tummy?" and the like. Moreover, during these early months the infant will readily imitate gestures reflected in such games as peek-a-boo.

Benton was one of the first to construct formal tests intended to determine both the accuracy as well as the speed with which children can identify body parts as they mature. The Benton test requires that a child point to the body parts in a picture in making identifications (Benton, 1959). Ilg and Ames in early studies began to illuminate some of the ways in which children begin to identify body parts as they mature. By the age of 5, over 80 percent of the children they tested were able to identify parts of the face, and the arms and hands. Parts of the hands are identified beginning at the age of 5, when the thumb is discovered; the process continues until the age of 7, when the elusive ring finger is finally detected (Ilg and Ames, 1966).

More recently, Kuczar and Maratsos (1975) explored the child's acquisition of the concepts of front, back, and side. Among other qualities they tried to illuminate is whether or not children must become aware of their *own* front and back before they can detect the same qualities in objects external to the body. It is interesting to note that the children they evaluated, ranging in age from 30 to 49 months, seemed to acquire front-back concepts both for themselves as well as for objects at about the same time. This finding is in contrast to the often-stated hypothesis that children must first somehow perceptually organize their body and its parts before being expected to make complex judgments about visual space. These researchers found that front and back concepts were far easier to acquire than notions about the side of the body and of objects. However, the children they tested also seemed to discover the concept of side both on themselves and on objects at about the same months of age.

As a result of this assessment, Kuczaj and Maratsos concluded that the children they polled, ranging in age from 2.5 to slightly over 4 years, exhibited the following sequence when asked to identify side, back, and front:

1. First, children can place objects in front and in back of themselves with accuracy. It was also found that these concepts of front and back were equally difficult for the children tested.
2. Next, children are able to touch the fronts and backs of objects that obviously have a front and back, such as a typewriter.
3. Third, the child can place objects correctly to the back and front of "fronted" objects, those having delineated fronts and backs.
4. Next, the child becomes able to understand the concept of side, both within himself or herself, as well as connected to objects in space.

More work is needed to explore in greater detail the acquisition of these concepts with reference to the body, as well as similar qualities possessed by other people and objects in the child's space field. Studies are needed that determine whether various kinds of motor training using verbal cues will heighten and accelerate the acquisition of these kinds of concepts in nursery-school-age youngsters.

Left-Right Discriminations

Major efforts have been made during the past twenty years to ascertain the child's acquisition of left-right concepts relative to body parts. It has been hypothesized that this judgment, when accurately made about the body, will transfer to space. It has also been suggested the child's early reading efforts will be impaired unless he or she is able to discriminate accurately between various asymmetrical letters, the correct placement order of letters in words, and the correct (left in English) end of the line from which to start reading.

In early studies, Ilg and Ames (1966) again provide some guidance as to how younger children begin to acquire the idea that different sides and parts of their body have different names, one group called "right," the other named "left." For example, after pointing to a hand or body part, the investigators asked, "What is the name of this to you?" If was found that 74 percent of the girls and 66 percent of the boys at the age of 5 failed to identify correctly their left and right hands; by the age of 6, 62 percent of the girls and 56 percent of the boys still failed to make this kind of discrimination. By 7 years, however, only 14 percent of the girls and 16 percent of the boys were unable to identify their left and right hands correctly.

The reasons children gave for making these left-right discriminations were classified by the experimenters. The most frequent was that the hand was connected with a motor function of some kind: "I use it to salute the flag, to eat with, to write with."

Ilg and Ames requested other right-left discriminations to be made in relation to other body parts. It was found that the left ear and eye were identified correctly (or were accorded consistent opposite identifications) by about 50 percent of the 5-year-olds and by about 68 percent of the 6-year-olds. (By chance, children can be expected to give correct responses concerning left and right about 50 percent of the time!) By the age of 6, 64 percent of these children were able to identify correctly the left and right hands of the examiner; by 7 years 74 percent were able to do so; and by the age of 8, 95 percent could successfully project themselves into the reference system of the examiner.

Although the development of unilateral hand use is seen as early as the seventh *month* of age according to some authorities, it seems that cognitive awareness of the body's left-right dimensions is gained considerably later, at about the age of 6 or 7 *years*.

Binet suggests that this kind of left-right recognition occurs at about the age of 7; Terman places it at 6 years, and Piaget agrees with him. According to Gallifret-Granjon (1959) the recognition of a child's own left and right occurred at 6 years of age in 86 percent of the cases he surveyed, and the recognition of left and right in an observer did not occur until the age of 8. The recognition of the relative position of three objects, using Piaget's test, does not occur before 10 or 12 years of age (Hacaen and Ajuriaguerra, 1964).

Cacoursiere-Paige has investigated the importance of a number of variables, including intelligence, the ability to draw the human figure, and figure-copying tests, in relation to left-right discrimination. In this 1974 study, chronological age was found to be more predictive of left-right discrimination in children than other variables studied (Cacoursiere-Paige, 1974). Moreover, it has been found that left-right discriminations in children are reflected in several stages:

Stage I: The child cannot distinguish between the two sides of his body; from birth to about 3.5 years.

Stage II: The child becomes aware that his left and right limbs are found on either side of his body but is unaware of their location, which body parts are called "left" and which ones are "right." This stage usually occurs between the ages of 4 and 5 years.

Stage III: The child realizes that the left and right limbs and organs are found on opposite sides of his body without knowing that they are right or left parts; between the ages of 6 and 7 years.

Stage IV: During the fourth stage the child comes to know precisely which parts of his body are right and left; between the ages of 8 and 9 years.

It is becoming increasingly apparent that children's judgments about the left-right dimensions of themselves and of others (things and objects) continues to undergo evolution throughout childhood and even into adolescence. Illustrating this important concept is information obtained by Long and Looft in their 1972 study. They used 140 children and 125 items in a comprehensive testing effort encompassing seven age levels. It was found that the following qualities emerged from the ages of 6 to 12 years:

1.   At age 6, the children were able to mirror or imitate the movements made by another, using one side of their body. These movements could easily be made across the midpoint of their bodies.

2.   By 7, children exhibited more refined laterality. They could project spatial judgments to objects by correctly placing a coin between, or in the middle of, two objects when asked to do so. Further, they could make reference to both sides of the body. They could, for example, respond correctly to such requests as "Show me your left hand and your right eye."

3.   At year 8, a marked increase was seen in the laterality scores obtained in the children when contrasted to those of 7-year-olds. They could, for example, exhibit what the researchers called "decentration" by freeing judgments about space from their bodies; at this age the children could grasp that "the key is to the right of the coin" without reference to the left and right of their own bodies.

4.   At 9 years, even more flexible spatial judgments could be made about the location of objects in space, and about their placement relative to each other. Children could easily process more and more information and react accurately to such directions as "Draw a line from the upper right-hand corner to the lower left-hand corner of the page." Judgments that required them to cross their body were possible at this age. They could, for example, react properly when asked to touch their left ear with their right hand.

5.   More and more freedom from a personal bodily orientation was seen at the age of 10 years. The children could correctly identify the left and right of an individual facing them. This and other qualities at this age indicate that children are becoming increasingly able to free themselves from a personal reference system.

6.   By 11 and 12 years, the children had become able to employ more than one reference system at the same time, and to use such concepts as "The sun is rising in the east."

These data are often referred to as evidence of body image development. However, these judgments are heavily dependent on both conceptual and linguistic abilities (Kuczaj and Maratsos, 1975). Moreover, if the child is given directions to carry out some complicated spatial judgment and/or to respond in a complicated manner, both motor planning and auditory memory are brought into play. For example, if a child is asked to "touch your left eye with your right hand," at least seven bits of information need to be perceived in the correct order, stored in short-term memory, and then executed as a complicated motor plan.

Some inroads have been made concerning whether or not these kinds of body image and related spatial judgments may be improved through tutoring. Employing operant conditioning, Spionnek has demonstrated that by 5 years of age children can be taught to correctly identify their left and right body parts. This is two years before children could normally be expected to make these kinds of judgments. Data from an unpublished study by the author and one of his students also demonstrated that left-right discriminations in children classified as minimally neurologically handicapped could be significantly improved through training in various movement activities that incorporated left-right decisions on the part of the child ("Roll over your left shoulder," "Jump and turn to your right"). In experiments in which choice answers are required (left or right), it may not be assumed that "correct" answers are being elicited unless a population of children responds with accuracy about 75 percent of the time. It is thus apparent that not until about the age of 7 can normal children correctly identify their left and right body parts and sides with consistency.

Finally, it should be emphasized that these so-called tests of body image, and of the resultant spatial judgments, are invariably performed more poorly by children lacking academic abilities and high measures of verbal intelligence. It should not therefore be assumed that a poor body image score (gained through testing involving verbal responses) somehow causes learning disabilities, and that all one must do is simply raise the body image score to improve reading. It is more valid to conclude that lack of awarenesses of the verbal-cognitive dimensions of body parts, and of spatial judgments related to these, is simply another confirmation that the child needs academic and intellectual tutoring in a broad way. Simply correcting a purported body image deficit will not inevitably increase scores on academic and reading tests.

Imitation of Gestures

Within the last several decades, several clinicians (Ayres, 1969; Kephart, 1964) have developed tests and subtests purportedly evaluating body image that require the child to correctly imitate the gestures or positions of the examiner. One of the more sophisticated of these was produced by Berges and Lezine and translated into the English from the French in which it initially appeared. The children's bodily awareness is hypothetically evaluated in this instrument by noting the accuracy with which they can imitate the hand and limb gestures of the examiner (Berges and Lezine, 1965).

The test has been divided into two sections including both simple and complex gestures. In the initial portion of the test, simple hand and arm positions are assumed by the examiner, and the child is scored according to the proficiency he exhibits when imitating them. In the complex gesture section, the child is asked to imitate more difficult finger and arm gestures, some of which require imitation of the tester's movements.

In the simple-gestures portion of the test, it has been found that 3-year-olds are able to perform only about half as well as 6-year-olds; at the age of 4 years, the children evidence about 75 percent of the proficiency of children two years older. When responses to complex gestures are evaluated, the 3-year-olds are found to be only one-third as proficient at copying these more complicated patterns, several of which involve movement, as are 6-year-olds.

The simplest gestures for the children to copy were those in which static positioning was involved, usually employing the arm and/or hand. More difficult were gestures in which two body parts were employed at the same time, such as "raise right arm and extend left horizontally." The most difficulty was encountered when children were asked to imitate gestures in which the limbs positioned in two planes, such as "parallel hands in different places with left hand forward."

Ayres has produced data in a similar test which indicates that marked changes in ability to imitate gestures in children occur at each six-month interval from 4 to about 8 years. After that age, a deceleration of scores seems to occur, but even at age 8 errors continue to be made in the imitation of relatively simple gestures. For the most part, these tests involve simple motor planning, but they do not sufficiently tax youngsters' abilities to process information that may be gradually added to, until a "topping off" effect is reached. Some of the tests and qualities examined in the section on motor planning in Chapter 9, titled "special qualities," permit a more thorough evaluation of the ability of a child to first perceive and then to organize and produce movements at various levels of complexity.

SUMMARY

Physical maturation does not proceed evenly throughout childhood and adolescence. Growth rates of both boys and girls decelerate after the ages of 1 and 2 years and show acceleration again during adolescence.

Sex differences in rate and the nature of physical growth include (a) the earlier onset of the adolescent growth spurt in females, (b) greater percent of body fat in females, and (c) a tendency for females to be smaller than males at all ages.

Individual differences in body build and in rate of maturation are important consideratons when evaluating how children and youth feel about their bodies. For the most part, a muscular physique is valued more highly than a thin or a fat one in most cultures of the world when youngsters' opinions are evaluated. Moreover, the difference between what a youngster views as ideal and the measurable physique of the child is often an important index of adequate self-acceptance.

Body build and body image measures range from those based on objective measures of fat, bony girth, and height/weight to those reflecting a psychological orientaton. For the most part it is at about the age of 8 to 9 years that youngsters begin to perceive (a) that various body builds exist, and (b) that theirs may be acceptable, or less than acceptable, to them. Both positive and negative feelings about body build are often heightened during adolescence.

Perceptions of the body and accurate verbal identifications of body parts are often unrelated qualities. For the most part, verbal identification of body parts and left-right dimensions reflect vocabulary and cognitive abilities. The left-right identifications of the body, and of other spatial qualities (front-back) of both the body and of things in space, undergo regular changes throughout childhood and early adolescence.

Physical development programs intended to improve various physique qualities should contain measures intended to objectify the physical size, shape, and performance capacities of the youngsters served, as well as their measures of the ways in which they may perceive their bodies.

QUESTIONS FOR DISCUSSION

1. What kinds of psychological distortions of the body image may emerge in late childhood or early adolescence?
2. What kinds of individual differences may be seen in how the body matures physically? How might these differences modify the child's emerging body-concept?
3. What cultural-ethnic influences may there be on adolescents' body images in various countries of the world?
4. How may the body image be evaluated? What are some of the advantages and disadvantages of some of the various measures available?
5. What stages may be seen in how children identify left and right body parts, and the various left-right and front-back dimensions of objects in space?
6. What are relationships between body build and performance capacities in a large group of average boys and girls? Do these relationships change if one employs Olympic athletes in the comparison?
7. What sex differences may be seen in measures of physique, physical maturation, and body image?
8. What advantages might an early maturing boy or girl enjoy socially and athletically? What about a late maturing boy or girl?
9. What does the research say about relationships between left-right discriminations made on the body and reading, letter reversal, and the like within an academic context?
10. How do children seem to become able to identify their body parts' left-right dimensions? Do judgments of this type about the body occur before or at the same time as similar judgments about objects are formed?
11. Contrast and compare the concepts of genotype and phenotype.

STUDENT PROJECTS

1. Pay a visit to a playground and observe possible differences in the way children with various physiques react emotionally and physically within game contexts. Can you score or in some way objectify these differences?

2. Discuss, in a case study approach, with a 10-year-old how he would like to perform, how he does perform, and his perceptions of his present and future body build. Do the same with a girl of from 10 to 12 years. What variables in family and home environment might modify their responses? How does their inherited physique influence their responses? What differences can you detect between their physical bodies and their ideal or desired body type?

3. Survey the manner in which a variety of left-right judgments are made by a child of 4 and one of 7. Use object qualities in your evaluations ("What is the left and right of that box?") What differences do you find? How do the data you obtain compare to what is said about these qualities in the literature?

4. Apply one of the contemporary somatotyping techniques (Heath-Carter) to an adolescent. Formulate predictions about how the youngster feels about his or her body, and about the potential and present performance capacities of the youngster.

CHAPTER FOUR
VARIABLES INFLUENCING MOTOR DEVELOPMENT

Many things can influence the unfolding of movement capacities in infants and children. These variables may be roughly classified into two main groups including (a) qualities that cause normal variations in movement qualities such as inherited size and bodily conformations, and (b) influences that produce pathological conditions, reflected in atypical action patterns.

The first part of the chapter contains how "normal" variation in actions may be elicited by differences in learning opportunities and in racial-ethnic backgrounds. Secondly, a brief survey is made of some of the more prevalent pathological conditions that may influence movement and the formation of a healthy fetus. The chapter concludes with a section covering intervention programs.

It is believed important for the movement specialist to become reasonably well grounded in this kind of information for several reasons. Awareness of the factors that cause individual differences, both normal and atypical, help the movement specialist to become a more sensitive evaluator and observer of the action patterns of the youth being served. Often the movement specialist in a nursery school setting is the first to observe that "something may be wrong" with a child, an observation that should prompt early and appropriate referral. More and more atypical children are being mainstreamed into programs containing "normal" youngsters. Those who are responsible for such programs should be aware of the limitations and problems of various kinds of "atypical" children and youth. And finally, movement specialists are increasingly being called upon to provide special remediation programs for motorically handicapped children.

RACIAL-ETHNIC DIFFERENCES

For decades, relatively consistent racial-ethnic differences in motor development have been identified when children in various parts of the world have been surveyed and compared. Typically, children within the black race have evidenced superiority, starting with an apparent advantage at birth and continuing into the first year of life. Black children both in the United States as well as abroad have been found to be better able to run (Hutsinger, 1959), to throw farther, and even to balance better than white children with whom they were contrasted (Bonds, 1969).

Black infants abroad have similarly been shown to be superior in motor development when compared to norms obtained on white children in the United States. The Gesell scale was a favorite instrument early in the history of such studies. Werner (1972), in a survey of these investigations prior to 1970, points out the remarkably consistent superiority of all children born within what she identifies as "preindustrial societies" when contrasted to infants born within more modern communities.

Werner's survey disclosed that infants born within preindustrial societies in several parts of the world, including Latin America, Africa, and India, at birth equaled the sensory-motor development of infants born in industrialized societies at from 3 to 4 months of age. These precocious infants seemed to be less hypertonic at birth and were not apparently restricted by the presence of such reflexes as the Moro. They seemed equipped to begin to move voluntarily much earlier than infants born within more modern settings. Even evidence obtained from electroencephalographic evaluations of the nervous systems of these infants revealed maturity in advance of that of children from more industrialized cultures (Gerber and Dean, 1957, 1964). Other data suggested that differences in bone density and the appearance of ossification milestones appear when the races are compared even at birth (Seale, 1959; Kelly and Reynolds, 1947; Masse and Hunt, 1963). At times even premature babies born to some African and to Central American mothers may evidence motor development similar to that of children who are born at full term within more "favorable" circumstances (Werner, 1972).

The findings from more recent studies, however, suggest that differences in child-rearing practices may contribute to differences in motor precocity that were previously attributed to race or ethnicity. For example, children reared in a preindustrial setting enjoy the benefits of several practices that are likely to hasten motor development. These include: (a) The child is more likely to be breast-fed. (b) An extended family often affords the infant a great deal of physical contact and handling during the first year of life. (c) The infants are usually toileted and fed upon demand, instead of according to more rigid time schedules. (d) Their clothing is often sparse and thus not likely to restrict early efforts at movement.

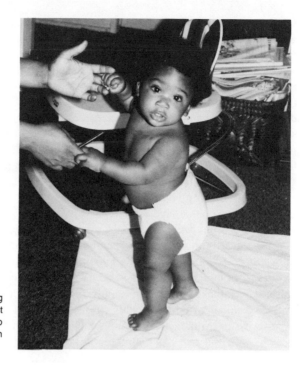

FIGURE 4.1
This motorically precocious young lady, whose parents are from West Africa, is easily able to pull herself to her feet at 6.5 months, and to walk with some assistance.

Additionally, it is often highly desirable for infants in a preindustrial setting to sit up, crawl, and walk well before the first year of life is completed. It has been found recently that mothers in these settings make special efforts to teach their youngsters important developmental skills that lead to walking at young ages (Super, 1978). In some African subcultures, it has been found that over 80 percent of the parents make the effort to teach their children to sit, stand, and walk. On a visit to West Africa a few years ago, I was introduced to the practice some village women had of actually "planting" their infants in an upright position, buried to the waist, in the earth beside the fields, in order to hasten the acquisition of an upright stance. It has been noted that some African languages contain specific words denoting this type of early motor training by parents (Super, 1978). Current findings (Hennessee and Dixon, 1984) suggest that the more mature gait characteristics seen in black African children, when contrasted to these qualities in Caucasian children, are the result of maternal training efforts.

It has also been found that often the apparent early acceleration in motor development noted in preindustrial societies may disappear toward the end of the first year, when such youngsters are weaned. Thus, both physical handling plus breast-feeding correlate with early acceleration of motor qualities. When good or adequate nourishment from the mother is withdrawn and a less nutritious diet is substituted, previous gains in movement capacities are negated (Werner, 1972).

However, in recent studies, efforts have been made to sort out the influence of various cultural and racial variables as they might influence so-called superiority of various racial and ethnic groups. Lee (1980), for example, studied the motor abilities of both white and black children raised in either a permissive or authoritarian manner. She found that independent of the child-rearing practices engaged in by the mothers, black children evidenced superiority in both running and jumping. Solomons studied some of the possible causes behind infant motor development in children in the Yucatan. Solomons believes, for example, that the infants in the group she studied tended to use their hands rather early in life because of the nonavailability of toys. She argues, as have others, for norms of infant development that are in line with specific subcultures, rather than applying so-called averages in an indiscriminate manner (Solomons, 1978).

Kilbride recently (1980) found that infants within two African subcultures lagged behind comparable American white infants in signs of motor development (sitting, creeping, walking). In the African subcultures studied (the Baganda and Somia), early motor training by parents was not stressed. Kilbride suggests that rather than accepting the simple hypothesis that African infants overall are somehow precocious motorically, it is better to formulate models that take into account cultural variables, rather than simply race and/or ethnicity.

A number of other possible causes have been hypothesized for the apparent superiority of children from various racial and ethnic groups. Schultz (1926), for example, finding that black children possess longer arms and legs, suggested that better leverage may be applied in certain tasks as a result. It is clear that the body sizes of youngsters in various parts of the world differ even at early ages. Meredith (1970), obtaining the results of 170 investigations of children from every continent and from numerous countries of the world, found that average differences in body weight by the first year were as much as 9 pounds. Differences in body lengths and in chest circumferences between children at one year of age in various parts of the world also were great.

As Figure 4.2 indicates, children from various countries of the world were found to differ markedly in size. Data of this type make it difficult to recommend that infant motor development norms obtained from one culture or subculture be applied indiscriminately to infants in another part of the world, as has frequently been the practice in the past. The available data thus indicate that while there are apparent racial and ethnic differences in motor development milestones evidenced by youngsters during the first year of life, the reasons for these differences are likely to be varied and complex. Child-rearing practices, coupled with possible structural and genetic differences, are likely to combine in ways not completely understood to cause some of the acceleration and delays evidenced in the available literature.

Overall, the data cited indicate that the blanket application of so-called norms for infant motor development should be tempered with the knowledge that the numerous racial and ethnic subgroups within the United States are likely to be influenced by the degree to which child-rearing practices from the child's original culture are continued in the home. Moreover, ethnic subgroups in the U.S. often differ as to adherence to previously valued nutritional habits, as well as to the degree to which the children are integrated at play with children of other races and

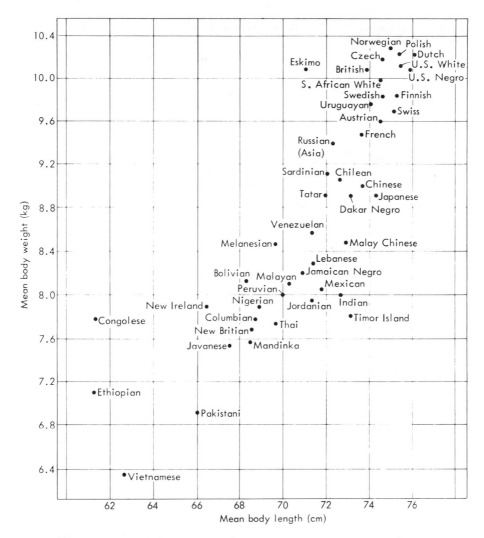

FIGURE 4.2 The relation of mean body weight and mean body length among contemporary groups of 1-year-old infants. From H. W. Meredith, "Body Size of Contemporary Group of One-Year-Old Infants Studied in Different Parts of the World," *Child Development,* 41 (1970), pp. 576-80. With the permission of the Society for Research in Child Development.

ethnic subgroups, both factors that can influence motor performance and learning tendencies.

MATURATION VERSUS LEARNING AND EXPERIENCE

In several decades of this century researchers have published studies exploring the roles of maturation and learning in the formation of movement qualities early in life. One of the more popular strategies was to employ a set of twins, giving one some kind of motor training and leaving the other as a purported control. It was assumed that if the trained twin evidenced accelerated movement capacities as the result of training, learning was demonstrated to somehow override the effects of maturation. If the trained twin evidenced no advancement in movement abilities, maturation was shown to exert more influence than training.

Often the results of these early efforts were mixed, possibly because the twins often were not kept apart, and the untrained child might have become a teacher of the other. Gesell and Thompson (1934), for example, found that an untrained twin of 46 weeks progressed more than the one given special help in both block handling and climbing activities. Hilgard (1932) also found that maturation seemed to exert effects that failed to overcome special training of one twin in locomotor tasks and in climbing activities.

At times, differences in this kind of study depended upon the tasks trained for. Minerva (1935), for example, found that special training of several sets of twins elicited improvement in complex throwing tasks, while more basic locomotor functions were not significantly influenced by special training. McGraw (1935), upon training one twin, found that he evidenced superiority in selected locomotor tasks and in climbing abilities, despite the fact that both twins began walking at the same ages.

As time passed, studies of the "co-twin" control type diminished in popularity, and investigations in which groups of children and infants were taught and stimulated took their place. The children and infants in this second type of study served as their own controls. It was usually assumed that if some group of infants, due to stimulation of various kinds, progressed more rapidly than some kind of norms against which they were compared, the training or stimulation had exerted a positive effect, and thus the normal maturational progress was somehow overpowered by teaching and learning. Again, however, the trained groups did not always improve. Hicks and Ralph (1931), for example, produced no improvement in a maze drawing task among 2- and 3-year-olds with special training. Werner (1974), on the other hand, was able to demonstrate acceleration of balancing, kicking, and jumping activities in young children through what he termed "guided instruction."[1]

As time progressed, investigations involving more subjects, and with conditions more precisely specified, have appeared in the literature. Another related trend is studies in which a single movement quality is concentrated on. Training in walking (Thelen, 1982; Zelazo, 1983), reaching behaviors (White and Held, 1963), as well as crawling (Lagerspetz et al., 1971) and the stages leading to standing (Pikler, 1972), have been among the more popular qualities researched in this manner. For the most part, investigators in the 1970s and 1980s reported positive training results for the skills they concentrated on. However, one wonders how much of the observed improvement recorded was due to the well-known experimenter effect, an

---

[1]Dennis has reported one of the few studies in which infants were intentionally limited in motor and social stimulation. For obvious ethical reasons, this type of investigation is not carried out with frequency (Dennis, 1935).

effect that often contaminates the best-intentioned investigator's perceptions of what infants do. Indeed, one observer has even referred to the twitchings of the human infant often recorded in such studies as evidence of a kind of experimenter Rorschach effect. That is, the scientist at times seems to project his or her personality into the data at what seems to be an almost alarming rate.

White and Held (1963), for example, reported that the handling of infants by carrying them around a room accelerated various reaching responses, even though within their own data it was clear that the infants given more opportunities to view their environment began to view their own hands about three weeks *later* than infants who were not given the same opportunities. Emma Pikler (1972) attempted to make it quite clear that institutionally reared children with a minimum of adult supervision progressed in a manner similar to those reared in the home. However, she may have been unduly influenced by the fact that her study was conducted in a country (Hungary) in which state-supported child care centers abound.

The physical restriction of infants may not always produce motoric delays. Dennis (1940), in studies of Hopi Indian children several decades ago, found that despite their restriction to cradle boards on their mothers' backs for the first three months of life, the children evidenced normal locomotor development when these apparently restrictive conditions were removed.[2] It is possible that the close maternal contact the cradle afforded, as well as the upright position in which they were maintained during these early formative days of life, produced more positive benefits than negative ones.

At the same time, contemporary data do make it clear that under certain conditions special stimulation of motor functions may have a positive effect—for example, the work of Thelen (1981) and Zelazo (1983) in which the stepping response was exercised, resulting in earlier and more pronounced pseudowalking and real walking. Lagerspetz, Nygard, and Strandvik (1971) also report that 11 infants under one year of age, when given exercise in creeping for 15 minutes a day, exhibited earlier evidence of this response voluntarily than a set of controls.

But even the results of these recent efforts should be carefully weighed, both scientifically and philosophically. Thelen makes it quite clear that the ratio of leg weight to leg strength influences whether some kind of stepping response training is likely to work. Philosophically, the question should be asked whether or not early stimulation of a single function or two contributes in general ways to useful exploratory behaviors, or whether such acceleration in walking and other locomotor responses is more likely to create a real safety problem in the infants exposed to this kind of training (Thelen, 1982).

Most caretakers and parents are, to varying degrees, informal teachers of motor tasks to infants during the first years of life. Thus their characteristics and attitudes are important to explore. The material contained in Chapter 7 dealing with

---

[2] In recent follow-up studies it has been found that Hopi Indian children evidence even more precocious motor development in recent years, probably due to improvement in nutritional status (Harriman and Lukosius, 1982).

social variables outlines the roles of these potential parental influencers on the ac-quisition of movement qualities early in life. Birth-order differences in infancy probably produce differences in levels of parental stimulation and attitudes about risk-taking in ways that influence later motor abilities (Schnabl-Dicky, 1978; Alberts and Landers, 1978). First-borns, presenting a unique and interesting train-ing experience for the parents, may be encouraged to walk earlier, but also may be more limited in risk-taking by parents. Later born infants, having the additional stimulation of siblings, plus a reduction of the parent's tendencies to overprotect, may evidence different motor development patterns than do first-borns (Samuels, 1980). In any case, studies of training of motor qualities need to take into account the qualities of the social situation that interact with such training and stimulation.

Infants during the first months of life are seldom inactive. Pikler, for example, found that infants within the first six months averaged only 2 minutes in a single posture. After that time, the "resting time" was reduced to 1.5 minutes in duration. Caretakers' reactions to that kind of incessant motion are as likely to exert effects upon subsequent efforts by the infant as are formal efforts to teach the child to move in various ways (Pikler, 1972).

It is with some frequency that I have evaluated children evidencing motor re-tardation from homes containing a single working parent. It appeared that the move-ment opportunities of these youngsters had been extremely limited. Indeed, the lit-erature documents the adverse effects of too much mothering (smothering) on infant and child development (Levy, 1943; Beller, 1959). Often children from homes in which either extreme of stimulation has occurred prove to be candidates for pro-grams of motor development.

BLUNTERS OF MOVEMENT CAPACITIES IN INFANTS
AND CHILDREN

A multitude of variables have slight to profound negative influences on early move-ment capacities. These factors range from medical conditions of various kinds through genetic and chromosomal anomalies. Included in such a list are those that affect central nervous system functions and peripheral structures of the body, as well as biochemical and physiological processes underlying the acquisition of aver-age movement capacities.

Some of these "insulters" arrive in subtle, internal ways, while others are the obvious outcomes of environmental conditions, including poor maternal and child nutrition caused by depressed economic conditions. Some of the conditions to be discussed have a relatively positive and optimistic prognosis for change, while oth-ers do not. However, the degree to which the movement specialist can understand some of these causes for poor development should influence how well he or she can cope with infants and children who are somehow "special."

A thorough discussion of all these negative factors is well beyond the scope of this chapter. Indeed, sorting out and identifying these possible blunters of motor qualities often tax the competencies of a large team of medical and developmental experts. What we will attempt here will be to (a) briefly classify some of the factors that limit adequate motor development, and (b) formulate useful guidelines for those interested in understanding movement qualities in young children and in planning for their enrichment.

Virtually any kind of mechanical or biochemical stress placed upon the maturing fetus is likely to produce limitations in overall motor development, depending upon the severity of the imposition, the time of life at which the insult occurs, and the part of the nervous system affected. Generally the developing child's nervous system is most susceptible to injury and insult during the time of the "spurt" in the maturation of the brain described in Chapter 2. To an increasing degree, however, the biochemical health of the mother while carrying the child has been found to be an important influencer of early and later development of the infant and child.

Some of these insults happen over time, and thus their influence is likely to be greater than if a problem (a nutritional deficiency, for example) occurs during a relatively brief period during the child's life. At the same time, the specific time period in which the problem occurs may be critical, as well as its duration.

Nutrition

Nutritional problems reflect themselves in many ways in the manner in which infants and children begin to move. Quantitative differences in body build size may be caused by deprivation of essential nutrients during the prenatal period. Accompanying body-build and size differences are both quantitative and qualitative modifications in the nervous systems of infants deprived of essential nourishment early in their lives. For the most part, prolonged deprivation of essential nutrients is likely to have more pronounced effects than a brief period during which essential nourishment is not received by the maturing youngster.

Nutrition merges maturation of structure with adequate physiological supports in the maturing child. The term *chemical anthropology* has been used to denote the internal form and composition of the body. Nutrition represents the most important single influence upon both pre- and postnatal physical development (Barness, 1975). Malnutrition has been considered to affect functions at two levels: (a) Primary nutritional problems occur when one or more nutrients are missing in the diet, thus producing alterations in functions and neurological as well as structural growth and maturation. (b) Secondary nutritional problems are those that alter the mother's and infant's capacities to process food, placing increased demands upon both to provide energy and to maintain and process structures and bodily systems. These problems may cause genetic anomalies, as well as infections, metabolic problems, and chronic or acute illnesses, all of which may lead to retardation of motor functions as well as of physical growth.

The nature of specific dietary deficiencies varies from country to country. Iron deficiency anemia is one of the most common nutritional diseases found in surveys of populations within the United States (Interdepartmental Committee, 1963), whereas worldwide, inadequate intake of riboflavin (one of the B vitamins) may be the most common dietary problem. Much of riboflavin is lost when grains are processed for bread and cereals. Another source of riboflavin is meat, often an expensive food in a developing country.

The mother's child-bearing customs, as well as her age, may combine in various ways to influence the kind of nutrition afforded her developing fetus and infant. For example, some teenage mothers may be less likely to have adequate diets during gestation. Mothers who themselves are still growing are also less likely to have adequate nutritional stores than are more mature child-bearers. Mothers whose nutritional status may be depleted by frequent child-bearing may also provide inadequate nutrition for the fetus (Eichorn, 1979). In a recent study infants from mothers over 40 years of age were five times more likely to exhibit coordination problems than those from younger mothers (Gillberg et al., 1982). Chronic malnutrition is likely to have long-term effects upon children's later mental and motor processes. Hoorweg and Stanfiel (1976), for example, followed the progress of protein-deficient babies in Uganda from infancy through childhood. They found that even by the tenth to twelfth years these children displayed measurable losses in coordination when compared to norms established by well-nourished children. Gilliam and her colleagues have also reported important work delineating the relationship between early malnutrition and the later appearance of both motor problems, as well as school learning deficiencies in children (Gilliam et al., 1984). The survey included 101 children malnourished during their first year of life, in contrast to a similar number of children who were adequately nourished. The malnourished youngsters displayed slow motor performance in a number of tasks, including rhythmic tapping and actions of the arms and hands. Additionally, this poor motor performance was correlated with attentional deficits, low verbal performance on standard IQ tests, and delayed physical growth.

Researchers throughout the world, particularly since the 1960s, have focused on socio-cultural as well as economic conditions reflected in food production and consumption that are likely to produce malnutrition in children and infants. For the most part, they suggest that nutrition and later behaviors of infants and children are relationships that are not always easy to untangle. Several types of variables are likely to influence food-intake to quality-of-behavior relationships. For example, the food consumption habits of various ethnic groups and socioeconomic subdivisions often interfere with the consumption of proper foods by children and by pregnant mothers, thus producing infants that may not thrive. Junk food snacking by members of some of the lower socioeconomic subgroups in the United States, as well as by higher socioeconomic groups in developing countries, are likely to sabotage the best efforts of educators and food producers to explain nutrition and to provide nourishment to the world's peoples (Owens et al., 1974).

Interesting paradoxes exist when contrasting economic conditions, life styles, customs, and the motor development patterns of children in various parts of the world. For example, it is not unusual to find youngsters in conditions that seem relatively harsh who perform well in tests of physical fitness. Children exposed to apparently poor diets, but who somehow remained vigorous in Europe during World War II, outperformed American children of the same period in tests of muscular strength and flexibility, prompting the establishment of the first President's Committee on physical fitness in this country (Kraus and Hirschland, 1954). It is sometimes found that children in some Latin American countries living under apparent poverty conditions in the *favelas* (slums) surrounding larger cities are apparently more physically fit, because of vigorous life styles imposed upon them, than are middle- and upper-class children in the same countries who suffer from diets promoting obesity (Matsuda, 1982). However, children evidencing this kind of early physical precocity within nutritionally harsh circumstances often encounter a variety of health problems rather early in life. For example, dental health among such populations is invariably poor. Thus, even a vigorous early life style will not overcome the prolonged effects of nutritional deficiencies in the diet.

A Ten State Nutritional Survey (TSNS, 1972) was published in the 1970s dealing partly with familial conditions that might contribute to poor nutrition. It was found that mothers in more comfortable economic circumstances seem to have more time to (a) adequately monitor the eating habits of their children, and (b) prepare nutritionally sound meals and keep up with current dietary information. In contrast, mothers from less favorable income groups, although at times able to afford nutritionally adequate food, seemed to have less time to carry out nutritionally sound child-rearing and cooking practices. It is probable that the pressure of economic circumstances contributed to the problems seen among the economically less advantaged in this study. However, it seems apparent that both in the United States and abroad adequate nutrition will come about when (a) adequate, nutritionally sound foods are available, and (b) education in sound nutritional practices is disseminated through populations that are currently malnourished.

The Mother's Condition and Habits

Both the level of the mother's health and habits that might add or detract from that health influence the health of the fetus, and thus the early developmental history of the child. Use of substances including alcohol, drugs, and tobacco all have been found to affect the infant's movement and intellectual competencies.

Before the turn of the century, it was found that women alcoholics in prison were likely to deliver infants with developmental difficulties (Rosett and Sander, 1979). However, it was not until the 1960s that carefully documented evidence led to the coining of the terms *fetal alcohol syndrome* or *FAS* (Lemoine et al., 1968). Work at the University of Washington in the 1970s further delineated the possible outcomes of the mother's use of alcohol (Streissguth, 1976). Offspring from an alcoholic mother may evidence a variety of symptoms, depending upon the time in pregnancy the alcohol influenced maturation and development. As is true with other so-called causes of developmental lags, it is difficult to pinpoint alcoholism as a single cause in the case of many mothers. For it is usual to find that alcoholics evidence a variety of other problems, including nutritional deficiencies, emotional difficulties, and tobacco use. Essentially, however, infants born to alcoholic mothers evidence disproportionate tendencies to exhibit hyperactivity, poor coordination, and weak muscle tone. Structural conditions encountered in these children include skeletal abnormalities, including hip dislocations and lack of maturation of the facial bones. Other physiological signs of this syndrome include heart defects. At the present time alcohol, according to some, is the third leading cause of birth defects (Licht, 1978), surpassed only by Down's syndrome and spina bifida. Alcohol in the mother's blood can pass directly through the placenta to the fetus, as biochemical screens are absent between the two. Research continues in an effort to determine just how much alcohol of what types influence birth problems when induced at various times within the development of the fetus.

Tobacco use is also a suspected modifier of birth weight in children (Pasamanuck and Knoblach, 1968). Even a pack a day has been found to produce infants who are smaller than the infants produced by nonsmoking mothers. These same infants rate lower on behavioral assessment scales, composed mostly of motor items (Strauss, 1975). Moreover, they are less likely to be socially and emotionally compatible with their early caretakers than are infants whose mothers ignore cigarettes during pregnancy. The effects of smoking appear to be relatively transitory in the case of the pregnant mother. It has been found, for example, that mothers who stop smoking before the fourth month of pregnancy are not more likely than nonsmoking mothers to produce an infant of an unusually low birth weight (Butler et al., 1972).

The mother may also be the source of several other infectious conditions as well as hormonal and chemical imbalances that may limit the early and later developmental progress of the infant and child. The infant born to a mother infected with German measles (Rubella) will display a variety of severe sensory and motor problems, including marked problems in coordination. Another example is the child born with congenital syphilis. He or she too will display a greater incidence of prematurity, coupled with a variety of negative developmental conditions. In a similar manner, a mother whose thyroid is not functioning normally may produce an infant with congenital hypothyroidism; poorly managed diabetes in an expectant mother may also produce offspring with physiological problems, as well as behavioral disorders reflected in poor motor function and mental retardation.

One of the main causes of cerebral palsy in children and also mild forms of coordination resembling the traditional types of cerebral palsy is incompatible Rh qualities in the blood of the mother and of the child. Often, an Rh negative mother will not influence the birth and development of her first Rh positive child. However, as antibodies continue to multiply in the mother between pregnancies, they may have a profound effect upon later infants. Medical intervention at birth usually corrects the condition in infants; chemical neutralizers may be applied to the mother between pregnancies. At the same time, this condition in areas of the world lacking modern medical facilities and personnel will continue to produce children with obvious motor problems.

Other Maternal and Perinatal Conditions

Numerous other medical problems, as well as perinatal stresses, can influence the early developmental history of the newborn. Drugs given during the birth process may be rapidly absorbed across the placenta, having an adverse effect upon the newborn (Goldstein et al., 1976; Blackbill, 1979). For the most part it is believed that these drugs may heighten the chances for birth anoxia. Drugs taken habitually by the mother are important modifiers of early development. Drugs in the form of various mind-altering abusive substances as well as medication taken for legitimate health problems have been shown to have potential adverse effects upon the newborn (Houston, 1969; Harbison and Mantilla-Plata, 1972; Litch, 1978).

Labor that it is prolonged or too short heightens the probability of developmental delays. Quick expulsion of the fetus with contractions of the uterus seems to somehow traumatize the newborn in ways that are not completely known. At the same, the position the infant may be assuming as he or she enters the world will significantly heighten the probabilities of later motor problems. Infants born in the breech position, buttocks first, like those born in a cross-wise position, are more likely to suffer some kind of trauma reflected later in delays of various kinds. These positions often heighten the possibility that the umbilical cord will become tangled, causing birth anoxia. Thus effective delivery care is important.

Undue mechanical pressures upon the infant, particularly the head, during delivery raises the chances for the child to display developmental problems. When forceps were used a decade or two ago, their use often proved disruptive to development. Today a birth canal that has not dilated enough, perhaps due to the fact that it is the mother's first pregnancy, is more likely to produce problems in the child.

Fetal Health, Size, and Prematurity

As the previous discussion makes clear, the human fetus prior to birth is not somehow isolated and protected from worldly stresses. These stresses, ranging from physical blows to nutritional insults and even including the emotional environment of the family, all may cause the fetus to become unhealthy before birth and cause the premature delivery of an underweight child.

In the past, low birth weights were considered those below 5.5 pounds, with a normal birth weight of 7 pounds used as the comparison. More recently, however, a birth weight of 4.5 pounds (2,000 grams) has been the criterion. However, as is pointed out in the following paragraphs, more specific benchmarks than merely birth weight are increasingly employed to describe the premature infant.

Overall, the various conditions described here, either in combination or alone, may have one or more of the following results:

1. The ability of the mother to carry the fetus to full term may be impaired. The child is born prematurely, resulting in the heightening of possible developmental deficiencies, including motor ineptitude.
2. The size and/or development of the fetus prior to or at birth may reflect immaturity

and/or lack of size. These low birth weight infants should be thought of as consisting of several subclassifications.

a.   One subgroup may be designated as "small for date." This includes two subclassifications (1) Those born at full-term (40 weeks gestational age) whose sizes are diminished (usually less than 2,500 grams), and (2) a second group born prematurely (at 37 weeks or less of gestational age) and who are small for their gestational ages. It is assumed that both these subgroups have suffered intrauterine growth retardation, reflecting inadequate nourishment in the uterus.

b.   The second major classification of low birth weight infants is those born before their expected date, but whose body weight is *appropriate* for their gestational ages. Some members of this subgroup may be born more prematurely than others. In any case, members of this second group who may be collectively labeled "normal birth weight for date," have apparently received adequate intrauterine nutrition. Their prognosis is sometimes better than for infants within the "small for dates" group relative to developmental problems, including delays in the assumption of adequate motor qualities.

Pre-term: Weight Appropriate for Gestational Age.   Children born prematurely are actually a multifaceted group. It is not inevitable that all will display later developmental problems, including motor delays. Some appear healthy and remain so, particularly with newer methods of pre- and postnatal care of such children. Others are born so early, or are apparently so stressed at birth, that prognoses must be made with care.

Improvements in newborn intensive care now include more sophistication in the control of nutrients and body temperature and the monitoring of many physiological functions. These advances, however, also have probably combined to produce more survivals, and thus more problem children overall appearing later in the schools. However, it is apparent that the chance of a great number of children from this kind of infant classification with serious problems is diminished (Francis-Williams and Davis, 1974).

It appears that the pre-term infant whose birth weight is normal for gestational age is more likely to display movement characteristics that are near normal, or normal, than are infants whose weights for gestational ages are low, and who are also premature. There are even some indications that pre-term (normal birth weight youngsters) who have had longer opportunities for visual experience than the infant born at term may be visually and perceptually precocious (Gesell and Amatrude, 1945; Saint-Anne Dargassies, 1966).

Intrauterine growth retardation: pre-term or full-term.   Infants small for dates (or small for gestational age) may be reduced in birth weight for several reasons and thus are a varied group. They may be small because of inadequate nutrition during prenatal life, or because of genetic or chromosomal problems. Small for dates infants are classified as having birth weights 2 standard deviations below the mean for a given gestational age (Ounsted and Ounsted, 1973). The mechanisms that underlie this condition include impairment of fetal oxygen, the transportation of nutrients to the fetus, and/or the exchange of the waste products of metabolism (Vorherr, 1975).

The conditions that may cause these mechanisms to malfunction are numerous and can range from infections, structural features of the uterus restricting transport functions, smoking, and drug use, as well as edema or thrombosis. Small fetal size is also associated with general health of the mother, her ethnic subgroup and social class, and placement of the residence in a city (Ounsted and Ounsted, 1973).

In general, small infants born at term are found to be superior developmentally to those born prematurely who are also undersized (Fitzhardinge and Steven, 1972). As is true when contrasting the sexes of other low birth weight groups, males seem to have a more difficult time catching up to their normal peers than do females (Fitzhardinge and Steven, 1972a, 1972b).

At birth these undersize infants may display poor head control and extraneous arm movements. Differences are also seen in the manner in which they execute the stepping and asymmetrical tonic neck reflexes (Michaelis et al., 1970). They may display less responsiveness to stimulation and poor muscle tone. Moreover, they may appear agitated when handled by their mothers (Als et al., 1976). However, many of these infants by the first year of life display behaviors comparable to those evidenced by peers with no previous birth difficulties or prematurity. Their sizes, however, are often permanently influenced by their early histories. They usually remain children of small stature (Davies and Davis, 1970; Bjerr, 1975).

Various programs have been carried out exploring later performance, mental, perceptual, and motor, of children low in birth weight. Often the results obtained are dependent upon the measures used and the criteria for what constitutes low birth weight. Although some reports have noted a marked reduction in mortality without an increase of serious handicaps among such children, when the infant is of a very low birth weight (VLBW), long-term behavioral, motor, and educational problems often are seen (Astbury et al., 1983). For example, Astbury and her colleagues (1983) reported recently upon the developmental performance of over 100 children having a birth weight of under 1,500 grams (a mean birthweight of 1,248 grams). Psychomotor development scores of the group lagged considerably behind normals at both 1 and 2 years of age, while one-third were later classified as hyperactive.

The problems encountered by suspect infants may produce negative influences upon their interactions with parent caretakers. Some caretakers of these youngsters may later report that they are unpredictable, too active, or intense (Rosenthal and Jacobson, 1968). These later behavioral inconsistencies may in fact be real, or may, as some have suggested, be the result of a self-fulfilling prophecy. That is, parents of these youngsters, expecting later problems as they interact with them, subtly influence their youngsters to be different. It was not uncommon in a clinic program I administer to observe the problem of infantilization. That is, a child might be brought for help whose developmental delay amounted to about a year, but whose parents had apparently so positively reinforced immature behaviors that the child actually evidenced delays of two or more years in language, motor, and social-emotional as well as cognitive functions (Cratty, 1975). Others have presented case studies documenting the tendency of parents of children whose start in life is somewhat shaky to distort child-rearing behaviors, distortions that lead to further delays (Solnit and Provence, 1979).

Genetic and Chromosomal Problems Causing Developmental Problems in Infancy

The possible genetic and chromosomal causes of developmental problems in infancy are numerous. They can range from gene-based disorders affecting metabolism to chromosomal problems influencing virtually every functioning system of the newborn. Often mutant genes trigger spontaneously terminated pregnancies during the first weeks after conception. However, in the case of some conditions, among them Down's syndrome, the infant is carried to full term.

One gene-based disorder is known as phenylketonuria (PKU). A recessive gene triggers its appearance. It involves an excessive buildup of a dietary amino acid related to the formation of protein. PKU affects the central nervous system, resulting in mental and motor retardation. This condition, like many in infancy, is not always apparent at birth. Its symptoms, however, may begin to appear within the first three or four months. It has been found that when treated early, infants with this condition are less likely to display later motor dysfunctions than are infants whose condition is discovered and treated later (Steinhausen, 1974).

Down's syndrome.   One prevalent chromosomal problem is Down's syndrome. The collection of symptoms include many that impede the development of normal motor behaviors and capacities. Characteristically these children are born with poor muscle tone. They tend to gain weight easily unless their diets are closely supervised, and they display the results of a lack of myelination to several parts of the nervous system. Variations of Down's syndrome include children whose motor problems are less acute (the Mosiac type). However, most benefit from early and carefully planned remediation of both motor and intellectual deficits.

The normal infant toward the end of the first year characteristically exhibits what has been described as an "explosion" of visual, emotional, and intellectual growth. During this same period, the Down's child's behaviors begin to depart markedly from those of normal infants (Carr, 1975; Dicks-Mireaux, 1972). It has only been recently that studies have indicated that useful changes may be achieved in such children if they are exposed to well-designed programs of motor development. Help in motor tasks needs to be accompanied by careful dietary supervision, help in self-care skills, as well as academic enrichment.

Unlike other conditions that may result in motor impairment near birth, the attending physician can easily identify the Down's child by unique conformations of the eyelids. It appears, however, that early intervention can achieve positive results and aid these children to reach their potentials in middle and late childhood. Remedial efforts have been shown to improve not only motor competencies, but also academic abilities in these children (Clunies-Ross and Graham, 1979).

Muscular Dystrophy.   Muscular dystrophy is a condition whose precise genetic causes are still somewhat murky. Its symptoms, however, are well known. It is a progressive disease whose prognosis at this writing is not very promising. Essentially it involves progressive muscular weakness due to the displacement of muscle cells with both fat cells and fibrous tissue. It is often not until the second to third year of life that the condition may be diagnosed. In fact, some of the early signs viewed by the nursery school teacher may trigger suppositions that the child is suffering from more popular conditions such as minimal neurological dysfunction or learning disabilities.

The young nursery-age child may evidence an enlargement in the calf area that at first appears to be an increase of muscle tissue. In fact, however, this swelling is false (pseudohypertrophy) and is evidence that fat cells are replacing useful muscle cells. Early signs of this condition in early childhood may include (a) running with an awkward flat-footed gait, (b) tiptoeing, due to an early weakness in the muscles that pull the foot up (dorsiflexors of the ankle and anterior tibial muscle), and (c) a sway back (Lordosis) due to an early weakness in the abdominal wall. The increase of muscular weaknesses may affect the upper legs, so that the child has problems rising from a prone or supine position to the feet. The preschool child beginning to show this condition will evidence what has been called a "growers sign." They use their arms and hands as aids when assuming an upright position by pushing on their thighs as they arise, while locking the knee joint.

Muscular dystrophy is only one of a score of possible degenerative muscular and neuromotor conditions that may affect infants and young children. These conditions are often progressive in nature, and may during the first years of life be masked by positive progress involving normal maturation. Thus the careful and sophisticated observer of the preschool child may be an important source of initial discovery of these conditions. Moreover, after problems of this type are discovered and correctly diagnosed by medical personnel, the motor development specialist may play an important role in their remediation, or in the maintenance of what capacities the child is likely to exhibit during what is sometimes a slowly descending performance curve.

Birth deformities.   Numerous so-called birth deformities may cause movement problems. Many of these are in fact caused by conditions occurring quite early in the fetal life of the infant. Some involve peripheral problems, including what is euphemistically called congenital amputations, or what is more simply a missing limb at birth. One of the more common conditions is discussed below. Its symptoms arise from abnormalities affecting the central nervous system as well as portions of the peripheral nervous system.

Spina bifida is a failure of the neural tube to close completely early in the prenatal period, causing portions of the spinal cord to protrude at the lower end of the spinal column (Chapter 2). Spina bifida produces a number of other symptoms, including increased pressure in the cerebral spinal fluid, which without proper early surgical intervention may cause an enlarged head, and intracranial pressures leading to a number of unfortunate behavioral characteristics. These include problems in motor planning and motor awkwardness, accompanied by a failure of the eyes to move in concert.

Often the availability of early medical intervention will influence the degree to which various symptoms persist. The movement characteristics of these children vary, but all evidence lack of adequate control of the lower limbs, coupled with a lack of good sensory awareness in the legs. Thus care must be taken to ensure that their braces are not causing injury that they cannot feel. Their intelligence as young children may be superior or equal to that of their normally moving peers. However, many cannot walk without assistance in early and late childhood. Their upper limbs often are relatively unimpaired, and activities used to strengthen the arms are often useful. The condition is not progressive, and most spina bifida children, if properly dealt with educationally and socially, are reasonably well adjusted and can compensate for problems caused by their condition.

Central Nervous System Problems Influencing Patterns of Movement

Many of the conditions discussed in the previous sections can lead to relatively stable, nonprogressive damage to the parts of the central nervous system controlling movements and coordinated patterns of movement. Although some newborn infants and young children merely evidence overall delays of motor development in ways that resemble action capacities that are less mature, other youngsters will display *qualitative* differences in actions when compared to their peers. The most common of these is cerebral palsy.

The term *cerebral palsy* conjures up visions of severely handicapped individuals often confined to wheelchairs with obvious and profound movement difficulties. In truth, however, mild forms of the typical types of this disorder are not uncommon within nursery school age children that have not been designated as "handicapped." Cerebral palsy is actually a group of movement conditions caused by insults, usually at birth, to portions of the central nervous system that plan and execute coordinate movements. It is nonprogressive in nature, and may even stem from an accident early in the life of the child. Its usual causal mechanisms are degrees of anoxia at birth, which in turn have been triggered by some of the conditions previously discussed relative to prematurity and low birth weight.

There are several subtypes of mild cerebral palsy sometimes seen within preschool populations. As is true when discovering the possible signs of progressive neurological and muscular disorders, often signs of mild to moderate cerebral palsy unfold gradually in early childhood. Therefore it often takes the most astute diagnostic skills by pediatric neurologists to classify the infant and the problem correctly.

Some of the types often observed include these:

1. The mild spastic. This child may have problems with relaxed slow movements that must be made with precision. The child may, for example, often be seen to knock over a glass when it is reached for, hitting it instead of slowly grasping it. Line drawing from point to point will evidence overshoots, as the hand somehow flashes by the ending point in such movement tasks. Undue toe walking (either on one or both toes) is sometimes a sign of this type of cerebral palsy in mild forms.

2. The ataxic. This child may be seen to evidence a slight tremor in his or her movements. Drawing a circle may be correct, but the quality of the line reflects a tremor. When walking, this type of child may be seen to move in an uneven manner, and seem to bounce when the ball of one foot hits the ground, instead of giving with the action in a relaxed way. This type of cerebellar ataxia may influence the lower OR upper limbs. It should not be assumed that because the legs seem unable to act with precision that the hands will not do so, or vice versa.

3. The athetoid. In its severe form, this type of cerebral palsy is perhaps the most dramatic. Individuals afflicted with it, often nonambulatory, engage in a constant symphony of "out of tune" actions, often resembling some of the birth reflexes discussed in Chapter 3.
   Early signs of this condition often involve a lack of muscle tone during the first 2-3 years of life. The child may lack good muscle tone in the eyelids, and seem to observe the world with a sleepy expression. In truth, however, the child may see quite well, but is evidencing a hypotonic muscular condition that later evolves into the irregular movements of a mild or moderate athetoid. This shift from hypertonia to athetoid actions is often first seen when the child is able and willing to grasp a pencil. The first efforts to draw will begin to reveal the irregular movement characteristics of the athetoid.

4. Mixed types. In the case of more severe forms of cerebral palsy, the so-called pure forms discussed above are not always observed. Often a mixed type will be seen, combining, for example, spastic characteristics with those involving ataxis or athetosis. The same is true among children evidencing mild forms of cerebral palsy. The teacher or motor development specialist should not expect that a given child will be highly predictable in terms of symptoms reflecting mild cerebral palsy. What such professionals *should do,* however, is refer such children to the proper medical diagnosticians. After such diagnoses, it will often fall to the movement specialist to formulate useful remedial movement strategies in order to improve such youngsters.

INTERVENTION PROGRAMS

The problem of poorly developing infants has long been with us. In England during the 1800s for example, it was estimated that about 75% of all children born failed to reach their second birthday. Data from the State of New York early in this century indicated that about 42% of all infants died before their first birthday, while for those born to foundling homes during this period the death rate was over 60% before their second birthday (Bremmer, 1971).

During the middle of this century it was found that poorly developing infants were often in social and emotional environments (including foundling homes) that were less than desirable (Spitz, 1945, 1950; Bowlby, 1951). In many countries of the world including Iran and Lebanon it was found that infants raised in bland surroundings often evidenced moderate to severe retardation in developmental signposts including motor maturation (Dennis, 1960; Dennis and Najarian, 1957).

It has only been within the past twenty years, however, that enlightened opinions about how infants can be influenced by their early environments have encouraged the initiation of programs designed to elicit positive modifications in behaviors and abilities. These programs have been organized in many different ways. Some focus on improving parenting skills and competencies; others bear directly upon the infant or child. Most employ the child's tendencies to behave actively in various ways. At the same time, goals emphasizing solely improved motor development are rare, and indeed such a focus would be superficial. The most successful of these programs usually emphasize movement as a form of exploratory behavior, which when combined with the encouragement of speech and language skills will make positive changes in later academic and intellectual behaviors exhibited during the first years of formal schooling.

The emphasis often includes helping the parent or offering direct help to the infant, emphasizing that the child is a capable individual and with effort is likely to succeed at tasks ranging from the concrete to the abstract. The focus is often on what is termed *proactive* planning for change. That is, the programs tend to encourage looking ahead in time by preparing the child with basic skills, often motor skills, that will enable successful participation in various tasks encountered in the home, neighborhood, and school (Hoke, 1968). As these programs have been applied over the past fifteen or twenty years, data have emerged that has shed light on the variables likely to promote positive changes in infants and children suffering cultural-social deprivation and/or lags in various aspects of development (Beller, 1979). At the same time, their continued use in the United States has depended on the social philosophies of those wielding power within the federal and state governments.

Motor tasks permeated these programs in several ways. First, intellectual and emotional growth was often encouraged by helping the child to engage in stimulating exploratory behaviors involving locomotor activities as well as manipulative operations. Self-efficacy was promoted by helping the child *do* things, rather than simply becoming a passive observer in social and play situations. Movement qualities were often an important part of the assessment evaluating program outcomes. The Hunt-Uzgiris scale for evaluating manipulative behaviors was sometimes employed to reflect change, as were numerous infant scales including the Bayley, which contains numerous motor items (Gray, 1977; Guinagh and Gordon, 1976).

Among the findings that have relevance for the stimulation and improvement of movement competencies in young children are the following:

1. Whether or not the program of improvement is beamed directly at the child or is somehow administered indirectly through parent education is not as important as its duration when change is evaluated (Huntington, 1979).

2. There are some data that indicate it is better to focus on younger children than those in middle childhood. The most important finding is that duration of program application is more important than whether it is initiated early or later within the preschool years. That is, children exposed to such enrichment programs for two to three years between the birth and age 5 are more likely to exhibit positive changes than those given the program early, but terminating it after a 12-month or 18-month period (Huntington, 1979).

3. The lack of simple correlations between the children's early signs of movement competencies and later verbal intelligence was not considered as important as the finding that signs of early pleasure in tasks were relatively good predictors of later

intellectual performance. For example, Birns and Golden (1972) found that the amount of pleasure elicited by infants from 18 to 24 months of age when engaged in the Cattel and Piaget object scales was predictive of their later intellectual performance on the Stanford Binet at 3 years of age. This and similar data reflect the importance of using early movement experiences as vehicles to promote positive attitudes toward exploration and what has been termed *competence motivation* by some (White, 1963), and *pleasure in mastery* by others (Hendrick, 1943).

Issues and Problems

There are numerous issues that the currently available data are beginning to bring to the forefront. For example, the effectiveness of different variations in treatment, as well as different ways of delivering such treatment, still needs sorting out. For the most part, however, movement tasks, when combined with verbal-linguistic and cognitive skills in ways that help the infant obtain feelings of success, seem more important than just who administers the program and in what setting the intervention effort occurs.

Data are lacking concerning how a program containing a predominance of motor tasks, with the effort made only to improve movement qualities, seems to affect movement abilities. Indeed, this type of restricted program would seem to be a waste of time. It appears that a program designed for motorically delayed infants must not only contain movement tasks, but movement tasks combined with qualities that encourage active hypothesis testing by the child in order to maintain high levels of motivation and effort (Brown, 1981).

SUMMARY

A vast number of variables cause individual differences in the manner in which youngsters move. Some of these factors correlate with normal variations in size, motor abilities, and motor performance. Other variables may cause anomalies in infant maturation and development of movement capacities.

Ethnic differences in children include obvious differences in body builds and structures, as well as more subtle attitudes toward movement experiences. For the most part, infant precocity in preindustrial societies, a continuing theme in the literature, in fact reflects a number of variables in addition to ethnicity. Child-rearing practices that include maternal training of movement skills within the first year or two of life, for example, are likely to produce superior scores on infant scales when children in some developing countries are surveyed.

Recent training studies indicate that various splinter skills may indeed be positively influenced. These have included training designed to accelerate crawling and to prolong and exercise the stepping response in infants. At the same time, this kind of piecemeal acceleration needs to be examined both practically and philosophically. Is it indeed important or even safe for a child of 8 to 10 months to become highly mobile?

A number of interacting conditions can cause moderate to severe movement problems in the infant. These can include those impinging upon the unborn fetus, as well as stresses that impinge upon the developing child after birth. As is true when examining ethnic differences, social and cultural factors are important to include when inspecting the nutritional, biochemical, and mechanical stresses sometimes placed on infants and children. Malnutrition may be caused not only by the lack of available nutrients in the diet of a culture or subculture, but also by cultural attitudes toward what foods should be eaten and when meals are appropriate throughout the day. Similarly, cultural attitudes toward child-bearing influence the quality of the diet available to the fetus and infant. Young mothers, or those bearing children too frequently, may lack adequate stores of appropriate nutrients.

Unhealthy or inadequate prenatal care, including dietary considerations, may result in children born too early and/or infants of low birth weight. Often low birth weight infants possess inadequately developed central nervous systems that in turn blunt the emergence of adequate movement qualities both early and later in life. Moreover, prolonged malnutrition during the first years of life may have irreversible outcomes, including mental and motor delays lasting into late childhood and adolescence.

A number of genetic and structural deficiencies can limit the movement capacities of young children. These include variations of Down's syndrome, degenerative problems, as well as mild, moderate, and severe kinds of cerebral palsy. Those supervising programs of early childhood education should be familiar with symptoms of these pathological conditions, as reflected in movement qualities, so that early medical referrals may take place.

Intervention programs intended to reverse negative developmental trends are effective in so far as they are prolonged in nature, provide a happy emotional environment, and combine motor interventions with those intended to stimulate verbal, social, and intellectual growth.

QUESTIONS FOR DISCUSSION

1. What are the interactions between child-rearing practices and differences in motor abilities seen in various ethnic groups around the world?

2. What effect might nutritional deficiencies during the prenatal period have upon the maturing nervous system and the development of neural mechanisms, as discussed in Chapter 2?

3. What movement deficiencies are seen in the Down's syndrome child?

4. What evidence exists that early and prolonged nutritional deficiencies cause later motor retardation?

5. Discuss the labels "low birth weight for date" and "adequate birth weight for date." What implications do these labels have for later physical maturation and motor competencies?

6. What symptoms may be seen in the movement behaviors of a preschool child

evidencing mild forms of cerebral palsy? Might various types of cerebral palsy result in specific atypical motor patterns?

7. Discuss the roles of maturation versus early training in various developmental milestones expected in children during their first 18 months of life. In what ways have the roles of maturation versus learning been studied?

8. What are some early signs of muscular dystrophy in a preschool child?

9. With reference to Chapter 7, what social influences are likely to positively affect the emergence of movement attributes in early childhood? What social conditions are likely to retard motor development during the first two or three years of life?

STUDENT PROJECTS

1. Visit a school for young handicapped children. Can you identify those with some of the anomalies discussed in the latter parts of this chapter? What are their movement characteristics?

2. Contrast the movement behaviors, as well as child-to-child contacts and/or interactions, among children in two playgrounds containing youngsters from diverse ethnic groups. What conclusions can you draw about ethnic differences in interpersonal relationships and the movement behaviors you saw, and that are reported in the literature as characteristic of various ethnic subgroups?

3. Observe the parental interactions among a family group containing a newborn. What can you conclude about the roles of the parents, the amount of stimulation they seem to be giving, and the later movement attributes of the infant you observe?

4. What does a library search of some type of special child discussed in this chapter reveal to you about (a) movement attributes, and (b) the prognosis for improvement of motor abilities as the result of enrichment and/or remediation?

5. Visit a program of infant stimulation. Record the kinds of interactions encouraged by those administering the program. Find out what evaluative methods they employ. What results do they claim for their interventions? Do their stated objectives, program content, and evaluative criteria correspond?

6. Formulate an ideal way to work with a normal newborn in order to optimize present and future movement qualities. What practical and philosophical considerations should you keep in mind?

CHAPTER FIVE
THE BEGINNINGS
OF MOVEMENT
IN THE NEWBORN
Reflexes and Stereotypies

To the casual observer the newborn infant presents a puzzling picture. Loud and apparently meaningless shrieks are accompanied by unusual twistings and twitchings of the arms, legs, and trunk. In the first months of life the child seemingly engages in random movements whose only main intent seems to be getting sources of nourishment to the mouth. For decades, however, astute scholars of human development have taken close looks at what infants do during the first six months of life, and why they seem to act in the ways they do. As the final decade of the twentieth century approaches, the careful observations and interpretations of these scientists have begun to paint a reasonably coherent picture of the meanings and uses of early perceptual as well as motor behavior emitted by the newborn.

Infants begin to exercise their movement capacities prior to birth, and levels of fetal activity are roughly predictive of later motor competency. For example, in 1938 Richards and Newberry recorded fetal activity in twelve infants from one to two weeks prior to birth for five- to six-hour periods and found moderate and positive relationships between the measures obtained and indices of motor development obtained at six months. Etta Walters, in a study completed in 1965, also found that prenatal movements, in both duration and intensity, were predictive of motor measures obtained up to the fifth year of life (Richards and Newberry, 1938; Walters, 1965).

It appears that general level of activity is a highly individual matter in infants. Irwin, for example, found that the activity levels measured in the more active of 73 infants during the first two weeks of life were 290 times greater than in the least active children within his population (Irwin, 1932). Most interesting have been recent attempts to codify and draw meaning from the numerous types of rhythmic movements engaged in during infancy. Careful classification of these actions of the trunk, legs, and arms has served to provide a more complete understanding of how early motor behaviors serve as important bases of later voluntary actions, and how reflexes, rhythmic movements, and other sensory and perceptual processes are interwoven into the fascinating fabric constituting the motor personality of the child during the first twelve months of life.

In the first part of this chapter we present a survey of some of the primary types of reflexes. Next we look at the variety of rhythmic and stereotyped movement behaviors seen in infancy. Next, the manner in which these two types of actions, reflex and rhythmic, combine in various ways to produce early voluntary behaviors is discussed and illustrated.

INFANT REFLEXES

The earliest movements that can be elicited in newborn infants consist of *reflexes,* involuntary actions triggered by various kinds of external stimuli. Reflexes may be classified in various ways: those involving the total body and its orientation to gravity versus various head and limb movements in which the labyrinths (balance mechanisms of the inner ear) are not involved; those that are the evolutionary remains of actions seen in animals lower in the phylogenic scale versus the movements that are later incorporated into the voluntary movement patterns of older children and adults; and those that differentiate between so-called normal and pathological motor behavior.

After an infant is born, it is important to determine whether the nervous system is sound by attempting to elicit the expected reflexes. If the reflex is uneven in strength when elicited on both sides of the body or is too weak or too strong, some kind of neurological dysfunction is usually suspected. If a "normal" reflex continues to be evidenced for too long a period of time during infancy, or fails to appear at all, the examining physician will probably suspect some type of neurological impairment.

Various *pathological* reflexes also indicate the possibility of some kind of irregular neural function. Many of the initial reflexes seen in infants are necessary to sustain life processes between the time the child is no longer nourished within the mother's amniotic fluid and the acquisition of useful voluntary actions. For example, the rooting reflex enables the infant to obtain nourishment: the child reflexively turns toward a tactual stimulus applied to the cheek and thus reaches the mother's milk. Other reflexes resemble later voluntary activities. For example, when infants are placed in certain positions, they will demonstrate a walking pattern. These reflexes usually disappear well before their voluntary counterpart is seen.

The study of the nature of infant reflexes is made difficult by the variability with which they appear and disappear. In a 1971 study, Touwen, for example, concluded that both the palmar grasp reflex as well as the Moro show great variability with regard to the time of their dissolution. This same researcher found, upon surveying 50 infants, that the onset of walking could not be predicted by knowing when the Moro and palmar grasp reflexes disappeared. The appearance of voluntary grasping was also found to be unrelated to the disappearance of the neonatal grasping response (the palmar reflex) (Touwen, 1971).

On the pages that follow, only a few of the numerous infant reflexes will be discussed, and passing reference will be made to various pathological reflexes. For a more thorough treatment of this topic, see the texts by Pieper (1963) and Illingworth (1967).

The Moro Reflex

The Moro reflex (Figure 5.1) was first elicited by striking the pillow of the infant; subsequently it was found that if the head was shaken quickly, the reflex would appear. Infants spread their arms and fingers and legs somewhat weakly, and return both limbs and fingers to a flexed position against the body. At times, they elicit the reflex as they cough or sneeze. Sudden movement initiated by the child can also trigger the Moro reflex. The beginning of the Moro reflex is opposite to the startle reflex, which is only a flexion without the prior extension pattern. The Moro reflex can be brought about rapidly and in succession, whereas the startle reflex needs some kind of recovery-from-fright time prior to its being triggered again. Touwen demonstrated that the apparent "disappearance" of the Moro reflex seems to depend on the method employed to elicit it. At times, when the Moro had appar-

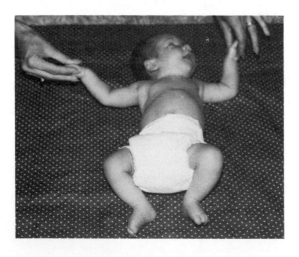

FIGURE 5.1 Moro reflex may be elicited by pulling the arms away from the body as shown.

ently disappeared it would seem to return when another method was used to trigger this type of behavior (Touwen, 1971).

The Moro reflex is seen in the fetus as early as the ninth week after conception and is always present in infants during the first three months of life. Persistence of the Moro reaction(s) impedes the onset of other useful reactions and voluntary movements. Unless the hands are able to come away from the body and this rigid fetal position is reduced, for example, it is unlikely that the child will begin to use the arms and hands in either support functions or in manipulative activities during the third to sixth months of life.

Tonic Neck Reflexes of the Limbs

If the infant's neck is turned, the stretch of the neck muscles triggers an increase of tonus in the limbs on the side toward which the head is facing (Figures 5.2 and 5.3). The limbs on the other side, in both animals and human infants, usually assume a flexed position.

The asymmetric tonic neck reflex may be triggered prior to birth and may be used to deliver the child. For example, as the child emerges and the head is turned, it is likely that a hand will emerge toward the face side, permitting the delivering physician to assist the delivery by grasping the hand. If the infant persists in

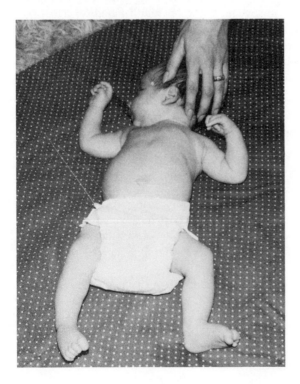

FIGURE 5.2
The asymmetrical tonic-neck reflex, infant evidences increased tonus on the side toward which the head is turned. Arm on the "skull side" flexes, and child assumes what has been described as a "fencer's position."

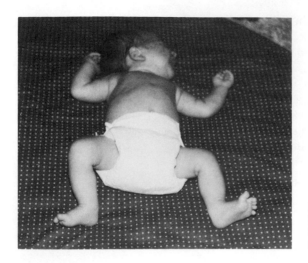

FIGURE 5.3
Infants often rest or sleep, in asymmetrical tonic-neck reflex position on their stomach or back.

evidencing a too-strong tonic neck reflex for too long a period of time, interference with a number of voluntary actions will occur. For example, the tonic neck reflex, if elicited, will act as a brake as the child seeks to turn from the back to the front. Stable positioning in a hands-and-knees crawl position is also impeded if strong and persistent neck-arm linkages remain by the third and fourth month of age.

A symmetric tonic neck reflex is also described in the literature. For the most part, this reaction is usually described as pathological. This symmetric tonic neck response consists of a flexion of both legs at the hip and knee joints when the head is bent forward. The actions of the legs and arms are reversed when the head is flexed backward.

Palmar and Plantar Grasp Reflexes

Touching both palms of the hands and the front part of the bottom of the toes tends to cause flexion of the hands and feet, respectively (Figure 5.4). This reflex in the hands usually results in a grasping action that excludes the thumb and may be strong enough to support the infant's weight for short periods of time. This reflex has been elicited as early as the eleventh week of gestation. It continues in the newborn and becomes progressively stronger between the twelfth day and the third month of life. This reflex usually becomes weaker by the sixth month, disappearing entirely by the end of the first year.

This reflex evidences a progression, as discussed in Chapter 8. Generally it is first elicited strongly, with the entire hand. Next a gradual reduction is noted, with it finally being evidenced as individual fingers are touched, resulting in their closures. The prehensile reflex is linked to the tonic neck reflex (asymmetric). It is elicited more strongly on the skull side than in the hand and arm facing the face when the child is in an asymmetric tonic neck reflex position.

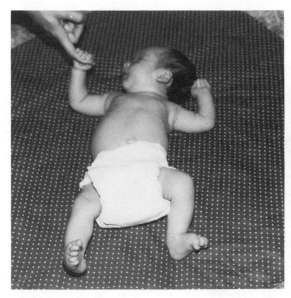
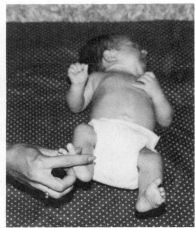

FIGURE 5.4 Prehensile reflex showing a grasp reaction when palm is stimulated or touched. Second picture shows plantar-flexion reflex.

These reflexes are probably the rudimentary remains of the grasping activity needed by primate ancestors. Confirming this supposition is the fact that it can be elicited by stroking the palm with a bit of hair. In the palmar reflex, if the infant's hand closes and elicits pressure of much less than 40 gm or more than 120 gm, some kind of neurological dysfunction is usually suspected.

Twitchell has found that the grasp reflex is multifaceted. That is, a grasping reaction may be elicited in an infant in a number of ways, including by extending the arm. Furthermore, he found that if an object is placed momentarily in the hand and then removed, the infant will manually search for the object; this search-and-grasp reaction is unaccompanied by visual attention (Twitchell, 1965). The strength of this reflex must fade out during the first year of life in order for precise voluntary grasping actions to take place. An additional discussion of this reflex is found in Chapter 8.

Righting Reflexes of the Head and Body

Two related reflexes seen during the first year of life in normal infants probably contribute to the achievement of later voluntary turning movements in the crib. One is the neck-righting reflex of the body, which is elicited by turning the head as the infant is on his back; the trunk will reflexively turn in the same direction (Figure 5.5). The opposite action, the body-righting reflex of the head, is elicited by turning the hips in one direction, as the child is prone, and eliciting a head-turning movement in the same direction.

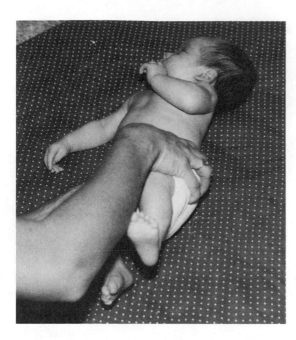

FIGURE 5.5
One aspect of righting reflex shown as hips are turned, head tends to turn in the same direction. The opposite is also true. When the head is gently turned, the hips shortly follow in the same direction. These are also called body derotative responses.

These reactions are also called body-derotative responses and are used to trigger turning actions in children suspected of evidencing developmental delays. The reaction is probably a precursor of turning reactions—from supine to prone and from prone to supine. This reaction, coupled with support reactions of the arms, prepares the child for important substages of locomotion.

The Labyrinthine Righting Reflex

The labyrinthine righting reflex is seldom seem in the newborn, but it becomes stronger during the middle of the first year. It contributes to the assumption of an upright head and body position and to the child's movement forward during the end of the first year.

Generally the infant evidences this reflex by a tendency to attempt to maintain upright position by lifting the head upward when the body is tipped downward (Figure 5.6). Similarly, if the upright infant is held by the shoulders and bent backward, the head will move forward, still attempting to maintain its original position with relation to gravity. The reflex may also be seen if the upright infant is angled to the left or right. The head tends to maintain the original upright posture with relation to gravity.

The reflex is first seen in about the second month after birth as the infant attempts to look upward while on its stomach. Later the head is aided by the supportive reaction of the arms to the same stimulus as they push on the surface of the crib to permit the head to remain up for increasing periods of time.

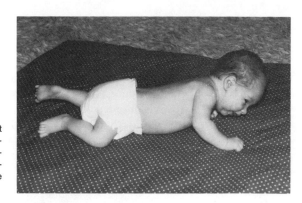

FIGURE 5.6
Even during the first month the infant will begin to lift the head toward the upright as shown. Also seen here is a partial support reaction of the right hand-arm, preparation for later more vigorous support reactions.

The first of these righting reactions is seen in the first and second months, as the infant looks up and orients the head to gravity. Later a stronger support reaction, together with better orientation to gravity by the head and body, enables the strong hand-knee position seen at 6 months (Figure 5.7).

The labyrinthine righting reaction(s) are a group of important gravity reflexes needed during the first weeks, months, and year of life. These reactions contribute to the assumption of an upright head position as the infant is in a prone position. They are also called righting reactions. The absence or extreme weakness of this response is a sign of neurological impairment.

FIGURE 5.7
A strong hand-knee position at six months, aided by a strong support reaction together with adequate labyrinthine reactions and orientation of the head to gravity.

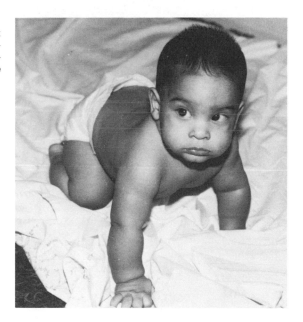

Support Reactions of the Arms and Legs

Similar to the reactions seen in cats, the human infant at about 4 months will react when brought toward surfaces by reflexively extending the arms, indicating a readiness to support himself (Figure 5.8). Moreover, this supporting reaction is useful as the child begins to reduce the friction between the body and the surface on which the body is resting in order to accomplish other tasks, including (a) better visual inspection of the world, (b) turning over, and (c) crude creeping (Figure 5.9).

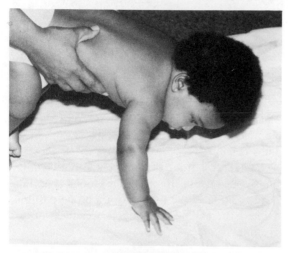

FIGURE 5.8
A support reaction occurs as the infant is brought slowly toward a surface, as shown.

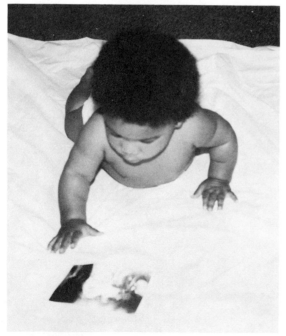

FIGURE 5.9
Infant shown evidences a strong support reaction with one hand (the right), while reaching with the left for an object.

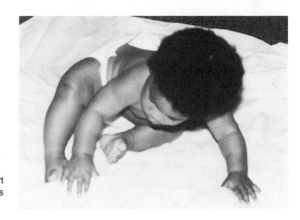

FIGURE 5.10
Infant shows a sophisticated support reaction with the left hand as she tilts forward.

This support reaction takes more advanced forms as the child gains a seated position. If the body is displaced to one side, the arm will reach out on the other side to maintain support and the body will "bow" toward the side to which the child tilts (Figure 5.10). The legs will tend to extend, if the infant is lowered toward a surface, at about the ninth month of age. This modification may indicate the infant is ready to stand, with assistance. Its absence during the first 6 to 7 months indicates that the infant is not ready to stand. The reaction will persist for longer and longer periods of time during the final fourth of the first year. Moreover, the reflexive stepping reactions often terminate as this support reaction phases in.

A more complex and advanced support reaction is seen in the parachute reaction needed when the child may gain an upright stance for the first time. The reaction consists of a reaching out by the hands, coupled with a knee bend, as the infant quickly ascends (or falls) from the first attempts to stand.

Tilting Reactions

Reactions similar to the support reactions described in the previous section are termed *tilting* reactions. They are triggered when the surface upon which the infant is placed is tilted to either side. When this is done, the infant will reflexively extend the arm and evidence increased tonus and a curve of the spine in a C toward the upward side of the tilt in order to regain balance. This response is usually seen at about the fifth month and may be elicited while the infant is lying, sitting, kneeling, or standing.

Pull-Up Reactions

Actions of both the arms and hands result in a pull-up reaction. This secondary reflex, incorporating a palmar grasp, appears only after several months. It may be elicited as the infant is seated, or when standing, as shown in the illustrations here (Figure 5.11). The reaction, when the infant is moved to the side, is probably accompanied by a modified tonic neck reaction as asymmetric tonus occurs on the side of the flexed arm.

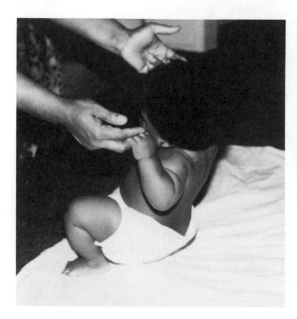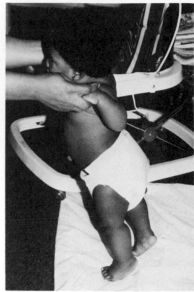

FIGURE 5.11 Two illustrations of pull-up reaction, one as child is drawn from a seated position, and the second when child is tilted backward in a standing position. In the latter case the infant flexes her arms to maintain an upright position.

REFLEXIVE LOCOMOTOR, SWIMMING, CRAWLING, AND CLIMBING MOVEMENTS

A number of complicated reflex patterns that can be elicited in infants after the first weeks after birth resemble to a marked degree later voluntary attempts to proceed forward or to climb upward. It has been demonstrated in animals and in humans that these movements are controlled by the spinal cord, with no involvement of the higher brain centers. There seems to be no direct connection in time between these reflexive movements and the infant's later attempts to assume voluntarily an upright posture to walk, to swim, and to climb. For example, the so-called walking reflex described below terminates in about the fourth to fifth month, whereas voluntary walking does not appear until some time between the ninth and fifteenth months. However, the presence of these interesting reflexes apparently indicates how deeply locomotor activities are ingrained within the human nervous system.

The Walking Reflex

By the end of the second week of life many (about 58 percent) infants will "walk" if held in an upright position with their feet permitted to touch a level horizontal surface (Figure 5.12). This walking pattern involves a distinct knee tilt, but does not involve other body parts, e.g., an arm swing. The child can be made to "climb" stairs while supported in this manner and can also be made to "walk"

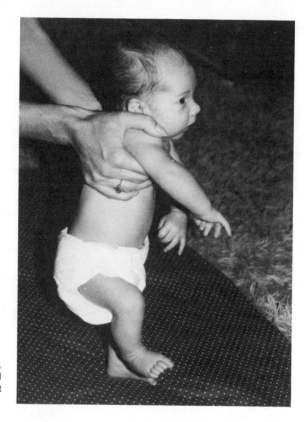

FIGURE 5.12
Stepping reaction shown at 3 weeks, with infant held upright. The usual right-reference is shown in this first step taken.

while upside down, indicating the lack of involvement of the righting reflex of the labyrinths. As the higher brain centers mature, this reflex disappears; it is usually gone by about the fifth month.

Although it was formerly assumed that some kind of training in the walking reaction would have little or no positive effect, data from a 1953 study refute this assumption. Exercising infants in this walking response on a daily basis, Andre-Thomas and St. Dargassies (1952) found that "secondary" or voluntary walking was greatly accelerated. Other reflexes that in various ways resemble voluntary movements which are separated in time, relative to their onset, may be related in ways not commonly assumed by many child development specialists. Zelazo et al. in a 1972 study with 24 infants also found that daily stimulation of the walking reflex during the first nine weeks of life led to a high rate of responding to stimulation of the reflex by the eighth week, and to an earlier onset of walking unaided. Infants in two control groups did not evidence walking behavior at the same time as those receiving this type of "reflex exercise."

Controversy, however, surrounds the question as to whether true walking is or should be facilitated by somehow exercising this stepping response. Zelazo, for example, continues to present studies in which this response has been stimulated and prolonged (Zelazo, 1983). He contends that walking is an important accompaniment to the emergence of cognitive abilities also surfacing at about the first year of life. Others believe that not only does stimulating "infant walking" not serve any useful ends, but that this type of "exercise" may have harmful effects. Pontius (1973), for example, believes that this kind of infant walking when stimulated may even retard neurological maturation, insofar as the infant's nervous system is not given the time it needs to mature because of overstimulation. Thelen and her colleagues, in a 1982 investigation (Thelen, Fisher, Ridley-Johnson, and Griffin, 1982), demonstrate quite clearly how infant walking increases when the infant is aroused and probably terminates toward the middle of the first year of life as the bulk of the leg increases faster than does the muscle strength needed to move heavier legs in this cyclic type of response.

I believe that a logical explanation of the emergence and disappearance of this stepping reaction depends upon the interaction of maturational processes, coupled with the increased gain in the bulk of the legs. Standing and later walking, I believe, are dependent upon relationships between body weight and length, neurological maturity, and muscular strength, coupled with balance abilities. More important than the continuation of a stepping response are various rhythmic actions while sitting and standing in which the infant engages just prior to standing and walking. A picture of these interacting movement qualities, together with the presence of support reactions needed when standing, is found at the end of this chapter.

The Crawling Reflex

If the infant is placed face down on a surface and pressure is alternately applied to the bottoms of the feet, he or she will perform a crawling pattern with the upper and lower limbs (Figure 5.13). This reflex can be seen at birth and has been elicited in a fetus of seven months' gestation. It usually disappears sometime between the third and fourth months after birth; there is a distinct time interval between its disappearance and the emergence of voluntary creeping, which occurs sometime between the seventh and ninth months.

Some clinicians have speculated that this reflex is the remains of a phylogenetic action needed by the primate to crawl up the mother's stomach to reach her breast. Whether these reflexive crawling movements are precursors of true voluntary creeping and crawling is controversial. For the most part, they disappear at about the fourth or fifth month in normal infants.

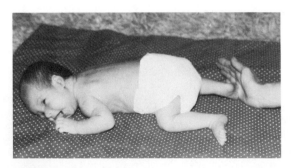

FIGURE 5.13
Crawling reaction elicited by pressure to the bottom of each foot in an alternating manner.

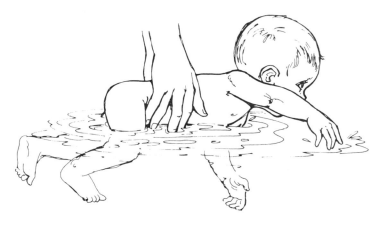

FIGURE 5.14 Swimming reflex. Swimming movements are elicited when the infant is exposed to water. Most of the propulsion comes from movements of the trunk and legs, with the arms remaining relatively stable in a high-guard position.

Swimming Movements

One of the most interesting reflexes seen in infants is a swimming movement when they are held in or *over* water (Figure 5.14). These swimming movements have been filmed by McGraw (1966) in infants 11 days old. If infants are placed in water, the head must be supported, because they are unable to maintain the head above the water level. These movements are more rhythmic than the previously described crawling movement and usually disappear by about the fifth month of age. The same reflexive swimming movements have also been noted by several experimenters in a number of mammalian species.

These movements are not as distinct in the air as they are in the water. In the newborn these movements are accompanied by reflexive breath holding; however, a month or two later the infant may incur great distress when the head is immersed. By the age of 2, however, the head must be supported if any kind of swimming or psuedoswimming is attempted or encouraged in the child. Real swimming needs to be learned several years later, when the child may cognitively acquire an awareness of the demands of the action, may acquire the strength and coordination to breathe correctly, and may otherwise understand the rigors and possible dangers of a swimming experience.

Climbing Movements

In addition to reflexes that resemble later voluntary attempts to move in a horizontal plane, newborn infants manifest a reflex similar to vertical climbing (Figure 5.15). With the infant held vertically, some observers have elicited an alternate upward arm movement and the palmar-grasp reflex in one palm. Some experimenters have noted that reciprocal movements of the legs occur under these circumstances. Others have suggested that this reflex is a remnant of the movement needed by the primate infant to reach the mother's nipple from a position on her lap. Most observ-

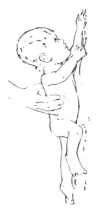

FIGURE 5.15
Climbing reflex. Climbing movements are seen when the proper stimuli are present.

ers usually place this climbing reflex toward the end of the first year of life and into the second year. It is seemingly associated with the assumption of upright gait and early attempts to walk voluntarily.

There is disagreement, however, as to what constitutes evidence of this reaction. Many have described "contraction" waves in the body, as the infant grasps upward and the trunk periodically flexes in an effort to keep up with the upper body. However, not all researchers can elicit this motion. The inconsistency of reports of this phenomenon may be due to a variety of climbing tasks that have been presented to infants.

RHYTHMIC MOVEMENTS OF INFANTS: STEREOTYPIES

One may trace research on infant reflexes back to the first decades of the last century. However, it has only been within the last decade that observers have begun to codify and try to explain actions which are at least as pervasive within the motor personality of the infant. These motions consist of rhythmic actions and occur in ways that are unvarying in nature, or that in other terms are *stereotypic*. These actions consist of kicking, waving, banging, rocking, and swaying movements of the arms, legs, and trunk. They are also characterized by the absence of any observable goal. The infant seems absorbed and motivated to participate in these actions for their own sake.

These rhythmic actions sometimes occur in conjunction with various other reflexes. At other times, they are seen by themselves. They are pursued with diligence and vigor by normal human infants during the first year of life. Some infants have been observed to engage in these flappings, rockings, and wavings for as much as 40 percent of their waking hours.

These actions first attracted the attention of those studying atypical children. They are seen to an abnormal degree and later in life in populations of the emotionally disturbed and of the blind, for example. Their presence in both these groups of children and in normal infants has been explained in many ways. Piaget, observing them, sometimes described them as "secondary circular reactions" consisting of feedback systems involving the body and parts of the environment. However, most early observers of these actions in both normal and abnormal groups are not in close agreement as to their causes and effects. Among the various explanations they offered are these: (a) They represent attempts by the infant to re-create prenatal experience. (b) The motions represent the exercise of satisfying experiences that are precursors to intellectual development. (c) The actions are important to the early balancing of the flexor and extensor actions of the muscles in infancy.

During the early 1970s, some researchers began to suspect that these frequent and interesting events served more straightforward purposes that are related to motor development. The actions were seen as evidence that the child was attempting to do something, but could not quite manage it. Moreover, these rhythmics seemed to take place in ways that resembled various kinds of important movement milestones, including kneeling, crawling, standing, and even walking.

Thelen (1979) was among the first to conduct an investigation which attempted to (a) classify the occurrence of these movements in infants, and (b) propose a reasonable explanation for their appearance. Thelen's investigations consisted of longitudinal studies of infants from 2 weeks to 1 year of age. The behaviors were observed during home visits, during which the infants were carrying out their normal activities. The one-hour visits, every two weeks, resulted in the collection of over 16,000 "bouts" of these rhythmic behaviors.[1] Thelen and her colleagues had little difficulty classifying these behaviors into 47 distinct movements. The most frequently encountered rhythmic stereotypies included the following.

Movements of the Legs and Feet

These movements were the most common and occurred earlier than the other types classified. Six of the seven subtypes seen involved flexions, extension, and flappings of the legs while the child was in a supine or prone position. They consisted of alternate kicking actions, single-leg kicking, and one foot rubbing the other. A distinct type included a frog-kicking action, seen when the infant was on its stomach and the back was arched (Figure 5.16). Furthermore, these rhythmic movements of the legs and feet phased in strongly between the twelfth and twentieth weeks of life, and appeared in some infants as young as 9 weeks of age. These movements may be useful adjuncts and precursors to turning over and to head control, and to other preliminaries to standing. These studies have indicated that it is probable that the same spinal generators control both kicking and the reflex stepping reactions discussed previously (Figure 5.17).

---

[1]A single "bout" was defined as a movement of parts of the body, or of the whole body, that was repeated in the same form for at least three times at regular short intervals of about a second or less.

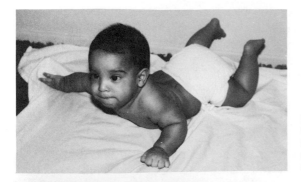

FIGURE 5.16
Child engaging in a body-rocking type of stereotypy, in this position leg stereotypies of various types are also often seen.

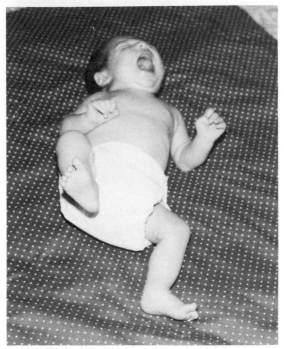

FIGURE 5.17
This three week old infant is engaging in alternate leg- kicking (Stereotypies) while angry.

Movements of the Torso

A number of important movements reflecting actions of the torso were recorded. These include those executed while the infant was prone, seated, kneeling (hands and knees), as well as standing. While prone, an arch-back rock was seen.

Hand-knee rocking was seen as the infant rocked back and forth in a hand-knees position. This action peaked around the third to eighth month of life and diminished after that time (Figure 5.18). In this movement the shoulders are over the hands at the forward position, and the arms remain straight during the action. A hand-knees back and forth sway, from side to side, was also recorded.

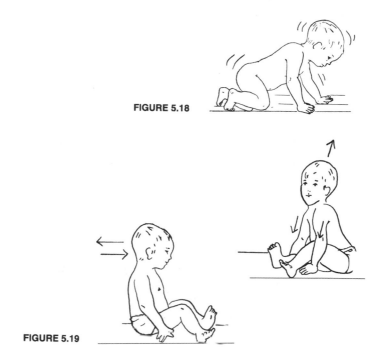

FIGURE 5.18

FIGURE 5.19

Seated Movements

In a seated position, the infants were seen to rock back and forth from front to back. They sometimes bounced up and down while seated; a side-to-side sway was sometimes recorded while the infant was seated. These seated rhythmics appeared about the twentieth week of life and increased in frequency from the twenty-fourth to the fortieth weeks (Figure 5.19).

Standing Movements

A standing bounce was a frequently recorded behavior. The infants moved up and down in one variation. Sometimes the infants moved from side to side, and toward or away from their supporting hands. In this movement, as was true of some others, the infants moved rhythmically in all directions possible, while maintaining a relatively balanced position, in this case on their feet (Figure 5.20).

This standing bounce and its variations appeared most markedly about the twenty-eighth week. The infants continued in this action during the remainder of the year they were observed. The numbers of these types of standing rhythmics increased toward the end of the first year. Less frequently recorded were rhythmic movements while the child was in a kneeling position. These were seen in only four of the twelve children and for a brief period of time, mainly after the thirty-fourth week of life.

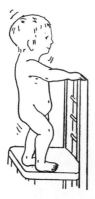

FIGURE 5.20

Movements of the Arms, Hands, and Fingers

All the infants in Thelen's study were observed to engage in rhythmic movements of the arms, hands, and fingers. Some of the time these actions included objects, as the children struck or repeatedly banged or shook hand-held objects of various kinds.

An often observed movement involved moving the arm in a waving action from the shoulder, with the elbow relatively straight. It was called *banging* if an object was in the hand and *waving* if no object was present. Sometimes the action terminated in the air; at other times the palm slapped to the ground (Figure 5.21).

This action was sometimes seen with one arm and sometimes accomplished with both arms. These actions of the arms were seen in some children shortly after birth. However, their peak age of occurrence was the time between the thirty-fourth and forty-second weeks. Arm-hand actions were far more prevalent than were movements of the torso during the first year of life among the children evaluated by Thelen (Figures 5.22 and 5.23).

A frequently observed stereotypy involved only the hands. Two types were recorded: one involving the rhythmic bending and extending of the wrist, and one in which the hands were also rotated. These actions were recorded for 18 of the 20 children observed, and were seen most between the twenty-fourth and forty-second

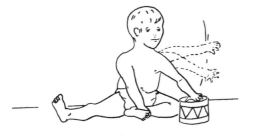

FIGURE 5.21

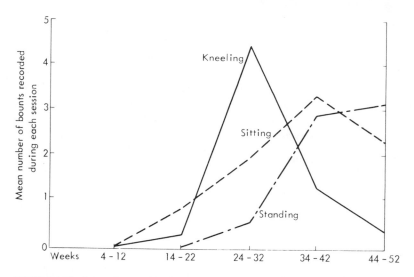

FIGURE 5.22 Comparison of three types of rhythmic stereotypies seen in torso movements: kneeling, sitting, and standing. Redrawn from data from E. Thelen, "Rhythmical Stereotypes in Infants," *Animal Behavior, 27* (1979), pp. 699-715, with permission of the author and the editors, Bailliere Tindall, London.

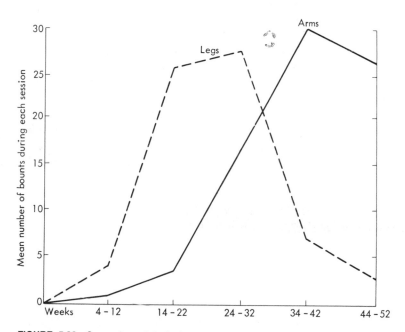

FIGURE 5.23 Comparison of rhythmic stereotypies seen in the arms and legs during the first year. Drawn from data from E. Thelen, "Rhythmical Stereotypes in Infants," *Animal Behavior, 27* (1979), pp. 699-715, with permission of the author and the editors, Bailliere Tindall, London.

weeks. A finger flex action was also observed throughout the first year of life. The four fingers and often the thumb were flexed and then extended in a rhythmic way. These finger twitchings were most often observed, however, between the twenty-fourth and forty-second weeks of life. Finger and hand movements occurred during the entire year, but the types changed as the infants studied matured. The nature of these actions are explored further in Chapter 8.

Other Rhythmic Stereotypes

Other rhythmic movements were also seen in the head and face. These less frequently recorded actions included shakes and nods of the head, small mouthing movements, as well as both side-to-side and in-and-out movements of the tongue. These other stereotypies, however, were seen in less than half the children surveyed.

Overall Trends

While over 50 movement types were recorded, some were very common and others were very rare. Kicking and banging movements, for example, were seen in all the infants observed; other movements were seen in only one or two infants. There were significant age trends in the appearance of various types of movements. Various of the movements displayed different patterns of appearance, peaking, and disappearance. Leg movements increased gradually to a peak at between 14 and 32 weeks, and then declined, so that only a few appeared at the end of the first year, while arm movements did not peak until about 10 weeks later. Rhythmic movements with the child seated and on hands and knees appeared rather abruptly at about the fifth month, and then peaked during the sixth and seventh months. These movements declined by the end of the first year. In contrast, twitchings of the fingers displayed a continuous appearance, from the first month to the twelfth. Standing and kneeling stereotypes appeared suddenly at about the ninth month and continued to the end of the year. Hand movements appeared at about the sixth month, peaking at about the seventh month. While a given type of movement sustained itself through the first year, often variations within types changed as a function of age. Different types of hand-finger movements appeared during the latter part of the first year, in contrast to those seen during the earlier months.

Another trend in the data, reflecting the appearance and type of these actions, is a tendency for them to proliferate in variety as the infant matures. Their numbers within each category and their overall appearance often tend to diminish toward the end of the first year. However, the *variety* of these movements increases markedly from the first to the twelfth month of age. This tendency for the movements to expand in kind as a function of age reflects some of the postulates in the previous chapter describing the diffusion effect in motor abilities as a function of age. Thus the infant's motor personality, just like that of the older child, adolescent, and adult, tends to become more complex and differentiated as the nervous system matures.

As can be seen, the appearance of various kinds of movements seemed to correspond to several developmental stages important in attaining various movement goals by the infant. Seated rocking appears at about the time children normally attempt to sit; standing rocking, during the month or two prior to the child gaining an upright stance. Rocking on the hands and knees appears at about the time the infant is preparing to crawl. Statistical verification of these associations was obtained by Thelen in her 1979 investigation. For the most part there were significant correlations between the onset of these rhythmic stereotypies and items in the Bayley Scale (1969) that reflect similar motor milestones. For example, when the children were scored as able to pick up a cube, they were also engaging in a marked number of stereotypies involving the arms (both waving and banging). When the children were scored able to sit alone with good coordination, they were also seen to engage in stereotypies of various kinds while in a seated position. The ability recorded on the Bayley Scale of pulling to a standing position was signaled by rhythmic movements in a standing position.

As a result of these close associations between various kinds of rhythmic actions and developmental milestones involving similar positions or actions, Thelen proposes that the appearance of these behaviors is dependent upon the maturation of proper neuromotor pathways. Further, Thelen contends these actions by the child are generally under conscious and central control. Their outward appearance seems rather random. However, the manner in which they appear in the infant's motor personality is predictable and highly orderly. This predictability of appearance, Thelen suggests, reflects specific stages of maturation of the nervous system components controlling specific movement patterns, actions, and positions. These actions, according to some (Lourie, 1949), consist of what might be termed *transition* behaviors, or behaviors needed within a muscle group and action pattern to somehow train and ready a more complex activity just as the infant begins to gain postural control of that action or activity. Fentress, observing these same actions in animals (1976), concluded that they represent what the animal "feels like " doing, but somehow does not quite know how to do in a precise way. He contends that in animals the neural processing circuits may become overloaded, often when the animals are under stress or in conflict. The animals, he concludes, perform rhythmic behaviors that require minimal processing capacities when in confusing stress situations.

Thelen suggests that these same rhythmic behaviors seen in human infants may also be due to immature temporarily overloaded neural systems. These actions, she concludes, reflect useful stages in "normal" maturation, actions that prepare the child for more complex use of the neural pathways involved, as well as for the actions these more primitive movements resemble (Thelen, 1979). There is some disagreement (Zelazo, 1983) with the maturational hypothesis advanced by Thelen. But I believe, along with Thelen, that neural maturation of rather basic kinds, reflected in the rhythmic movements discussed in this section, together with the interaction of reflexes, reflex suppression, and some of the basic responses discussed in the first part of this chapter, contributes in observable and logical ways to important and basic movements and postures needed during the first twelve months of life. During these same months, however, environmental stimulation, or lack of it, may also make moderate to marked modifications in the appearance of some of these milestones.

To fully understand motor development during the first year of life, it is necessary to illustrate how both maturational forces, reflected in movements, reflexes, and the like, and environmental stimulation may interact. To give one example, when the infant is preparing to crawl, numerous rhythmic preparations are necessary, together with the suppression of less-than-useful reflexes. First stages in the crawl may, in addition, be stimulated as objects are made available for the child to seek while in a hand-knees position. Thus rhythmic stereotypies involving hand-knee rockings, foot rhythmics, as well as suppression of hand-neck linkages harmful to the hand-knees balance required to begin the crawling action, are all necessary to provide a behavioral-movement base from which the child may proceed to crawl. Further illustrations of the ways in which reflex suppression, basic response patterns, and rhythmic stereotypes interact to prepare, instigate, and maintain useful movement patterns within the first year of life are found in the section that follows.

Work continues in an effort to determine what external and possible internal "events" may trigger these interesting rhythmics in infants (Thelen, 1981b). It has been suggested, for example, that much of the time they occur when the infant is at various stages of arousal, including a "fussy" stage. As a caretaker approaches an infant, the child often responds with kicks (Thelen, 1981b). If the caretaker seems to handle the child less, the child seems to seek more self-stimulation in the form of trunk movements. Thus the infant seems to seek vestibular sensation in the absence of movements of the trunk instigated by an adult. Also, from the twentieth week the presence of objects seems to trigger a great deal of arm waving by infants (Thelen, 1981).

Thelen has found that in the first half of the first year of life, the infant seems to be responding to external stimuli through the exercise of these movements. However, during the second year of life it seems as though the infant, when aroused, moves more in response to some kind of internalized drive. This same switching to an internal state when aroused was seen in studies of animals in earlier work by Fentress (1976).

Additionally, in recent work Thelen and her colleagues have determined that often the temporal patterns of these useless stereotypies remain the same when an infant changes how one may be used (Thelen and Fisher, 1983). For example, when the parts of a kicking stereotype were recorded before and after the leg movement caused a mobile to become activated, even though amplitude and duration of the kicking changed, temporal qualities of the movements' components remained similar under the two conditions. These findings thus indicate that similar neural pattern generators may be involved in both the early stereotypies as well as in corresponding voluntary actions that follow.

BEHAVIORAL INTERWEAVING AND THE ACHIEVEMENT
OF EARLY MOTOR MILESTONES

During the first year of life, the infant has been shown to be a remarkably perceptive organism, taking in large amounts of data from the environment. Learning to sort out and process that data will take a lifetime, but even during infancy the young human responds in ways which indicate that a remarkable number of important cognitive qualities are already making their appearance. The infant can recognize new and novel situations, people, and stimuli. Curiosity drives the infant to explore more and more novel actions, objects, situations, and people (Chapter 11).

As the information in this chapter indicates, the neonate's neuromotor system begins to express itself in ways which at times are both fascinating and seemingly unstoppable. Observation of an infant at about the second or third month of life reveals a never-ending mosaic of actions, reactions, twitching, and rhythmics. The sophisticated observer is able to identify various of the reflexes described, even though their appearance is often only transitory. Sustained and careful scrutiny, like that carried out by Thelen and others, reveals even more fascinating groups of motor behaviors, which appear and disappear at relatively predictable times during the first months of life.

The available evidence thus makes it reasonable to hypothesize that the appearance of early developmental milestones is the result of the interaction of at least three main types of actions within the maturing child. These consist of (a) the presence and emergence of various useful reflexes and response patterns; (b) the suppression by higher centers of some less-than-useful reflexes and reactions, and finally (c) evidence of the crude maturation of selected neural pathways as evidenced by the appearance of rhythmic stereotypies of the types described in the previous section. Additional contributors to the achievement of these selected motor milestones are environmental stimulation consisting of parent reactions, interesting sights and objects, as well as the nature of the clothing used, which may either encourage or restrict some of the actions mentioned above.

Several scholars during the past few decades have both observed and attempted to objectify and codify these interactive motor processes. Milani-Comparetti and his colleagues provided a testing instrument, based upon this rationale, in Italy during the 1960s. This assessment instrument, as well as others proposed over the ensuing years by Hoskin and Squire (1973), Molnar (1978), as well as Roberton and her colleagues (1977), has been based upon the observation that useful voluntary movements and positions early in life are dependent upon the interaction of reflexes and basic response patterns. They proposed that the appearance of useful response patterns and the disappearance (or suppression) of unwanted reflexes are both necessary occurrences when the infant first turns over, sits up, crawls, stands, and finally walks. These interactions have been carefully charted by these authors.

In the schema provided in this section, however, a third important dimension has been added to the processes described by Hoskin and Squire, Molnar, Milani-Comparetti, and their colleagues. The important work of Thelen describing rhythmic stereotypies provides a vital and useful adjunct to our understanding of how basic motor patterns and postures emerge during the first year of life. This interweaving of reflex suppression, reaction appearance, and rhythmic exercise, is illustrated below with regard to (a) turning over, (b) sitting (c) kneeling and crawling, and (d) standing. These important dimensions must be understood as they interact in order completely to comprehend how motor things happen during the first year, and also to begin to provide meaningful remediation and stimulation to the young child who may present developmental deficits reflected in motor delays.

Turning Over

It is likely that a number of basic responses must be present and contribute to the infant's ability to turn from the back to the front. The labyrinthine reflex, reflected in a head-up position evidenced in a controlled way, must be active and healthy. The asymmetrical tonic neck reflex must be at least partially suppressed so that it does not act as a brake as the child's head turns toward the intended direction of rotation. The righting reflexes or body derotative responses must be "in" and healthy. That is, as the head turns, the chest and hips must also rotate quickly and efficiently. Finally, various rhythmic stereotypies should be operative, probably those reflecting moderate maturation of pathways governing the actions of the legs, as well as a bowed back rocking motion with the child in a prone position. Both bilateral as well as unilateral stereotypies of the legs are probably useful. Figure 5.24 shows several of these influencers on the act of turning from back to front.

Turning from the back to the front may also be facilitated if the infant is able to watch and become interested in moving objects. Visual following responses, reflected in head turning, are likely to trigger some of the first almost accidentlike attempts and successes in making this back to front turn. Turning in the opposite direction also requires some of the same actions and responses as were necessary to facilitate rotation in the opposite way. A good positive support reflex should be in place before the child is able to turn front to back, in order to reduce friction between the stomach and the surface on which the infant is resting. The head should be under good control and reflect healthy labyrinthine function. Body-righting reactions should be operative, so that when the infant turns, either by accident or intention (perhaps to watch an object moving across the space field), a turning will occur. Turning actions on this long axis are usually preceded by rhythmic wavings of the legs, either separately or together.

Sitting

Several reactions and movements accompany sitting. Various rhythmic stereotypies involving rhythmic motions in several directions may occur if the infant

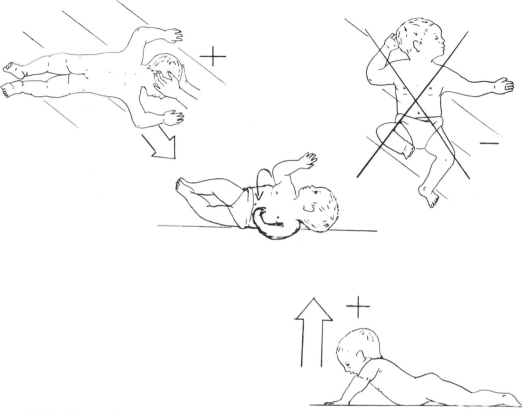

FIGURE 5.24 Contributors and detractors to rolling over.

is held or supported in a sitting position prior to the assumption of a nonsupported sit. Moreover, the infant must possess various support reactions if tilted either forward or backward, reflected in the tendency of the hands to reach out and catch balance, and the movement of the head to the direction opposite to that of the direction of tilt. The tonic neck reactions should be suppressed or suppressable, insofar as neck-arm linkages are not useful nor compatible with the support or propping reactions needed to maintain a sustained and balanced sit. About the time the infant is able to sit, the arms and hands are free to provide assistance other than their previous support functions. Therefore it is probable that prior to or during the time the infant is learning to sit, a series of rhythmic stereotypes will be seen, including arm waving and arm-hand banging. In Figure 5.25, propping reactions are seen in parts (a) and (b). Seating rhythmics are depicted in (c), and one type of arm rhythmics is shown in part (d).

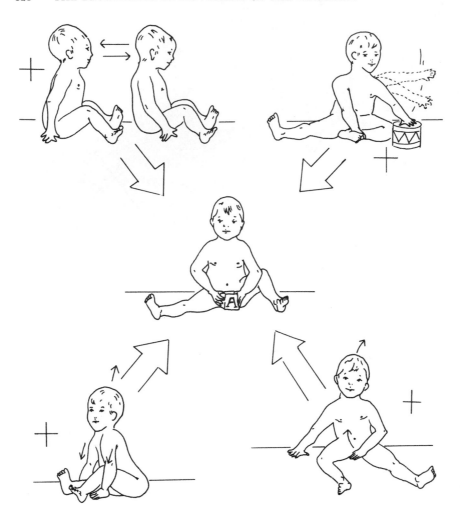

FIGURE 5.25 Actions contributing to and detracting from sitting up.

Creeping and Crawling

Usually crawling is defined as locomotion while the stomach remains on the floor; creeping involves locomotion from a hand-knee position with the stomach clear of the floor. Obviously crawling precedes creeping, and both are useful precursors of standing and walking. Creeping is facilitated if a creeping reflex is present—that is, movement will occur if pressure is exerted on the soles of the feet in alternating ways. Usually this progression of motion occurs on first one side and then the other, with the hand on the side of the knee inching forward, also proceeding forward.

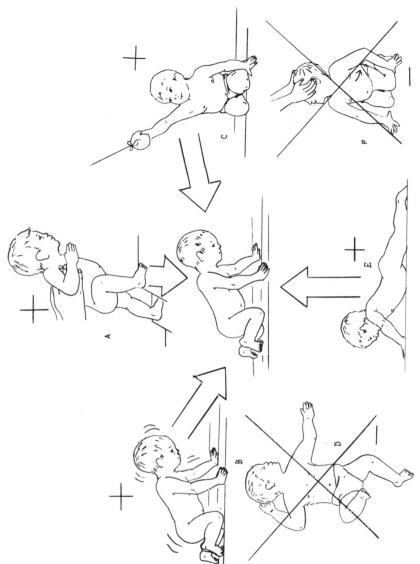

FIGURE 5.26 Actions contributing to and detracting from a balance position, in readiness to creep.

Both crawling and creeping depend upon the relative suppression of a strong asymmetrical tonic neck reflex, although primate forms of crawling may not be impeded with the presence of this reflex. Labyrinthine reflexes should also be healthy, and the infant should display good head control with regard to movement against gravity. In crawling, the arms and hands are used together with the elbows; in creeping, the hands are in a strong supporting reaction and begin to move out first independently and then in a pattern that reflects leg movement (an arm-leg opposition, with the hand moving forward as the knee on the opposite side progresses).

In Figure 5.26 the contributors to, and detractors from, adequate creeping are illustrated. For example, contributing to creeping, and to the support position illustrated, are (a) an alternate leg flexion seen first in the stepping reflex. Rhythmic rockings, as shown in (b), in a hand-knee position are useful precursors of the stabilized starting position needed. Part (e), a strong support reaction of the arms, is essential, together with a suppression of the tendency of the asymmetrical tonic neck reaction to appear in the arms if the head is turned (d,f), illustrating the presence of an asymmetrical tonic neck reflex. In contrast, the head and arms should be able to move independently, as the infant may reach for an object and thus be provided with an impetus to move, as in (c).

Crawling may begin in crude forms by the fourth or fifth month, whereas creeping begins three to four months later, and often accompanies upright locomotion for several months, as the child finds it easier and faster to get from one place to another, using efficient creeping, rather than unstable and inefficient early walking efforts.

Standing Unassisted

Standing is the infant's crowning achievement about the end of the first year. A case could be made for the fact that virtually all of previous reflex suppression, reaction formation, and rhythmic production contribute to this difficult balance position. Some of the main contributors and one detractor are shown in Figure 5.27. Initially the child needs to pull to an upright position, as shown in (d). The infant must have incentives (objects which provide incentives for this useful action), as well as the means, a ladder or pole, that provides handholds for this dangerous undertaking. The infant who has accomplished this will usually spend a month or two traveling or cruising around objects, holding on, while moving the feet sideways, as shown in (f). A stable base of support during these times is made possible by a suppression of the plantar flexion reflex, as shown in (e). Moreover, useful thrust or support reactions by the limbs, as the child is brought toward the floor, may help in the initial standing positioning. "Exercise" of neural pathways, as provided by various kinds of rhythmic stereotypies shown in (b), are useful and appear before and during the child's attempt to stand alone. These can consist of a variety of actions taken in all directions while the child is cruising, or while hanging on in the stable position illustrated.

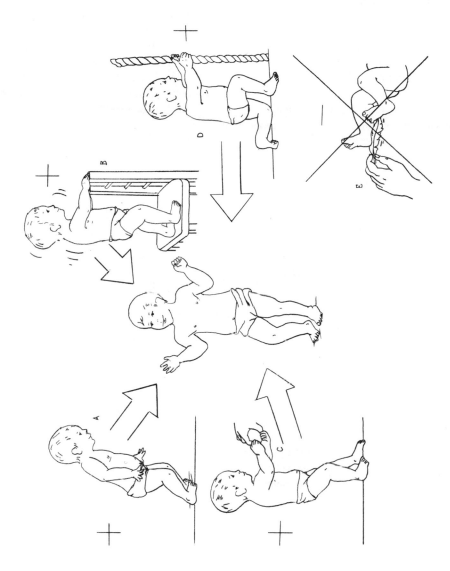

FIGURE 5.27 Actions contributing to and detracting from standing alone, in preparation for walking.

Finally, a complicated but essential parachute reaction is important. As shown in Figure 5.27(a), the child's neuromotor system should be mature enough to emit a response that permits the lowering of the body to the floor when it is desired to descend, or when balance is lost. This response involves a compensation of the head—forward if balance is lost backward, a quick bending of the knees, together with a reaching-out-for-support reaction by the hands, as shown. If repeated early efforts to rise are terminated by jolting returns to the floor because of the absence of this parachute reaction, it is unlikely that the child will incur further risks, and will not vigorously pursue further attempts to stand.

TABLE 5.1   Appearance of Reflexes and Stereotypes

APPROXIMATE TIME BEHAVIOR OCCURS	BEHAVIOR INDICATIVE OF THE ORIGINS OF MOVEMENT IN INFANTS
Gestation	Moro reflex appears Fetal activity prior to birth indicative of later motor competency and vigor
Birth	Birth reflexes, including Moro, startle, palmar grasp, rooting, crawling reflex Seeks novel stimuli, variable activity levels evidenced Walking reflex seen
30 days	Arm-supporting reflex seen Labyrinthine righting reflex appears
48 days	Leg rhythmic stereotypes maximize
60 days	Separate perceptual-motor and cognitive traits identifiable
90 days	Pull-up reactions in the arm (reflex) Walking reflex terminates Infant can turn over from back to stomach
4 months	Hand-knee stereotypes at maximum
6 months	Moro reflex terminates Voluntary creeping appears Swimming reflex disappears Voluntary crawling appears Crawling reflex disappears
8 months	Arm and seated rhythmic stereotypes peak
9 months	Supporting reflex in the legs seen Standing rhythmics seen Palmar and plantar grasp reflexes disappear Righting reflexes of the head and body disappear
12 months	Supported walking Can arise from a back-lying position to a standing position, independent locomotion

SUMMARY

This chapter focuses upon infant movements involving the trunk and limbs through a survey of some of the most prominent infant reflexes and some early and basic movement responses, as well as more recent literature reflecting attempts to classify and to explain what are termed *rhythmic stereotypies*. Analysis of these dimensions of early human action leads to models for understanding the ways in which the neuromotor system apparently displays maturational progression by suppressing unneeded reflexes. Furthermore, understanding the instigation of voluntary and necessary movements and positions is facilitated by surveying the manner in which various rhythmic actions occur in the trunk, the arms, and hands, as well as in the body in various support positions.

Several other motor qualities occurring within the first year of life include reflexes, reflex suppression, basic reactions, and rhythmic behaviors as they influence turning, creeping-crawling, sitting, and standing. Analyses of the beginnings of speech and manual abilities are found in later chapters. The interesting hand and arm wavings identified by Thelen, as well as movements of the face and tongue, are obviously supportive of early facial expressions, manual skills, and speech. In Chapter 6 the focus is on the child from 1 to 5 years.

QUESTIONS FOR DISCUSSION

1. Discuss the term "reflexes" as used in this chapter, as contrasted with the word used by sports writers when describing good athletic performance in mature adults ("the batter has good reflexes").

2. What advantages and possible disadvantages might reflex training (in walking, etc.) have when applied to the maturing infant?

3. What reflexes seem to prepare the infant to assume an upright position, i.e., to work against gravity?

4. What reflexes seem to prepare the infant for locomotion?

5. The prolongation of what reflex(es) might impede voluntary grasping behavior?

6. What reflexes seem important for survival of the infant during the first months of life?

7. What reflex(es) in the human infant seem to be the evolutionary "remains" of movements no longer needed?

8. How might a knowledge of reflex behavior assist in the teaching of sports skills? What sport skills seem to resemble (or be aided) by various reflexes? What sport skills and actions seem to somehow "work against" reflex patterns?

9. What might be the disadvantages and advantages of exposing an infant of 6 to 10 months of age to swimming lessons?

10. How might reflexes contribute to the apparent swimming of an infant of 8 months of age?

11. Discuss how certain reflexes must be phased out (disappear) prior to the onset of certain voluntary movements. Be specific: just what reflexes seem to impede the onset of what voluntary movements?

12. Discuss and describe the lead-up activities necessary to achieve a coordinated upright gait.

13. Observe a basketball player for a prolonged period during a game. Note what simple reflexes seem to contribute to jumping, running, and shooting skills. What reflexes might possibly impede certain of the basketball skills he or she evidences?

14. Observe a swimmer turning, stroking, and starting. What basic reflex patterns seem to contribute to or detract from optimum performance?

15. What programs of physical therapy require detailed knowledge of infant reflexes?

16. How might atypical reflexes be studied in children by placing them in water or by observing them on a trampoline?

17. Observe an infant within the third or fourth month and try to codify the nature of the rhythmic movements seen. How do these movements correspond to whatever developmental task (sitting, etc.) you see the infant engage in.

18. Review the literature on the recent controversy about infant stepping reactions (Pontius, 1974; Thelen, 1983; Zelazo, 1983). Identify the data and issues involved. Form a conclusion about the desirability of encouraging the stepping response.

CHAPTER SIX
INFANCY AND EARLY CHILDHOOD
Action Sequences and Skills Exhibited by the Larger Muscle Groups

Almost from birth, the infant begins to engage in various purposeful actions involving the larger muscles of the body. In addition to the patterns of movements involving the rhythmic flappings and reflexes discussed in Chapter 5, the infant and then the child reacts in purposeful and often powerful ways to objects and tasks in the environment. In addition, internalized needs and thoughts about actions become increasingly complex.

One major portion of these early voluntary movements involves subsequences necessary to assume an upright stance, and the postures and balances necessary to walk. Other efforts seem to involve reactions to gravity, but involve the assumption of stabilized positions from which the infant and child may first manipulate objects, and then when standing is achieved, engage in such skills as throwing, catching, kicking, and later even striking objects with bats, rackets, and paddles.

Thus the child seems to acquire two kinds of balance skills. One type involves the acquisition of the ability to stabilize in such positions as sitting, standing, and the like. The other skill involves the ability to lose balance in just the correct ways, and then periodically to restabilize, as is required to progress when walking, creeping, running, and skipping.

As the child enters the third, fourth, and fifth years, the skills expected grow more complex and often involve using extensions of the body, such as rackets and bats. Additional complexity also occurs as more and more subskills must be put together in ever-increasing wholes. Thus, for example, simply trapping a ball while seated is no longer considered useful in 4-year-olds; they must often please their parents by catching balls in an upright position, or even moving their bodies to the future locations of missiles coming their way.

A two-way classification system is also useful to consider within the context of this discussion. The action patterns of the maturing child are often separated into materials reflecting their biomechanical descriptions, in contrast to the *results* of the child's applications of force, speed, levers, and pulleys. Thus running may be analyzed according to the forces and velocities taken by the lower limbs, trunk, and other body parts, as well as by the consideration of simply how fast a child is moving. Throwing, to cite another example, may be analyzed by observing films of how and in what order various body parts are called in to participate in the movement patterns involved, or be looked at simply by measuring how far or how accurately the child is able to propel a missile.

In this chapter both types of approaches will be integrated. Actions will be described, and their biochemical characteristics discussed and portrayed in illustrations. Additionally, when available, the product of various actions will also be presented. These products can include how fast a child can run or how far a throw is made.

Marked individual differences exist not only in preschool children's physical abilities, but in the maturity of the mechanics they appear to use when performing various skills. Additionally, it is becoming increasingly clear that children at these young ages vary greatly in measures of the quantity of activity they evidence as well as in their exposure to formal physical education programs (Parizkova, 1984). One investigator recently found that children who ranked high in activity level raised their heart rates over 175/minute, four times longer each day, than did children judged to be low in activity level (Saris, 1980).

Reasonably accurate descriptions of the action patterns children acquire as they mature, as well as the results of these actions, are becoming easier to explain and understand. More and more useful filmed analyses are becoming available, together with developmental trends in how children improve in various tasks ranging from balance to ball striking.

ACTIONS AND POSTURES: THE FIRST YEAR

In addition to the rhythmic flappings and the reflexive behaviors discussed in Chapter 5, the infant during the first year is obsessed not only with the need to move, but to move in ways that will eventuate in standing and walking by the beginning of the second year of life. Rarely does the infant remain in a fixed position. Pikler, for example, has found that during the first year infants retain a fixed position for an average of about 2 minutes during the first six months. During the second half of the year, as movement capacities expand, the resting time diminishes to about 1.5 minutes (Pikler, 1972).

Actions during this first year seem often initiated because of some inner drive to action possessed not only by the human infant, but by the young of many species. As Garvin Maxwell has observed when studying playful sea mammals: ''Otters are extremely bad at doing nothing.'' At the same time, however, the infant displays the drive to get places in order to do things, and to obtain interesting objects that may be in view. Thus seeking behaviors, supported by adequate vision, are a second main impetus to move.

Several other progressions are taking place at the same time. One involves bunching the feet under the rear of the body while flexing the knees. This is preparatory to the assumption of a crawling position and then later creeping postures. As the legs move in the various ways described in Chapter 3, the infant, accidentally at first, and then later with purpose, may begin to push across the floor in rudimentary crawling actions. The stomach remains in contact with the floor, and the exact leg movements that accomplish this kind of action often vary from youngster to youngster. Indeed, the exact method discovered may have come about as the result of a happy accident, rather than because of any kind of precise developmental quality.

At this same time, the infant is learning to move from a position lying on the back to one lying on the stomach. This may be accomplished at first because of a

FIGURE 6.1(a)
Rolling from the back to front may be triggered by the infant's desire to obtain an object, as shown. The body-derotative response triggered by a head turn is then transferred to the hip and the infant rolls over. (b) Turning facilitated by desire to reach an object, in this case from back to front.

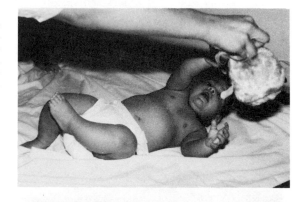

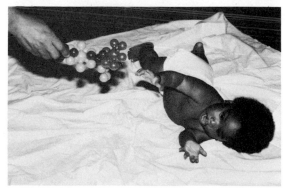

visual searching response that turns the head and then turns the body, as described in Chapter 3. This back to front turn, as has been pointed out, will tend to be impeded if there is an excess of tonicity within the movement make-up of the child, thus triggering a total or partial asymmetrical tonic neck reaction by the arm on the side toward which the head is attempting to initiate the turn.

Caretaker Influences

Toward the end of the third and during the fourth month, it is likely that efforts of interested caretakers may begin to play an increasing role in movements of the total body the infant tends to produce. Indeed, many so-called objective scales contain such items during these and later months as (a) "sits with support," or perhaps (b) "walks with aid." Pikler (1972) as well as others have correctly criticized the presence of this kind of evaluative criteria as being somewhat subjective. For after all, how much aid is "aided," and how much "support" is really being rendered by an interested mother or encouraging father? Parizkova has recently found that time taken by parents to stimulate preschool infants enhanced motor performance (1984).

At the same time, there are progressions during the third to sixth months that involve the assistance of others. For example, the pull-to-a-support group of responses is often found on infant scales. This involves a series of three responses reflecting how well the infant responds when being pulled to a seated position, using the hands, from a back lying (supine) position. As shown in Figures 6.2 and 6.3, the three response patterns involve first a marked "lag" of the head, as the infant is pulled forward and upward. Next, the head first lags back, and then the front of the neck flexes and the body is lifted as a single unit. Finally, during the most mature phase, the infant reacts instantly when touched on the hands, sometimes even when seeing the approach of a caretaker's hands, and flexes forward at the neck while being pulled upright. In this manner, the body moves upward in a single unit.

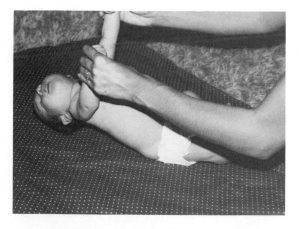

FIGURE 6.2
A head-lag shown at 3 months as the baby is pulled slowly to an upright position.

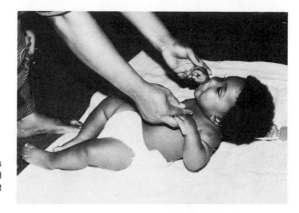

FIGURE 6.3
A more mature reaction at 6 months as the head is flexed forward and accompanies the body when the infant is pulled upright.

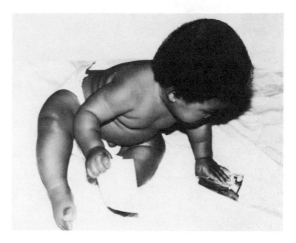

FIGURE 6.4
A stable seated position enables this child of 6.5 months to manipulate two objects, holding one while inspecting the other.

Still another caretaker-involved action is reflected in the assumption of seated positions with varying amounts of help and evidencing varying degrees of strength and balance on the part of the infant. These activities may begin at about the fourth month, and the first attempts to support the infant usually elicit a flaccid trunk posture by the youngster, with only moderate head control. The caretaker at this point is usually quite essential. However, as the next two months pass, less and less parental support is needed, and finally the infant is able to sit alone by the sixth or seventh month. This final unaided position is an extremely important developmental milestone, because the hands are now free to begin their important job of manipulating the environment.

Locomotion Continues

During the same months the caretaker may be attempting to help the youngster sit and to pull him or her to an upright position, additional efforts are beginning

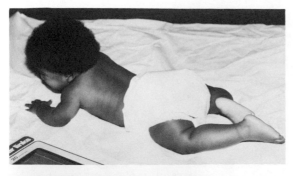

FIGURE 6.5
This infant has somehow learned to make progress with a breast-stroke-like extension of both legs simultaneously, propelling her forward.

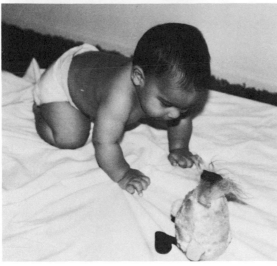

FIGURE 6.6
This six month old is now beginning to think about creeping to obtain a desired object.

to produce more and more vigorous and precise forms of locomotion. At times these efforts may occur in a seated position. An infant may, for example, adopt creative ways of moving called "scooting" in which the feet push the infant along in a seated position, back first.

Gradually, crawling and its modifications continue. The legs become stronger, head control improves, and between the sixth to eighth month the infant may begin to posture in an all fours position, in preparation for creeping. This position is often accompanied by rhythmic rocking, as discussed in Chapter 5. At the same time, first efforts to assume this position are often accompanied by failure. An arm may buckle, causing the infant to descend quickly. Movement out of this position, however, is first likely to occur when the infant wants to obtain an object just out of reach.

During these months activity levels pick up, and creeping progresses through several stages. The initial stage is marked by an unsteadiness; often only the arms move forward, and the legs drag behind. The infant is not aware of their actions, and is unable to incorporate them into the total movement. Next the legs and arms

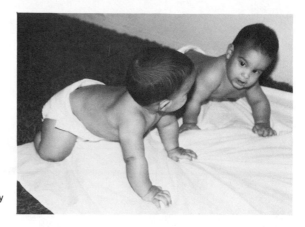

FIGURE 6.7
These advanced creepers seem only
to be awaiting the starter's gun.

move, but not in concert. They usually advance one at a time, almost at random. However, at this stage the infant is able to maintain the creeping position for prolonged periods of time. Finally, the creeping pattern assumes maturity. A cross-extension pattern is acquired, with the left hand placed as the right knee comes forward. Next the right hand advances as the left knee moves forward.

As the illustration indicates, this advanced pattern may be so satisfying that it is continued and accompanies the more difficult efforts of gaining an upright position and early walking patterns. The infant may, for example, learn to crawl over obstacles and up stairs with great vigor and high levels of motivation. However, it also should be remembered that many infants, usually more mature and linear youngsters, may omit an extended creeping stage altogether, or pass through it so quickly that a short time later a parent will scarcely remember its occurrence.

Onward and Upward

Although finding satisfaction in moving forward while creeping, the infant by the ninth to tenth month begins to evidence the desire to move upward. Usually this is seen first in linear children, and in more mature girls. At the same time, parental encouragement, as well as the presence of supports enabling the child to pull himself or herself to a standing position, tend to accelerate the assumption of an upright standing position. Also aiding these first efforts are improved head control, stronger legs, and a spinal column that is becoming stronger, and that assumes an S-shaped curve, enabling it to become a more efficient weight bearer.

Whether or not the child persists in this kind of somewhat unsteady undertaking depends upon how well a quick descent is managed. The presence of an adequate parachute reaction, described in Chapter 3, for example, will lessen the shock of a quick sitdown, and thus not discourage the child from trying to stand, time, and time again.

As it is most common for an upright position to be achieved by holding on to someone or something, the next stage in prelocomotive efforts involves what has

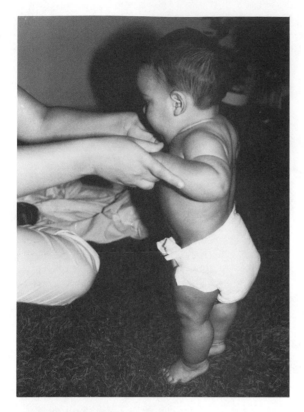

FIGURE 6.8
A child standing, or pulled to a stand, as shown here, will be secure and try again to the extent to which a safe descent is accomplishable via a parachute reaction, i. e., knee bend, and a controlled descent, with the arms reaching out for support upon arrival at the surface.

FIGURE 6.9
"Cruising" preceeds unassisted walking.

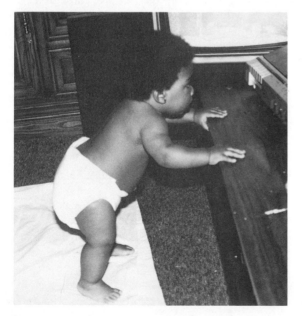

been labeled *cruising*. This involves lateral movement in a standing position, while retaining handholds on available supports. Often cruising first occurs around a convenient coffee table.

Cruising leads naturally to the assumption of a first unaided step or two. These unsteady efforts are invariably accompanied by excess tension in the arms, causing them to extend upward at the shoulders in what has been labeled a high guard position. Actually the label is a misnomer, insofar as the arms held in this position would seem to take longer to descend if the infant falls. Thus, rather than providing a guard, they are actually an impediment to a relaxed, safe gait. The arms in this position also tend to raise the infant's center of mass, a further impediment to stability in gait. The infant will lower the arms and hands to a low guard position sometime within the latter part of the second year of life (Noller and Igrisano, 1984).

THE GAIT CHANGES: THE SECOND YEAR

Over the next several months, the gait begins to become more prolonged, and in time more rhythmic and regular. The arms start to descend while walking, although the assumption of a mature cross-extension pattern in the walk is several years away. The most predictable quality in the infant's gait during the second year of life is its irregularity. The distance per step is dependent upon leg length, as would be expected (Rose-Jacobs, 1982; Beck et al., 1980). A more mature gait is not usually seen until the fifth year of life (Beck et al., 1980), but changes in the walking characteristics of children continue to be recorded up until the ages of 8 to 10 years (Nordlin et al., 1981).

By the age of 2 the child's gait will evidence increasing rhythmicity, with a pattern of about 170 steps per minute emerging (Espenschade and Eckert, 1967). The base provided by widely spaced feet during the first year gradually becomes narrower during the second year, as the feet begin to point straight ahead and are closer together during walking. In the second year the child will also evidence the tendency to "hurry" a walk, turning it often into a true run by the end of the second year or the middle of the third. Generally, however, the child during the midpoint of the second year will often be seeming to run without exhibiting a true run. A *true run* is one in which at some time during the gait cycle, both feet are off the ground at the same time. But children during this second year may "hurry" rather fast. In a recent unpublished study, we found that children midway in their second year could travel as fast as 5 to 6 ft/sec, with some moving even faster. In this study, both speed and efficiency of locomotion were moderately correlated to linearity of body build (evaluated using the ponderal index as a measure), as well as to leg length.

Gait characteristics of children undergo significant changes during the next two years (Fortney, 1983). Generally, the force and speeds generated in the limbs during running tend to differ significantly at 2, 4, and 6 years of age (Fortney, 1983). Thus even though some 2-year olds may apparently begin to walk and to run in a mature fashion, they will evidence significant changes during the next three to

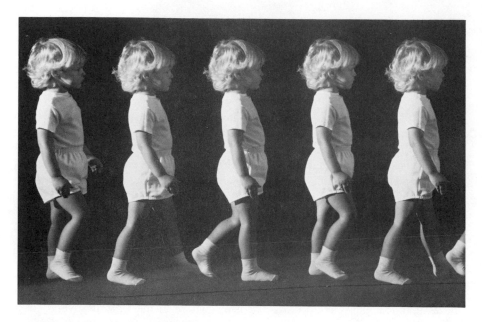

FIGURE 6.10 A relaxed arm-swing with mature arm-leg opposition will not usually be seen during the second year. However, during the third year this child evidences at times a cross-extension pattern, eg., the left arm swings forward when the right leg steps.

four years. By the age of 5 the child will become able to run twice as fast as was possible during the second year of life, or over 11 ft/sec (Jenkins, 1930).

These increases in locomotion speed during the years 3 to 5 are accompanied by several biomechanical changes. These include (a) the period of nonsupport becomes progressively longer, (b) the body leans forward more, particularly as the first support leg contacts the ground, (c) there is less up and down movement of the body; the center of gravity changes position less in an up-down direction, and (d) the portion of the foot touching the ground, and the order in which various parts of the foot touch the ground, change.

Overall, Seefelt, Rueschlein, and Vogel (1972) identified four stages seen as children gradually gain more mature running form from their third to sixth year of life. These include:

(a) Phase one is signalled by the arms being held high, the full sole of the foot contacts the ground, and the strike is short with little knee flexion.

(b) In phase two the stride becomes longer, there is more knee flexion, and a longer non-support phase occurs.

(c) The third phase is marked by contact being made first with heel and then toe; there is increasingly more vigorous arm action with the arms held lower; and tending to rotate slightly.

(d) Finally in stage four, at higher speeds the child will only contact the ground with the front of the foot, and there is a consistent and vigorous arm-leg opposition, with a vigorous thrust upward and forward of the right arm as the left knee comes forward and down.

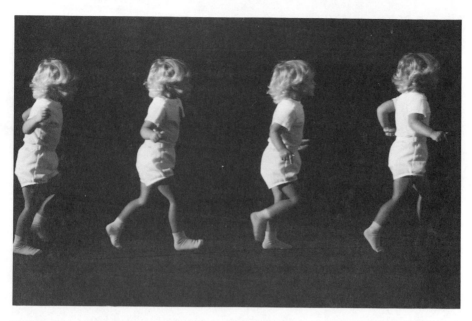

FIGURE 6.11 While some believe the "true" running occurs during the third year, many children do not leave the ground. Even when asked to run they hurry. Moreover, as is seen here, a cross-extension pattern is not seen in these early "hurrys" or runs. The left arm for example, does not thrust forward when the right leg comes forward, as will be seen at four and five years of age.

FIGURE 6.12 In contrast to the children in their third year, this five year old evidences a relatively mature running pattern, perhaps because he has older brothers and sisters to imitate.

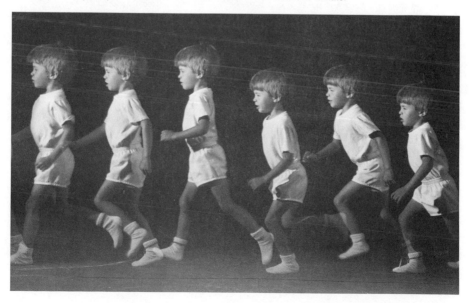

AN EXPLOSION OF SKILLS: AGES 3 TO 5

From the ages of 3 to 5, a number of skills begin to arise and expand upon the simple movement patterns seen as the child attempts to master walking and rudimentary running during the second year of life. Motorically precocious youngsters during these years often evidence body builds that are linear and relatively free of fat. At the same time, child-rearing attitudes and the presence of older siblings may be very influential in how fast various movement capacities explode during the next 3 to 4 years (Samuels, 1980; Schnabl-Dickey, 1978).

Two apparently contrasting tendencies emerge. (1) The child begins to evidence more consistency. When running, for example, more regularity and consistency of gait is seen. Indeed, it has been demonstrated that the running patterns of 3-year-olds may be more consistent than their walking efforts (Rose-Jacobs, 1983). (2) On the other hand, the young child begins to seek variations within a given family of movement skills. Backward and sideways locomotion may be attempted during the next two years. Gait variations seen in other children are similarly observed and copied, including jumping and hopping patterns.

The ability to balance begins to mature during these years, contributing to the expansion of movement skills. This apparently simple kind of task is actually dependent for adequate performance on the precise interaction of at least three different subsystems: (a) Vision, and its ability to stabilize the visual-perceptual field of the child (Zernicke, Gregor, and Cratty, 1982; Lee and Aaronson, 1974); (b) move-

FIGURE 6.13 Lateral movement is slow and thoughtfully executed during the third and fourth years, but in a year or two lateral movement is possible in a rapid and fluid manner. (See Chapter 13.)

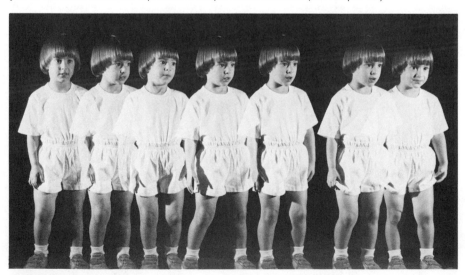

ment qualities involving the precise correction of imbalances when remaining in one position or when walking a balance beam; and finally (c) the mechanisms of the inner ear that act as integrators of visual and motor information impinging upon the maturing child. Defects in any one of these subsystems are likely to produce balance problems for the maturing child that in turn will impede the stability needed to exhibit new and emerging skills of the larger muscle groups, including kicking, throwing, and catching balls and other objects.

Leaving the Ground

As preschool age youngsters view others leaving the ground, they too attempt to jump. Usually efforts during the second year of life are unsuccessful; the child cannot get both feet off the ground at the same time. The lift provided by an appropriate arm action is not only absent, but the leg muscles may lack the quick strength and power needed to overcome the child's bulk.

The first time the child leaves the ground usually involves what is termed an *unsupported step*. A takeoff is made, pushing with one foot, while the other foot takes the shock of landing. This is of course easier if first attempts are made from a higher takeoff surface to a lower landing surface. Later this may be attempted on a

FIGURE 6.14
Efforts made to jump may or may not result in the child leaving the ground during the second and third year of life. As is seen here, a lift upward is achieved, but the child remains in contact with the ground.

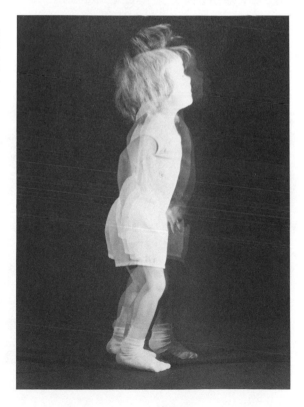

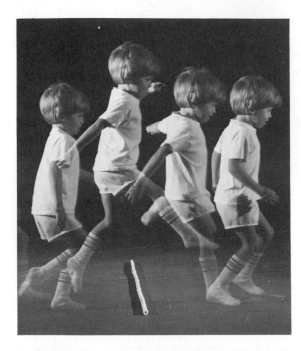

FIGURE 6.15
An unsupported step executed by a boy of 4.5 years.

FIGURE 6.16 In the beginning stages of jumping, demonstrated by a boy of four, the arms and legs are not synchronized, and the arms may or may not arise and extend forward as the legs extend at the knees.

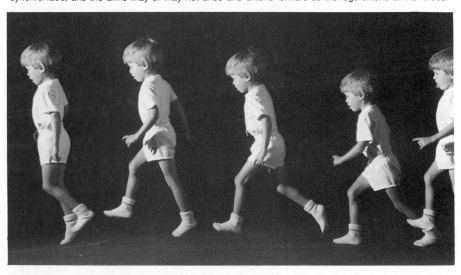

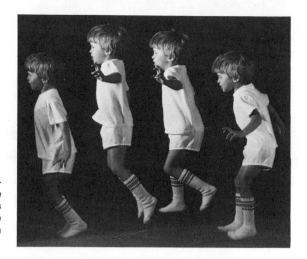

FIGURE 6.17
As the child matures, jumping is accomplished more and more with the arms and legs working in unison, as is shown by this boy of six. A still more advanced jumping pattern will be seen later in childhood (Chapter 15).

level surface, with landing and takeoff points at the same heights. Later a series of unsupported steps may be seen, and may be incorporated into a rudimentary one-footed skip—a step with one foot, alternating with a hop on the other.

A simple jump, with a two-foot takeoff and a two-foot simultaneous landing, is often seen next. Midway through the third year this is often possible, depending upon the maturity of the child, his or her body build, and what adult encouragement may be present (Schnabl-Dickey, 1978). Filmed analyses of the progression in this act also reveal several substeps. These steps involve an increasing tendency for the upper limbs to become properly involved in the jump.

Initially the jump occurs almost with the absence of any arm actions. The actions of the upper limbs that may be present are often simply inappropriate and tense flexions (see Chapter 9); or the opposite, weak and flaccid arms simply hanging by the child's sides as he or she attempts to jump, may be seen. A second stage involves a lift of the arms, together but not coordinated with the leg extension and thrust. The arms may, for example, be lifted upward and back of the body, with a flexion at the elbow joint, as shown. In recent work, boys have been found to be superior to girls in a standing broad jump, even as early as the third year of life (Morris et al., 1982)

Poe (1976) conducted a detailed filmed analysis of 2-year-olds' movement patterns as they jumped and reached for overhead balloons. Six difference maturity levels were identified in the jumping patterns. In general, the patterns she identified as more mature and ''better'' involved children moving from a deeper crouching position and using their arms through greater ranges of motion during the jump. However, it was interesting to note that (a) 6 of the 22 children analyzed did not leave the ground when attempting to jump, and (b) there was no significant relationship between the ''maturity'' of a child's jumping pattern and success. These findings led Poe to conclude that there are marked individual differences even at this early age in how fundamental movements are performed, and thus references to a "typical" jumping pattern are somewhat superficial and invalid. Moreover, her data also indicate that factors other than "good" or "bad" mechanics are likely to lead to success in various basic actions even at these early ages.

For example, in the task analyzed it is probable that body build, coupled with leg power, could have been at least as important as was the specific movement pattern used by the child in the jump-reach task analyzed. Thus, even at these early ages marked individual differences will be seen in the mechanics of movements in the same task evidenced by various children. Additionally, simply observing what seem to be "correct" mechanics may not afford complete insight into the relative success of youngsters in various basic movement tasks and in emerging skills involving missiles.

By the fourth and fifth years, in the presence of appropriate models and with the proper incentives, a marked improvement in the mechanics of jumping both upward and forward, as well as in the distances traveled, will be seen. Standing broad jump scores may more than double from the third to the fifth years of life in both boys and girls (Morris, et al., 1982). With maturity, more children will discover that the arms will tend to facilitate the jump, and will move them upward when attempting a high jump and forward when attempting a standing broad jump. At first, however, these arm actions will not occur at the same time the legs extend. With practice, later efforts will involve the arm-shoulder extension at the same time the legs extend. At first jumping height may not be closely aligned with correct biomechanics, but by later in the preschool years good mechanics involving arm-leg integration will contribute to increased heights or distances (Poe, 1976). Clark and Phillip's (1985) recent biomechanical analyses of the standing broadjump point to three distinct maturational stages.

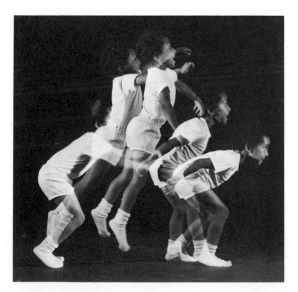

FIGURE 6.18

A hop or two is sometimes seen at four years, but a series is sometimes accomplishable by the end of the fourth or during the fifth years, as shown. Hopping with accuracy, however, is a task accomplishable by children in middle childhood (see Chapter 15).

Hopping is more difficult than jumping. Arising and descending on the same foot can be accomplished only from 1 to 3 times during the third year. A hopping series may be extended to around 7 to 9 at 4.5 years, and over 10 by the age of 5 (Wellman, 1937). Hopping speed for given distances improves with age, and by age 5 a child can hop 50 feet in around 10 seconds in the absence of any balance problem. As in jumping, the arms gradually become involved more and more appropriately as maturation occurs. Initially the arms may be either too tense or too loose. Later, the arms lift and aid in the balance required when hopping. If a higher hop is executed, the arms will lift appropriately also. With improved motor planning the child may become able to execute rhythmic hops from one foot to the other in a 2-2 rhythm, and later by middle childhood in a 2-3 rhythm (Chapter 9).

Several variations of gait aid the child to leave the ground, while evidencing more and more intricate patterns of movement, during the fourth and fifth years of life. A simple one-footed skip may be seen at 4 or 5. In this action a step is taken with one foot while being alternated with a step-shuffle with the second. It is a prelude to true skipping, usually seen by the age of 7 years. Generally these intricate gait patterns are seen earlier in girls than in boys. However, special training will often be effective with either sex.

Galloping (containing a lack-of-support phase) may also be accomplished by some of the more mature children during the later stages of the preschool years. In this task, as is true with skipping, girls are usually more proficient earlier in life than boys. Often this action is tense and performed in segments at first; later a fluid galloping pattern may be seen.

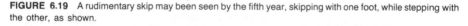

FIGURE 6.19   A rudimentary skip may been seen by the fifth year, skipping with one foot, while stepping with the other, as shown.

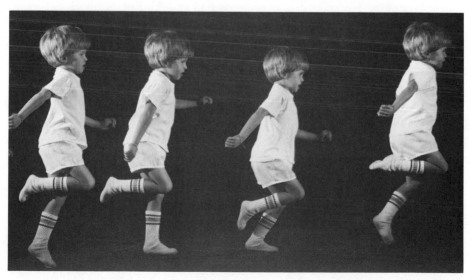

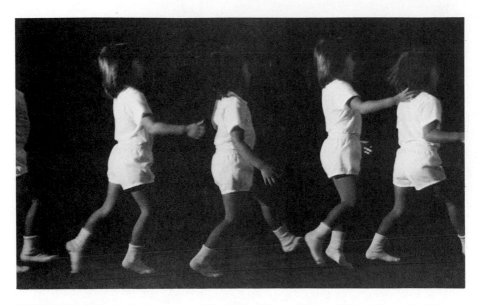

FIGURE 6.20 Although this five year old girl is able to skip, most boys and girls at this age find this task difficult or impossible. A one-footed skip is usual at five (see Figure 6.19).

Balance

Since the day of birth, the child has been confronted with the need to balance the body, or its parts, in relationship to gravity. Head control, in either a prone or supine position, for example, requires balance qualities. Unaided sitting and standing represent rather formidable balance tasks during the first year of life.

As walking is mastered during the second and third years, more and more balance tasks are imposed on the child. He or she is required to watch, catch, and throw balls while somehow keeping upright. Maintaining an upright position becomes even more difficult when various modifications of ball kicking are required during the fourth and fifth years. Later, when attempts are made to kick balls, even more demands are made upon the child's balance abilities.

Numerous balance tasks have been used to assess this complex quality in both young and older children over the years. At times, simple line walking has been used (Bayley, 1935). Both static and moving balance is often tested. Static balance in children is often evaluated by asking them to posture on one foot, sometimes for as long as they can (De Oreo and Wade, 1971), and at other times for periods of time ranging from 4 to 6 seconds (Cratty and Martin, 1970). Dynamic or moving balance has traditionally been measured by asking children to walk a beam. Sometimes the beam gradually narrows, and the measure used is the distance walked before the youngster steps off. At other times, a beam of constant width is employed.

One of the difficulties when drawing conclusions about changes with age, sex differences, and other dimensions of balance abilities in both younger and older children is the failure of investigators to control for important variables that may influence the score a child obtains. For example, walking a too-high balance beam may elicit feelings of fear. Thus the score obtained may reflect the child's general security rather than any basic ability to relate to gravity. Attention span, usually greater in younger girls, will influence the degree to which the child's eyes stabilize, and thus in turn modify balance scores on balance tests. DeOreo and Wade (1971), for example, comment upon the role of attention span in their task, which involves the ability to maintain balance on a tipping stabilometer. Asking a child to posture on one foot for "as long as you can," still being required by contemporary researchers, will probably elicit scores that reflect the child's pain threshold more than balance ability (Morris et al., 1982).

The most neglected variable, however, in research about balance in children involves directions that may affect the accompanying visual behaviors. Unless some attempt is made to have the child observe a target while balancing statically, the score obtained will likely represent (a) the child's stability of gaze, (b) the child's willingness to attend visually in a stable way to the environment, and/or (c) some exotic visual condition the child may possess that prevents him or her from fixing the gaze in a useful way when posturing (Zernecke et al., 1982).

Most of the time, if a young child is asked to fixate at a point at eye level and a few feet away, more stability of balance will be exhibited. At the same time, however, we have found that when testing children's balance abilities, some balance better with their eyes closed. It is apparent that in some cases, when the child's visual perceptual abilities are either immature or abnormal, closing the eyes produces more stability.

In general, balance abilities, however tested, improve with age (Ulrich and Ulrich, 1985). There is often a rather dramatic upturn in abilities from the fifth to seventh years. For the most part, sex differences are not always apparent, but in younger children it is sometimes seen that girls are superior to boys on static balance tasks (Winterhalter, 1974; DeOreo and Wade, 1971). However, all data do not reflect sex differences (Ulrich and Ulrich, 1985).

Children by the third year of life can walk a line from 1 to 2 inches wide for short periods of time without falling off (Bayley, 1935). By the age of 4, according to Wellman (1937), they are able to walk circular lines. Even at this age, however, duration and quality of attention to the line being walked are probably at least as critical as any balancing abilities the child may possess. Thus neurologically more mature children with longer attention spans, in the absence of any obvious motor difficulties, will appear to balance longer and better than will a less mature child, whose attention span is shorter and more diffuse.

Static balance may also be evaluated in younger children. However, asking a child younger than the age of 5 to balance on one foot will usually result in failure (Holbrook, 1953). Stott, in his test to screen out children with motor problems, uses

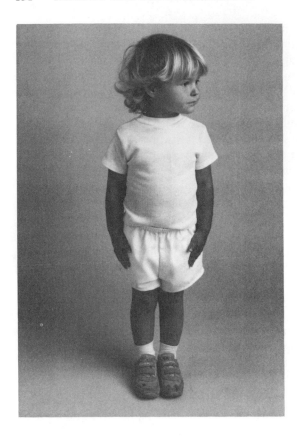

FIGURE 6.21
This girl in her third year is able to maintain a stable position, with feet together, even though her attention is distracted.

a one-foot balance at 6 years of age (1968). I would concur with Stott's placement of this task. Again, however, asking a child to fixate at a point will elicit better results than if no directions are given as to what must be done with the gaze and visual system. Likewise, even a one-foot balance, required for from 4 to 6 seconds, may evidence marked variations. One child may struggle to keep the foot on the ground, with arms waving and postures in constant flux. Another child, in contrast, may be able to retain a one-foot balance with relatively little body and/or upper limb actions. In the laboratory we evaluate differences in static balance postures of this type using a sensitive force platform (Ziernecke et al., 1982). In an informal school setting, however, the child may be asked to remain within a footprint, or to otherwise control extraneous movements.

Thus, prior to the age of 5, static balance must be evaluated by asking a child to posture with both feet on the ground, varying distances apart. As the child grows older, from 2 to 4 years, the distances between the feet may be reduced, with stability expected. By the age of 4 some children, for example, may become able to maintain an upright position with both feet together ''like a soldier.''

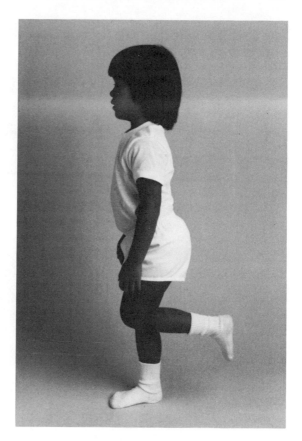

FIGURE 6.22
Although this girl of five can maintain a relatively stable one-foot stand, for the most part this task is able to be accomplished by those of six or seven years of age. Increased stability will be achieved, if the child is asked to focus upon an eye-level target a short distance away.

By the end of the preschool years, dynamic balance may often be evaluated using a balance beam. A 4-inch width is usually employed, placed about 6 inches above the ground. Faced with such a task, children of 4 and 5 will usually be able to traverse it in a shuffling manner, keeping one foot ahead of the other. More mature children at these ages, or those having received additional practice and thus confidence, may become able to walk the beam alternating their feet in a normal gait pattern. However, it is usually a year or two later that children will become able to traverse narrower beams with security (Keogh, 1965) and become able to lower to a kneeling position and rise on a beam 4 inches wide (DeOreo, 1975).

The motor systems of children are not usually mature enough by the age of 5 to permit static balances, using one foot, without the use of vision. Stable one-footed eyes-closed balances are not usually mastered until the ages of 7 to 8.[1] A

---

[1]Care must be taken when evaluating eyes-closed balances, insofar as a child with a defective motor system and poor feedback from muscle receptors may suddenly drop to the ground when deprived of stabilizing visual cues.

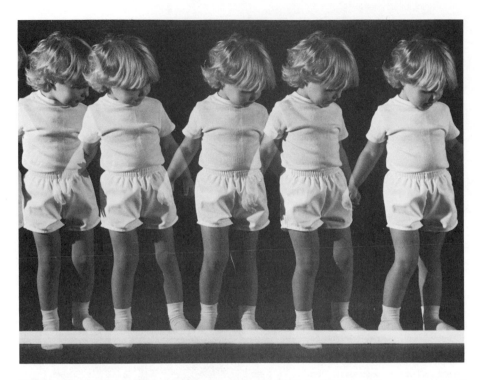

FIGURE 6.23 Children younger than five, as shown by this child in her third year of life, may traverse a 4″ wide beam sideways, using step-close-step action, not by crossing or alternating the feet.

FIGURE 6.24 This five year old boy can walk, alternating feet, along a 4″ wide beam with some ease.

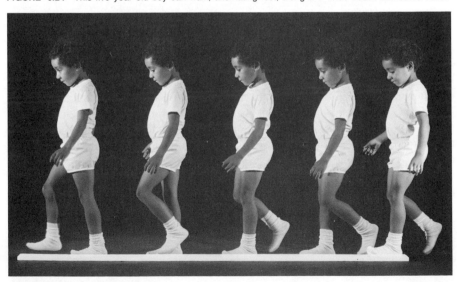

stable heal-to-toe position, with or without vision, is also a task too difficult for a preschooler to accomplish. This position (a Rhomberg position) is often used in neurological evaluations, but it is not an appropriate criterion for determining the presence of balance problems prior to the age of 7 years. Moreover, it is becoming increasingly apparent that balance performance is more closely related to the maturational level of a child during the preschool years than to absolute chronological age (Erbaugh, 1984). Balance tasks are important to include in any battery purporting to assess motor proficiencies. Ulrich and Ulrich (1985), for example, have recently discovered that balance ability is an important predictor of overall performance of fundamental gross motor tasks in pre-school youngsters 3, 4, and 5 years of age.

Ball Skills

Throwing.   Throwing is a highly prized skill within the United States because of its use in football and baseball. In other cultures, kicking is often a skill imposed rather early upon children. I recently witnessed an amazingly mature hand-held kick by the son of an Australian colleague. When I suggested it must have been an accident, father and son repeated the action, declaring that it represented preparation for Australian rules football.

The first time an infant throws it may be an accident, produced as a hand-held object pulls away from a rapidly swinging hand. Soon, however, the "accident" is repeated because of its satisfying outcomes. During the second to fourth years of life, children will evidence a variety of throwing patterns, as they apparently search for efficient ways of delivering missiles of various sizes, weights, and shapes. Often with appropriate stimulation and some training, a child will evidence a relatively mature and consistent throwing pattern by the ages of 5 and 6 years.

Throwing is analyzed mechanically by viewing its developmental stages from above the child, or while viewing the child from the side. Viewed from above, the child will be seen to improve as more and more rotation takes place around the long axis of the body. The shoulders will be seen to turn more and more toward the direction of the throw, in order to impart more and more velocity. Viewed from the side, the main observation will be that the child evidences more and more weight shift forward with age. This again will produce more and more speed and power on the ball. Biomechanically, the more velocity the hand achieves as the ball is released, the more distance the ball will travel. So more mature throwing patterns will evidence the fact that the arm-hand is made to move through longer and longer ranges of motion. Indeed, the *serape effect* is the term coined to describe the action of the throwing arm during the more mature stages of throwing.

Overall throwing proficiency has been found recently to positively correlate not only to muscular strength in preschoolers, but also to the time they are exposed to effective physical education instruction (Parizkova, 1984).

The first stage in imparting velocity and direction to objects starts with the pushing of a ball in a seated position. This may be accomplished first with one hand,

and later with two hands used together. During the last part of the second year and during the third and fourth years, having gained standing stability, children begin to exhibit rudimentary throwing patterns while in upright positions. Often at first these also will involve balls delivered with two hands at the same time, and with little or no weight shift forward as the release takes place. The child soon learns, however, that more velocity may be achieved with one-handed throws. Thus begins the first in a series of four stages in this more refined type of missile delivery system. These four stages were identified by Wild in 1938, and continue to remain useful benchmarks with which to evaluate throwing patterns in children (Williams, 1983). Generally, it is possible, using a 1 to 4 or 1 to 5 point scoring system, to score the maturity of children's throwing patterns using the following criteria (Cratty, Cortinas, and Kelly, 1973).

The first of these involves the projection of the ball primarily with arm thrust forward and elbow extension. The trunk may flex forward, but there is little or no rotation of the hips and trunk. Viewed from the side, the primary action is a backward and forward motion of the arm. Viewed from the top, there is shoulder rotation.

A second one-arm throwing pattern involves some rotation of the pelvis and shoulders. There is little or no transfer of weight forward, however. The third stage involves a weight shift forward, with the leg under the throwing arm sometimes

FIGURE 6.25 First throws, as seen by this child in her third year, consist of arm action unaccompanied by weight shift or shoulder rotation.

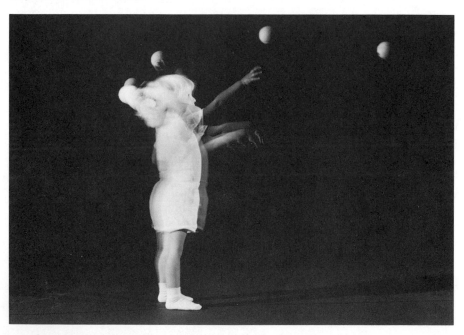

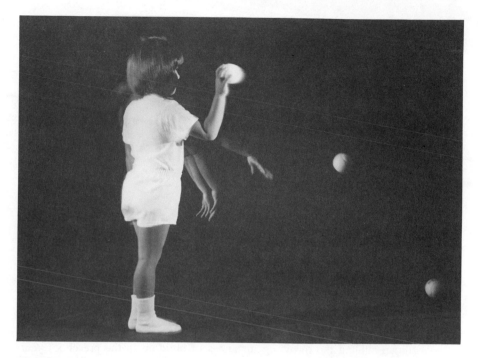

FIGURE 6.26 This second stage throwing pattern evidences some shoulder rotation, but little or no weight shift forward.

taking a step forward as this shift occurs. There is more rotation of the shoulders and pelvis, but the arm's range of motion remains limited. The final stage involves mature throwing and more range of motion of the arm, a step forward with the foot opposite to that of the throwing arm, and marked rotation of the shoulders and trunk during the preliminary stages of the throw.

At this stage, the child becomes able to vary the velocity of the throw well by exhibiting differences in the speed of trunk and shoulder rotation and of arm velocity. Placing a precise chronological age upon the assumption of this pattern is perilous. However, at times boys and girls as young as 5 years of age may exhibit this advanced type of motion. Usually, however, even with training, the final stage appears later in life.

It has been a consistent finding that boys not only throw farther, but exhibit a more mature pattern of throwing than do girls by the age of 5 years (Cratty, Cortinas, and Kelly, 1973). In a recent study one of my students attempted to elicit more advanced throwing patterns in 5-year-old girls whose throws were at about stage three. She found that with training some younger girls were seen to change to a more mature and efficient overhead throwing pattern, while others could not seem to do so (Goldstein, 1982). It is believed the useful recent work by East and Hensley (1985) detailing the influences of socio-cultural factors on the throwing patterns of children is a useful step in untangling the reasons children throw as they do.

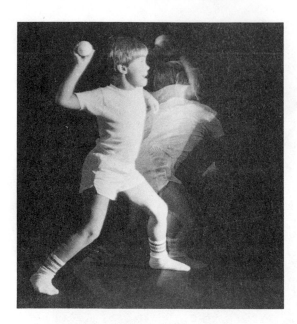

FIGURE 6.27
This remarkably mature throwing pattern was executed by a boy not yet five.

Wellman studied the throwing distances of children in the preschool years using a ball that was 9.5 inches in circumference. It was found that throwing distance at 2.5 years was from 4 to 5 feet. A year later, another 2 feet in distance was added, while after another year had gone by (at 4.5 years), the throwing distance had doubled to over 12 feet. A larger ball, having a circumference of slightly over 16 inches, was thrown on the average about 2 feet less at each age (Wellman, 1937).

Morris and her colleagues in a more recent study (1982) found similar age differences when asking children to throw a tennis ball for distance. Both boys and girls improved about 50 percent in distance between their third and fourth years. No distinct sex differences were obtained when the mean scores from 3 to 5 years posted by both boys and girls were surveyed. However, when average scores of a softball throw were contrasted, the means for 5-year-old males were significantly superior to those of females at the same age. This study indicates that sex differences that may appear in throwing competencies may be dependent upon the weight of the ball, as well as upon the throwing mechanics exhibited by boys and girls (Morris et al., 1983). Throwing accuracy and distance continue to improve after the preschool years. With improvement in skill, coupled with increases in leg and trunk strength, marked changes in throwing velocities, and thus in distances, are seen between the ages of 6 and 18 years.

Catching.   Catching may also start with the child in a seated position, attempting to "trap" balls rolled on the ground. Later, while standing, the child may or may not be required to change the position of the body to intercept a ball. Two

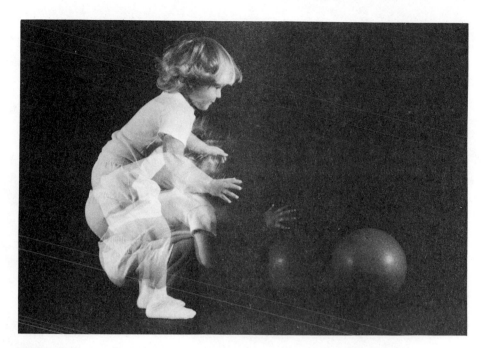

FIGURE 6.28 This girl of 2.5 years is able to bend and to intercept a ball rolled toward her at a moderate speed.

main variables influence success in catching a ball: the angle of projection of the ball, and the size and type of ball being used (Randt, 1985). Generally, larger balls are more easily trapped by the child than smaller ones, as might be expected. A more mature grasp is required when a tennis-ball-sized missile approaches than when the ball is 6 to 8 inches in diameter and filled with air (Wellman, 1937).

Children generally have more difficulty moving forward and backward to intercept balls than moving laterally (Bruce, 1966). Preschool schildren have difficulty judging the velocity of balls coming toward them. Thus bounced balls become easier to intercept, as might be expected. Generally, by the age of 4 or 5 years, we have found that most children can ''arm-catch'' an 8 inch air-filled ball when it is bounced to them 15 feet away (Cratty and Martin, 1970). It is interesting to note that the skills involved in catching and intercepting balls may be quite specific. We did not obtain a correlation, for example, between children's ability to touch a ball swinging before them on a 15-inch string and their ability to catch balls bounced to them. Thus the nature of the arch of the ball, as well as the plane the ball may be traveling in (in contrast to the child) all influence catching and intercepting ability (Cratty and Martin, 1970). Randt (1985) found that in general six-year-olds were twice as proficient in catching a ball than were children at four years of age.

Morris and her colleagues (Morris et al., 1983) scored the catching abilities of children from 3 to 6 years. They found that a large gain was achieved from the third

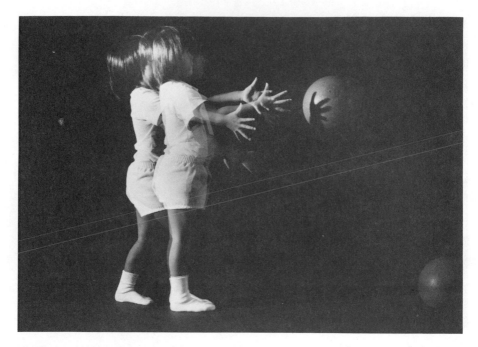

FIGURE 6.29   Stage 1 catching, with the ball being cradled against the body upon its arrival.

to the fourth year by both sexes. The boys in this study at 5 performed better than the girls. However, at the other ages no significant sex differences were recorded. It is difficult to interpret the data presented by Morris et al. in this catching test. They report using a 8.5-inch playground ball, but do not report from what distance it was thrown underhand, nor do they report the criteria used to score the quality of the catching actions observed.

Overall it is generally accepted that three stages exist in the standing and catching behaviors of youngsters. The first of these involves a basketlike waiting for the ball, the arms outstretched in advance of the throw, with the fingers stiff. When the ball arrives, the arms-hands and body are used as a single unit to trap the ball. If the ball comes too fast, it may simply bounce off the arms, as they are not likely to "give" when the ball arrives. The body and head remain stationary, and the child does not seem to watch the approaching missile. The head may even turn away in an avoidance reaction as the ball approaches.

Second-stage catching is more efficient. The eyes are likely to follow the flight, and the elbows may be slightly flexed and held to the front or sides of the body, with the fingers pointing to the direction of the incoming ball. The arms swing up as the ball is contacted and attempt to trap the missile.

The final and more mature catching pattern is seen at the age of 5 and above. The child awaits the ball in an expectant position, with the legs widespread,

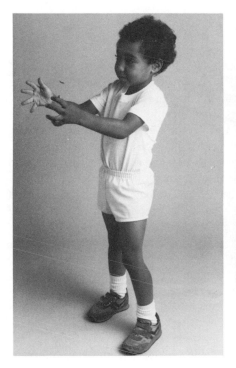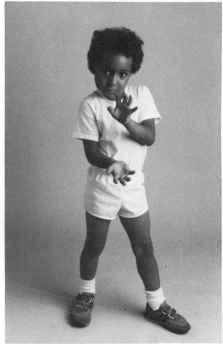

FIGURE 6.30 More advanced posture awaiting the ball will include the fingers outstretched, elbows away from the body, with the ball being intercepted with the hands, and not trapped against the body as it arrives.

permitting lateral movement if needed. The arms, hands, and fingers await the ball in a relaxed manner, with the fingers slightly cupped. When the ball arrives, the hands quickly adjust to the height of the ball's arrival, and both hands and fingers contact the ball. A primary characteristic is that the arms and hands ''give'' to effectively absorb the force of the ball.

Still more mature patterns of interception occur in several ways. (a) The child becomes able to determine how much lateral movement is required to position the body to a future location of a ball, and how to accomplish this motion (whether to turn and run sideways or to execute a side step while facing the ball). (b) The child becomes able to contact balls with extensions of the body, including bats, rackets, and paddles. At times, however, these more advanced forms of ball interception are beyond the capabilities of the preschool child, the subject of this chapter. At the same time, the more mature, and those with whom someone has worked even at the ages of 4 and 5, may begin to display moderate to advanced proficiencies in racket skills, as well as in the interception of missiles coming from some distance and with velocity. The acquisition of these and similar skills is dealt with more thoroughly in Chapter 7.

SUMMARY

The preschool years are a time during which rudimentary beginnings of a wide variety of physical skills are attempted. The child's maturing balance mechanisms during this period begin to enable the acquisition of ball skills, including throwing, catching, and kicking. Locomotor maturation is seen in the wider variety of ways children find to move their bodies from one point to another. Also during this period, the child begins to combine various subskills. Locomotion to a point accompanies getting the hands ready to trap or to catch a ball, to give one example.

Toward the latter part of this preschool period marked individual differences are seen, both in the velocity as well as the accuracy of movements expressed. Some sex differences begin to emerge, with the neurologically more mature girls often besting the boys in tasks requiring balance and precision of movement. The boys may evidence superior mechanical advantages when throwing and kicking. Additionally, children begin to show less intra-individual variability as the years progress; they decide upon a ''best'' way (for him or her) to throw or to catch a ball, rather than evidence a wide variety of projection and interception behaviors.

Even at the age of 2, however, several levels of maturity may be seen in various action patterns. Different levels of maturity, for example, may be seen in how children of these early years jump upward or forward.

Essentially the first year of life is a preparation for standing and walking. The second year permits the child to acquire a stable walking pattern, and to improve body and head balance when moving. However, by the third year an explosion of skills will take place with good encouragement from those in the child's environment.

QUESTIONS FOR DISCUSSION

1. Discuss the possible reasons for sex differences in motor abilities seen among preschool children.
2. What is intra-individual variability and interindividual variability? How do these concepts pertain to the emerging motor performance capabilities of the preschool child?
3. What implications does the concept of bonds have for explaining the complex motor behaviors emerging during the preschool years?
4. Why is sitting important to the emergence of hand control? What might a developmental specialist do in order to encourage hand-object manipulations in a child whose ability to sit is delayed?
5. What importance does the concept of diffusion have for the evaluation of motor competencies in 3-year-olds versus 5-year-olds?
6. What is cruising? What other steps are critical to the assumption of an upright gait?

7. What variables should be kept in mind when evaluating balance in preschool children?

8. What general changes in movement patterns are seen as children learn to throw and to kick?

9. How do running speeds improve from the age of 2 to 5 years? To what variables might you attribute this improvement?

10. Into what subdivision might a checklist for the evaluation of the gross motor abilities of preschool children be divided?

STUDENT PROJECTS

1. Observe a 6-month-old at play. Record the number of times the child assumes a static position within brief timed intervals (30 seconds to 1 minute). Contrast the data obtained to positions assumed by a 1-year-old during the same timed intervals. Do your figures correspond to those of Pikler's work relative to changes in activity level from the first to the second half of the first year of life?

2. Record the reflexes, stereotypes, and voluntary actions seen in a 4-month-old. Is it easy to separate these behaviors? What kinds of behaviors are easier to record? What kinds are more difficult to classify and to record? Why?

3. Observe the actions of a preschool group 2 to 4 years old at play. What kinds of behaviors seem self-initiated by the children? What kinds of behaviors seem stimulated by the presence or the actions of others?

4. What behaviors are likely to be seen in a child at 4 years (based upon the chapter's content)? Now visit a 4-year-old. Do his or her behaviors match a hypothetical average? Why might variations from the norm be seen in your subject?

5. Record individual variability in a throwing task by a 3-year-old and by a 5-year-old. Is the younger or older youngster more variable? Why? How does this correspond to common sense and/or to the material in this chapter (or to material in Chapter 10 on learning)?

CHAPTER SEVEN
MOTOR PERFORMANCE
IN CHILDHOOD
5 to 12 Years

In the United States, school starts for most children at the age of about 5. Thus, at a relatively early age the child is likely to feel pressure to begin to excel in sports and games. Often the first year of school is rather sheltered, but by first and second grades, the 6- and 7-year-old comes face to face with vigorous peers who are either joined in active play or who may elicit fear and withdrawal from active play.

During the elementary school years, a number of qualities emerge. Moral and ethical judgment becomes more sophisticated. Younger children at first seek games with structured rules and obey them to the letter, and then begin to formulate their own games and rule modifications without feelings of guilt. Most of all, the childhood years are the time to make definite skill commitments. Athletic skills are discovered and then refined. Often these years signal the beginnings of identification with sports heroes, emotional attachments that often linger into adolescence and even adulthood.

In general, virtually all motor performance data obtained between the kindergarden and sixth-grade years reflect upward trends. Plateaus sometimes appear between the seventh and ninth years, and often there tends to be some deceleration in improvement after the ages of 7 and 8. Sex differences, despite the previous assertion to the contrary, do appear with some regularity. Most of the time there are slight differences favoring males in direct and straightforward exhibitions of power, including such tasks as ball-throwing velocity and standing broad jump. Girls, on the other hand, sometimes excel in precise actions involving accurate hopping and balance. These differences may be caused by subtle contrasts in the rate of neurological maturation exhibited by the two sexes, and by the accompanying attentional differences this may bring about. A young girl, for example, may balance longer on one foot because her neurological maturity may permit her to attend visually and cognitively to such a task longer than the boy posturing and wobbling at her side.

Just as is true among younger children, youngsters during the elementary years continue to exhibit marked individual differences. Some of these variations reflect a blunting of physical skills, resulting in the labeling of some children as awkward. Generally, research about what children during these years are able to do with their bodies has taken several tracks during the past five decades. Numerous studies have been carried out using different children from 5 to 12 years in attempts to explore mean score changes at successive ages. Most often these studies have employed small samples, and seldom have they equated the children on the basis of the body-build characteristics known to be influential in motor performance scores (see Chapter 7, and Seils, 1951; Slaughter et al., 1980).

These cross-sectional investigations of successive ability changes by age using small, ill-defined samples often produce findings that defy explanation and conflict with common sense.

Helpful are studies that follow the same children throughout life. These longitudinal investigations, unfortunately, are few and far between (Clarke, 1971; Halverson et al., 1982). Problems in securing and retaining subjects, as well as in sustained federal funding, have undoubtedly limited their appearance in research journals.

Several investigators over the decades have attempted to identify groups of ability traits possessed by children (Carpenter, 1940, 1941; Vandenberg, 1964). Using factor analysis as a tool, they have extracted a relatively small number of basic qualities existing within a larger number of tests by determining what tests tend to cause children to vary in similar ways. Common sense and discretion also accompany the analysis and interpretaion of these results. The nature of the findings obtained are dependent upon the investigator's judgment when selecting tests and subjects. Naming the factors is more an art than a science, while the specific type of factor analytic technique employed may tend to distort the findings in various ways. The reader should keep these limitations in mind when reviewing some of the information that follows.

Researchers are also beginning to look at biomechanical changes in how children tend to, or prefer to, perform skills as they mature. However, even this research should be approached with caution. For example, it is typically found that at a given age a remarkable number of ways are used to accomplish the same task (Poe, 1976). Thus it is more useful simply to plot maturational changes in a given ability (such as broad jumping) than to attach precise ages to a given type of effort.

This chapter is organized as follows: First, we take a look at what general qualities seem to emerge in the motor personalities of children by reviewing some current factor analyses. Next we survey different movement tasks in order to determine some possible age trends as well as sex differences.

BASIC MOVEMENT QUALITIES

From the 1940s until the 1980s factor analyses have been carried out to identify facets of the motor component of youth's personalities. The findings depended on the nature of tests that interested them and that were used in their batteries. Further modifications of the results obtained were caused by the ages of the subjects, possibly by their intellectual endowments, by the region of the country from which they came, and also possibly by their race and sex.

Generally these investigations resulted in the identification of from six to eight basic abilities in childhood. These include the following:

1. Balance. This ability is divided into three or even more factors: (1) balancing objects (Cumbee, 1957); (2) statically balancing the body in one-foot standings of various kinds (Stott, 1972; Rarick and Dobbins, 1975); and (3) dynamic balance, usually evaluated by asking a child to walk a balance beam (Vandenberg, 1964). If one or more eyes-closed balance measures have been included in the battery, these tests may also group together and form still a fourth factor (Fleishman, 1965).

   Often in studies of younger children only two factors emerge, static and dynamic balance. In older children, and with the appropriate type and number of balance tests included, four separate balance qualities emerge (Fleishman, 1965).

2. Agility of the body. Tests that require the child to run while rapidly changing direction are likely to load into such a factor. Often a separate agility factor will emerge when vertical movements are required that involve rhythmic hopping, getting up rapidly, and/or vertical jumps of various kinds (Cumbee, 1957; Cratty and Martin, 1970). Generally one must carefully inspect the tasks the researcher has identified as contributing to an agility factor because they often vary markedly from study to study.

3. Body build qualities. These involve measurements of height, weight, physique, and age. This factor is often called *general maturity* in younger children or in retarded children. This factor is often accompanied by a number of other scores in tests of agility, strength, and the like.

4. Throwing abilities. Tests for these abilities include ball skills of various kinds. In earlier studies, catching qualities were included with throwing scores (Cumbee, 1957). In more recent studies, these seem to be separate qualities in children.

5. Speed. This quality is measured by tests reflecting foot and arm speed (Fleishman, 1965), and those involving the speed with which the total body can move without changing direction in such tasks as 30- and 40-yard runs (Rarick and Dobbins, 1975). So because a child can throw with velocity (arm speed) may not mean that the same child will show power and speed when running short distances. At the same time, developing velocity in both arms and legs is usually a common factor. Thus foot velocity (kicking for distance) will likely be correlated to throwing for distance (balls or javelins).

6. Precise movements of the hands. These virtually always constitute a factor (or factors, depending upon the number of fine-motor tests contained in the battery) separate and apart from qualities exhibited by the larger muscle groups (Rarick and Dobbins, 1975; Fleishman, 1965; Vandenberg, 1964). The scores obtained from a typical task such as asking children to drop pennies with precision and speed into a small opening (Stott, 1972) contribute to this factor.

7. Strength and power. Depending upon the number of strength tasks employed, this general classification may contain four or even more separate general qualities (Fleishman, 1961). Generally, measures of static strength involving pressure exerted

with a hand dynamometer are separable from scores obtained in tasks requiring children to move more quickly. Sometimes measures of sprinting for short distances will be grouped within a strength-power dimension (Rarick and Dobbins, 1975a). Often so-called strength scores elicited from younger children are difficult to interpret. It is often difficult to convince children of 5 to 6 years to display all-out effort in ways that will cause even momentary discomfort. Moeover, motivational conditions are seldom specified in such studies, despite the fact that the presence of others may exert a powerful influence on the children and thus on the scores obtained.

Factor Analyses: Purposes

It is important to consider just what the identification of so-called basic factors may do for those formulating evaluation programs and/or setting up motor development programs designed to change children in positive ways.

The information gained from factor analyses has aided, or should have aided, those developing batteries of tests designed to assess movement capabilities to construct what are called "factor pure" test batteries. Scientifically sound instruments should be composed of tests that represent main factors or qualities. Conversely, there should not be an abundance of tests in the same battery evaluating the same quality more than once. Thus efficiency in test-battery construction is one outcome of factor analyses (see Chapter 14).

A second purpose of factor analysis is to aid in the formulation of program content. If we want, for example, to formulate a broad, comprehensive program of motor remediation, we should consider tasks that represent a variety of qualities, not just a few. In this way it is more likely that a wide variety of skills will be positively affected.

More precise analyses of life's tasks will also reveal what kinds of basic qualities may contribute to each. One may thus proceed backward to information from factor analyses by first analyzing the basic qualities that are likely contributors to the task, and then proceeding to improve those abilities through tasks embedded in a program. To improve ball retrieving abilities needed in ball games encountered in late childhood, for example, a program should contain tasks designed to heighten lateral movement and agility, as well as those involving the interception of balls and precise finger-hand movements.

Still another use for information from data that have identified basic ability traits involves the sensible classification of children for competition and/or participation in physical education and recreation classes. To accomplish this, Rarick and Dobbins (1975b) statistically formed person clusters from factor analytic data. After first identifying four basic abilities in a group of children (strength-power, body coordination, fine coordination, and balance), they divided the children into groups whose ability patterns were similar. The groups ranged from those with mixed profiles to a group of children showing deficits in all four ability areas.

As Figure 7.1 shows, more boys than girls were in the two groups representing extremes of motor ability. The poorest group contained over twice as many boys as girls, while the best group also contained twice as many boys as girls.

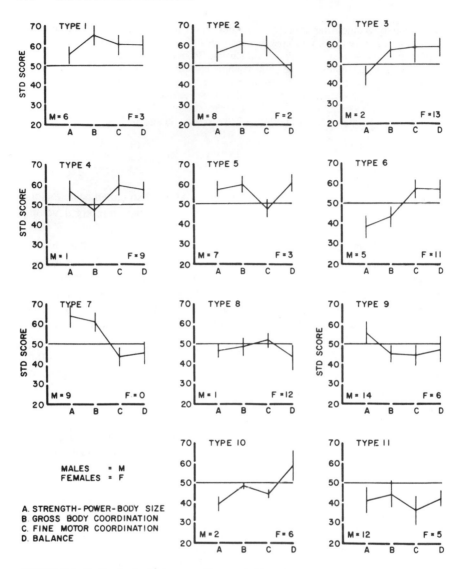

FIGURE 7.1 Profiles in standard scores of boys and girls on four components of motor performance. From G. L. Rarick and D. A. Dobbins, "A Motor Performance Typology of Boys and Girls in the Age Range 6–10 Years," *J. Mot. Behav., 7* (1975), pp. 37–43.

AGE TRENDS, SEX DIFFERENCES

Trends reflecting changes in children's abilities from 5 and 6 to 12 years of age are often found in research studies several decades old. The straightforward collection of scores from large groups of children is not today a highly respectable undertaking for reseachers. There is no apparent problem being solved in this kind of study, and thus it is often difficult for contemporary authors to obtain journal space for such information. The following material has been arbitrarily placed into two main sections. The first deals with so-called basic qualities and includes various locomotor activities, as well as jumping, balance, speed, flexibility, strength, and agility. The second section contains various actions the child must acquire in order to deal with balls and other missiles. Age changes during childhood in throwing, catching, kicking, striking, batting, and dribbling are discussed here.

Basic Qualities and Abilities

Strength and flexibility.   Strength and flexibility contribute to many physical tasks. Those requiring power demand what is termed ballistic strength, as well as the flexibility necessary to move body parts through wide ranges of motion. Short sprints, vertical jumps, and long jumps (standing and running) require leg strength; throwing and kicking demand high levels of flexibility.

Strength in children.   As children get older, they become stronger. This improvement may be due to a number of factors in addition to mere aging, including: experience at applying force and focusing attention upon the muscles or muscle contracted; improvement in the application of biomechanical forces; and increased willingness to undergo the mild to moderate pain associated with all-out efforts.

Motivation plays an important role when testing children's strength. The five-and-dime effect is often noted when such strength-endurance tasks as pushups are being tested. This effect is reflected in the large number of subjects likely to stop at multiples of five or ten rather than display maximum strength for a maximum number of trials.

Traditionally, physical educators and others interested in evaluating strength in children employed tasks that involve a series of movements, such as pushups or pullups. But a child's willingness to endure pain, as well as his or her endurance capacities, often interfere with the pure measure of strength the tester wishes to obtain.

When static strength is evaluated, on the other hand, the force of the hand grip has often been used despite the fact that grip strength does not correlate very well to other measures of muscular force exerted by other parts of the body, and that numerous biochemical factors, including the size of the child's hand, are rarely taken into account.

The best estimates of pure strength measured in a static fashion are obtainable from government reports. The data obtained are often used to design safe or usable products in industry. The information these reports obtain provides scientifically valid information, comprehensive in scope. Much of these data have relevance for those planning programs designed to improve the fitness qualities of children, including strengths in various parts of the body. These studies have employed highly sophisticated measures in recent years. Moreover, the subject samples have ranged from over five hundred to several thousand children.

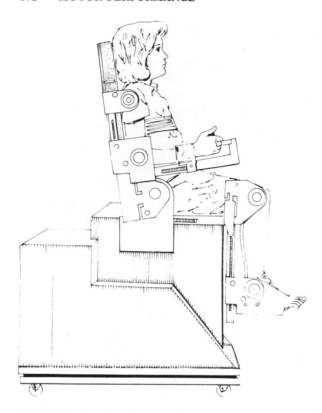

FIGURE 7.2   From C. L. Owings, et al., *Strength Characteristics for Product Safety Design,* report from the Consumer Product Safety Commission, Monograph, University of Michigan (1975). Reproduced with permission.

One of these reports contains information about 33 measures of strength from 500 children from 3 to 10 years of age (Owings et al., 1975). The data were collected using the testing chair shown in Figure 7.2. This enabled the researchers to isolate various joint actions and to obtain an exact printout of the pressure children could (or would) exert. The joint positions were carefully specified, and the measures of force obtained were expressed in kilopounds (kp). This may also be stated in kilogram force (kgf).

The amount of data emanating from this and similar reports is extensive. It has been found that:

1. Sex differences are not great, or are entirely absent, until about the seventh to eighth years, at which time boys slightly exceed girls in the ability to exert force in various parts of the body.

2. As might be expected, ability to apply force is greater around joints on which larger muscles act, such as the hips and knee, than around joints moved by smaller muscle groups (wrist, elbow). Age and sex differences should be interpreted with this in mind.

3. Overall from the third to the tenth year, children evidence the ability to multiply force from 3.5 to 5 times, depending on the muscle groups involved. On the average, the

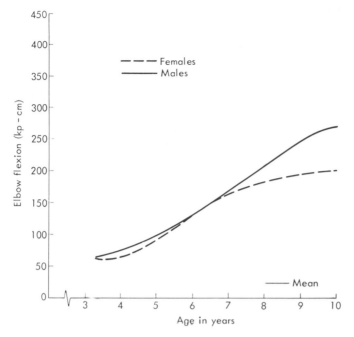

FIGURE 7.3 From C. L. Owings, et al, *Strength Characteristics for Product Safety Design,* report from the Consumer Product Safety Commission, Monograph, University of Michigan (1975). Reproduced with permission.

forces may be multiplied during this time span about 4.5 times when surveying most muscle groups.

4. While slight sex differences may be seen toward the end of childhood in these data, the variation among both boys and girls is great, and many girls exceed the strengths of boys during these same years.

5. In general, it appears that sex differences may be greater when measures of upper body strength are contrasted than when the measures are of trunk strength.

6. In these same data, contrasts of measures of rotation at the various joints—abduction versus adduction at the elbow, for example—show that sex differences virtually disappear, even in late childhood. This is partly due to the lesser forces that are able to be exerted in this manner than is true when straightforward flexion and extension actions are measured.

Although there are some data (Krogman, 1971) indicating that boys are superior to girls in early childhood, Figures 7.3 through 7.6 do not indicate significant differences prior to the ages of about 7 to 8, depending upon the strength measure depicted. The strength measure expressed on the vertical axes of these graphs is expressed in kilopound-centimeters (kp-cm).[1]

---

[1] A Kilopound or kilogram force (kgf) may be defined as the magnitude of force required to accelerate a mass of 1 kilogram at 1 g (acceleration due to gravity). A kilopound-centimeter (kp-cm) may be defined as the magnitude of torque generated around the axis of rotation due to the action of 1 kilopound occurring 1 centimeter away at right angles to the axis. *Note*: 1 kp-cm is only slightly less than 1 in.-lb (1 kp = 2.2046 lbs; 1 kp-cm = .8679 in.-lbs.

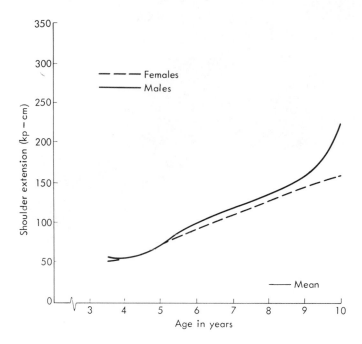

FIGURE 7.4 (a)

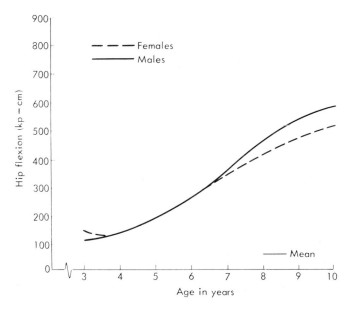

FIGURE 7.4 (b)   Both from C. L. Owings, et al., *Strength Characteristics for Product Safety Design,* report from the Consumer Product Safety Commission, Monograph, University of Michigan (1975). Reproduced with permission.

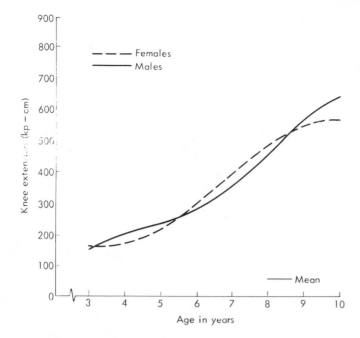

FIGURE 7.5 (a)

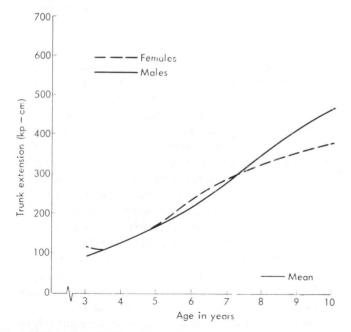

FIGURE 7.5 (b) Both from C. L. Owings, et al., *Strength Characteristics for Product Safety Design,* report from the Consumer Product Safety Commission, Monograph, University of Michigan (1975). Reproduced with permission.

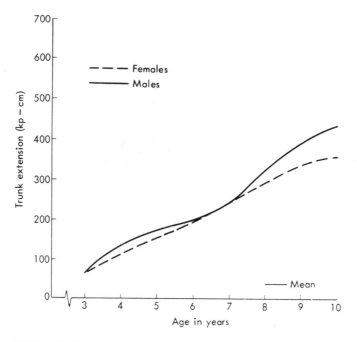

FIGURE 7.6 From C. L. Owings, et al. *Strength Characteristics for Product Safety Design,* report from the Consumer Product Safety Commission, Monograph, University of Michigan (1975). Reproduced with permission.

Flexibility. Relatively little data are available on flexibility changes during childhood. Not only can inherited joint characteristics cause individual differences in flexibility measures obtained, but obesity can severely limit the range of motion in children. Fleishman has identified two types of flexibility: dynamic flexibility, involving rapid movements through ranges of motion, and static flexibility, measures of actions done slowly and to fullest limits. Flexibility in some joints may decrease with age. Flexibility may tend to decline at about the eighth to tenth year in boys, and slightly later in girls. In general, contradictory findings from studies of the flexibility of girls in late childhood have been attributable to the fact that flexibility measures may be highly specific to the joint action being evaluated. That is, predicting how flexible a child will be in the shoulder region may not be possible by knowing how flexible his or her hips are. This regional specificity of flexibility in children may be seen in the data from Hupprich and Sigerseth (1950) shown in Figure 7.7. In general they demonstrated that while hip flexion can improve with age, thigh flexion may decline. Flexibility in the ankles and legs (knees) seems to decline, while trunk flexibility may gain in childhood, according to these data. It is probable that training aids flexibility, but studies demonstrating this are difficult to locate. Moreover, ethnic background may also be an influential variable.

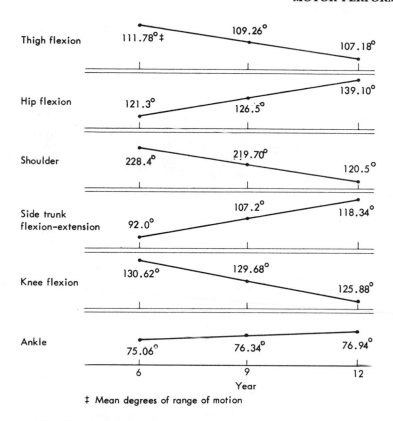

Thigh flexion   111.78°‡   109.26°   107.18°

Hip flexion   121.3°   126.5°   139.10°

Shoulder   228.4°   219.70°   120.5°

Side trunk flexion–extension   92.0°   107.2°   118.34°

Knee flexion   130.62°   129.68°   125.88°

Ankle   75.06°   76.34°   76.94°

6   9   12

Year

‡ Mean degrees of range of motion

FIGURE 7.7 Flexibility in various movements by girls. From F. L. Hupprich and P. O. Sigerseth, "The Specificity of Flexibility in Girls," *Res. Quart., 21* (1950), pp. 25–33.

Jumping. Jumping tests of a number of kinds have been employed to evaluate motor abilities in children. The most popular is the standing broad jump, but the jump reach and hurdle jump have also been used. In addition to jumping tests that tax leg power, there are those that require precision. Jumping with precision into squares is found on several batteries of tests, and has been the subject of some research.

Vertical jumping requires skill in summating the velocities of the leg extension and arm thrust upward. As was pointed out in Chapter 6 (Poe, 1976), even young children are likely to evidence a variety of arm-leg patterns. However, during childhood the method an individual child uses will become consistent, and a mature pattern involves a hard arm thrust upward as the legs extend.

Some vertical jumping tasks require reaching and touching a point as high as possible, after first being measured in the standing position with the hand over the head. Thus the measure looks at the difference of standing height plus reach, and jumping height plus reach. A measure of this type may tell the tester something

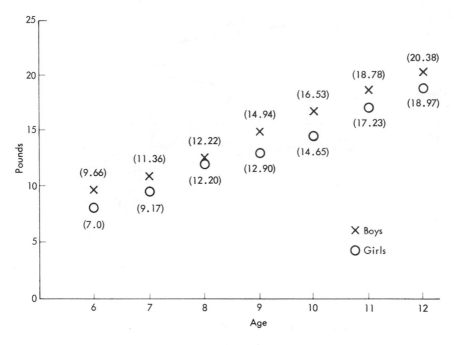

FIGURE 7.8 Vertical jump performance by age and sex. From R. D. Johnson, "Measurement of Achievement in Fundamental Skills of Elementary School Children," *Res. Quart.*, *33* (1962), p. 103.

about the child's ability to participate in vigorous games requiring powerful leg actions, including tennis, basketball, and football. As can be seen in Figure 7.8, boys usually beat girls in this task. By 7 children can usually jump about 7 inches over their heads, with improvement for boys in this study coming earlier than mean changes in girls. Between 7 and 8 years, for example, the boys improved about 25 percent, while the girls improved about 20 percent between 9 and 10, on the average.

In several studies, measures of both linearity and obesity in both boys and girls correlated with performance on this measure, as might be expected (Slaughter et al., 1977, 1980). Obese children do not project their bodies through space as well (Pissanos et al., 1983; Parizkova, 1984). Thus, linear girls and boys tend to jump higher, whereas those scoring high in the third component of the Health Carter Somatotype (fatness) score lower in this measure of jumping. I am unaware of biomechanical analyses of this action other than Poe's (1976). However, Figures 7.9 and 7.10 depict variations in the maturity of this action seen during childhood.

Hurdle jumps and other types of vertical jumping tasks have been used in research over the years and appear on various tests of motor ability (Cowen and Pratt, 1959; Stott, 1972; Carey, 1954). The hurdle jump involves a two-foot takeoff, a jump over the hurdle, and a two-foot landing. Mean scores improve at about the rate of 1.5 inches per year, with 5-year-olds able to negotiate a hurdle at about knee

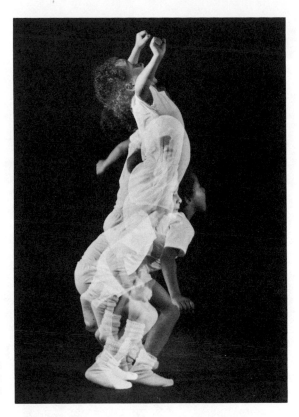

FIGURE 7.9
This six year old boy jumps upward well, but without the range of motion in accompanying arm action as is seen in the 10 year old in Figure 7.10.

height (Stott, 1972). Girls may excel boys at this task in early childhood (Hartman, 1943); however boys' mean scores are usually superior after the age of 7 years.

A hurdle jump may or may not correlate with body build; the available data are unclear on this point (Cowen and Pratt, 1959). However, mean scores from various studies vary greatly, and clear-cut norms are not available at this time. Stott uses other upward jumping tasks in his battery (1972). Among these are a standing upward jump accompanied by two hand claps, suggested as an accomplishable task at age 7. At the age of 10 in Stott's screening battery he believes that a hurdle jump at knee height should be possible with a two-foot takeoff and a one-foot landing. This task, however, like several in various often used batteries, may lead to knee injuries if given to a large group of children.

Standing broad jumps are often employed to evaluate leg power rather than a running broad jump in order to reduce the skill factor needed to take off at just the right time, as is required in the running broad jump (or long jump). This task, like the vertical jump, improves with age for several reasons, including the acquisition of greater leg power and the assumption of increasingly appropriate arm-leg mechanics.

As might be expected, better jumpers move their arms through greater ranges

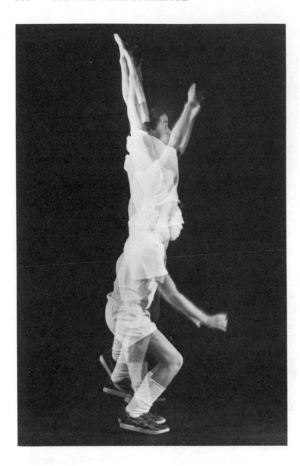

FIGURE 7.10
In contrast, this 10 year old jumps upward with a mature upward thrust of
the arms, involving an adult-like range
of motion.

of motion and bend their knees more initially than do the less proficient jumpers (Zimmerman, 1956). Average improvement at each age from 5 to 11 years is about 4.4 inches in boys and 4.1 inches in girls (Keogh, 1965). However, girls' scores average about 1 inch less than those of boys in early childhood (5–7 years), and from 4 to 5 inches less than boys in later childhood (8–11 years) (Keogh, 1965).

In a recent analysis of the arm and leg actions in the standing broad jump, Clark and Phillips (1985) identified the existence of four levels. This included Level I characterized by no arm action, or a "winging" of the arms out to the side. Leg action was usually a one-foot take-off. At Level II some shoulder flexion was seen, but the arms remained immobile during lower limb flexion. At Level III shoulder action was again incomplete, but does occur during lower limb extensions. The Level IV phase involves a jump after the heels arise from the surface, together with a complete and efficient arm action, characterized by shoulder flexion at the time of take-off.

In addition to measures of power jumping (upward and forward), precision of jumping actions has also been employed to assess motor abilities in children. Parts

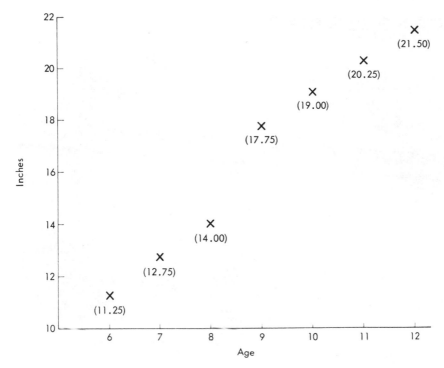

FIGURE 7.11 Hurdle-jumping ability by age. From E. Cowan and B. Pratt, "The Hurdle Jump as a Developmental and Diagnostic Test," *Child Development, 5* (1934), pp. 107–21.

of the Johnson test developed in the 1930s have involved hopping and jumping with precision onto mats containing grids. The job of the child is to make trips down the mat requiring increased precision, with the score for a successful trip containing no more than one error. In general, we have found that girls are more proficient than boys in this task. Children of 5 and below cannot successfully execute even a simple straight-ahead jumping pattern in each of the squares without making errors. However, by age 7, both boys and girls are able to jump and hop with precision in each square. Scores on this type of task tend to plateau at about 9 years of age in both boys and girls, according to our data (Cratty and Martin, 1979). Copying a demonstration of this task has also been used in research involving motor planning, specifically to evaluate trunk praxis or apraxia (Chapter 9) (Cratty and Samoy, 1984). Thus its use with younger children may also require qualities other than jumping precision. The ability to copy a complex demonstration may also contribute to relative success before age 5.

It is not to be expected that the various measures of jumping power and precision will correlate very well, although broad jumping and vertical jumping at times evidence moderate correlations. The sex differences that occur favor girls in the precision jumping tasks and boys in the power jumps. At the same time, when determining what kinds of jumping tasks may contribute to what sports skills and

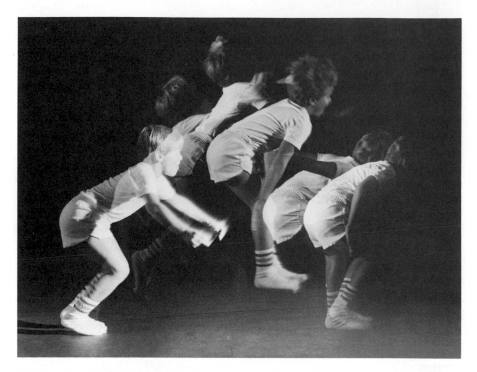

FIGURE 7.12 This boy in early childhood jumps forward well, but without the range of motion in the arm-thrust that is demonstrated in the 10 year old boy in Figure 7.13.

game prowess, careful analysis of the game's (sport's) demands should be conducted, rather than specific jumping training.

Gait variations.   Usually by early and middle childhood youngsters seek to learn and master various gait variations. Some are simply fun to do—skipping is an example. Others are imperative in many childhood games. Lateral movement is an example of an essential skill. At times, factors other than maturation and learning influence whether a child will exhibit galloping or skipping. Boys have informed me during evaluations of their abilities that skipping is "only for girls." At other times girls have apparently been unhappy with being asked to perform a galloping movement, which some may believe is appropriate only for boys. "Girls aren't horses" one snorted to me one day.

Skipping is often executed more precisely by girls earlier than this same pattern is seen in boys. Often learning to skip begins during the preschool years with a one-footed skip. Later the task is mastered in an alternating fashion, with quick transfers of weight from one side of the body to the other. By 7 the majority of children tested in various investigations are able to demonstrate a skip as was illustrated in Chapter 6. "True" galloping is often seen earlier than skipping, at about the fifth or sixth year. However, both are likely to be influenced by special

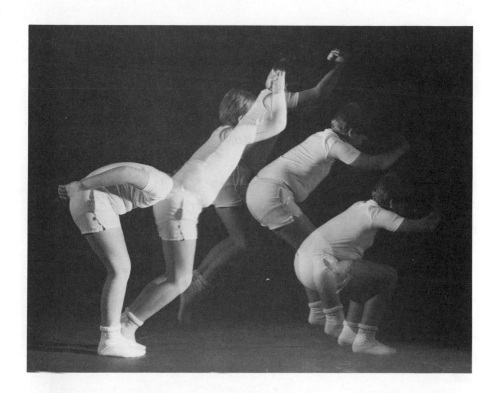

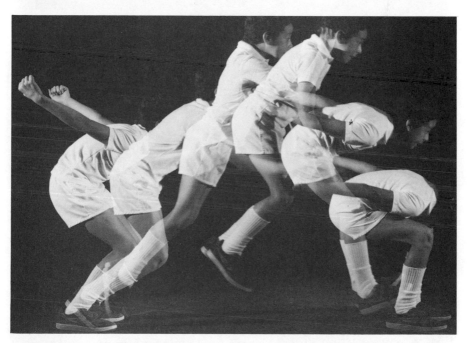

FIGURE 7.13 These photos show two boys of 10 executing a standing broad jump with slightly different styles, but with mature adult-like ranges of motion.

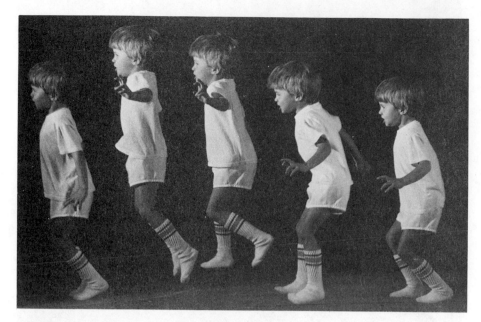

FIGURE 7.14 A boy of almost five can jump in succession, using both feet as shown, but is unable to jump with precision.

FIGURE 7.15 In contrast, this youngster in middle childhood may be expected to jump with precision into a gridded mat containing 1′ by 1′ squares, as shown.

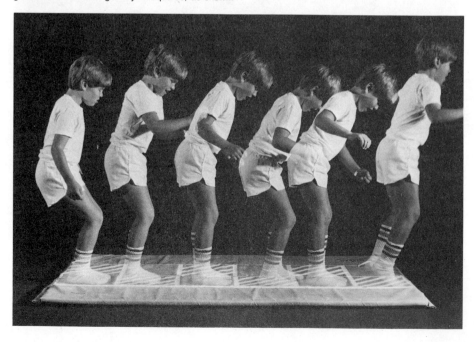

practice. First attempts at both galloping and skipping are likely to be accompanied by rather random arm actions. These can include the picture of loose arms flying in the air during the skipping and galloping actions. With maturity, however, both actions are accompanied by an approximation of a cross-extension pattern seen in running.

Lateral movement is often difficult for a child of 5 or 6 years. It is sometimes accompanied by excess tensions in the arms, and may also be difficult toward one side or the other. Moreover, during the early childhood years execution may be slow and cumbersome, rather than continuous and fluid. The task is an essential one, necessary when the child is confronted with defensive skills in many team games (baseball, soccer, football, basketball). Efficient lateral movement is also required when the child attempts to trap or to intercept balls that may be projected to either side. The maturity of the mechanics seen in this action is probably more dependent upon experience and learning than upon maturation during the childhood years.

Agility. Agility, like beauty, is different things to different people. Some researchers measuring motor performance have used a series of stunt-type tests that seem to them to have captured agility (Brace, 1941). Others have employed various zig-zag runs and used the scores to define the term. The Cable jump has also been used (Keogh, 1965). This requires a child to jump over a hand-held cable. In batteries of tests I have developed, we separated what we called locomotor agility, requiring children to jump and hop with accuracy into squares, from gross agility.

FIGURE 7.16 Lateral movement becomes smooth and vigorous by middle childhood.

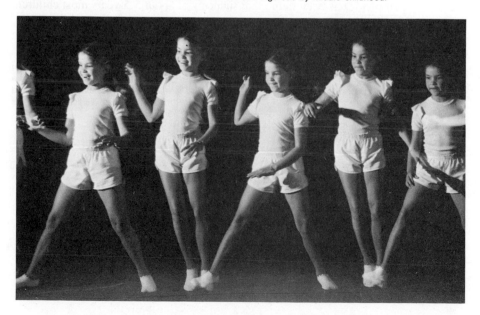

This latter term required children to move with accuracy in a vertical direction by responding to such directions as "get up as fast as you can" (Cratty and Martin, 1970). One group of measurers recently combined both upward and forward quickness with picking up a ball, terming the task a scramble (Morris et al., 1982). Perhaps the term *scramble* does indeed describe the problem of comparing scores from such diverse tests when trying to define agility and attempting to describe age and/or sex differences in childhood.

Generally, as would be expected, children improve in such tasks as dodge runs throughout childhood. Gallahue reports data from both tests given in Canada and in the United States (Manitoba Physical Fitness Test and the AAHPER). In both tests girls' mean scores leveled off at 12, while the scores of boys continued to improve (Gallahue, 1982).

Slight sex differences in leg power, reaction time, and movement speed favoring males during childhood could contribute to a number of differences seen in so-called tests of agility in which these qualities are required (Hodgkins, 1963). On the other hand, young girls are at times more flexible than males during childhood. Thus tasks that require hip flexibility, for example, may be performed better by females during the childhood years (Clarke, 1975; DiNucci, 1976). Therefore sex differences on so-called agility tasks may depend upon the type of task used to assess this elusive quality.

Overall, it appears that measures of agility are highly task-specific. It also seems that individual differences in basic movement qualities influence the scores obtained. For example, we found no correlations between two so-called gross agility items in our battery, one requiring controlled descending and arising, and the other a more rapid ascent ("How fast can you get up?"). In a fast ascent from the back, for example, it has been found that suddenly at about 5.5 years most children

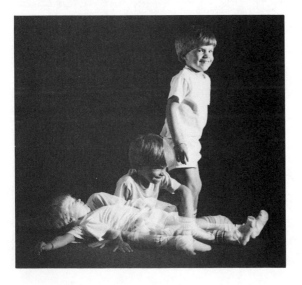

FIGURE 7.17
When asked to get up "as fast as you can" from a back lying position, a five year old will often turn to the side and then assume a vertical ascent, as shown.

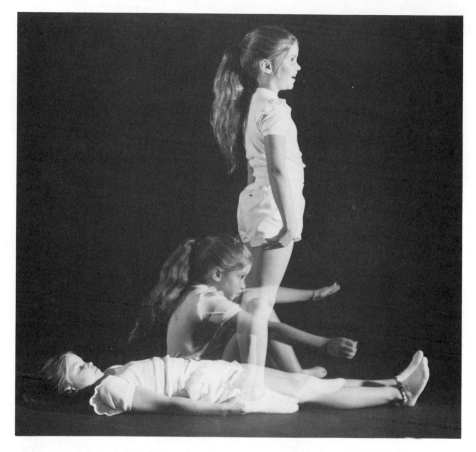

FIGURE 7.18 In contrast to the five year old, a youngster in middle childhood when asked to rise rapidly, will ascend quickly from the back and remain facing in the same direction.

can accomplish this without first turning to the front and using their hands to rise (Noller and Ingrisano, 1984).

Speed. Speed measures used with children consist of two major types: those involving arm or leg velocities and speeds with which the child is able to move the total body, usually in a dash of from 20 to 50 yards. These two qualities (limb speed and body speed) are not very well correlated in children during middle childhood (Hodgkins, 1963; Fleishman, 1965). The ways in which these two qualities are measured may influence the scores obtained. For example, children started in a short dash using a gun, and thus combining reaction times with movement speeds, may post quite different scores than if they are permitted to start whenever they are ready.

Keogh and Sugden (1985) have compiled and combined data from several studies of running in children, and based upon measures of feet/sec, it was found

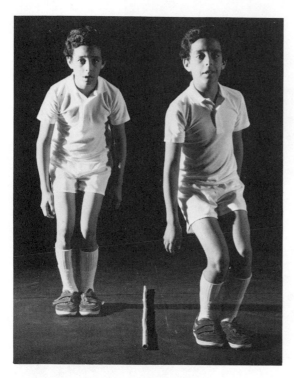

FIGURE 7.19
Lateral jumping for accuracy and/or
speed is sometimes used as an agility
task in some text batteries.

that (1) consistent sex differences in running speed existed at all ages, with the boys showing a linear pattern in scores from the seventh to the seventeenth year of life. The girls on the other hand tended to plateau in average running ability from about the thirteenth to the seventeenth year. Both boys and girls impoved 23 percent from the fifth to the twelfth year. However, the boys evidenced improvement of 49 percent from the seventh to seventeenth year, whereas the girls evidenced only slight improvement beyond age twelve.

Movement speed velocities that may be produced by a child probably influence performance in such tasks as kicking and throwing distances. Moreover, simply clocking a child's running-dash speed for short distances in a straight line is not likely to be predictive of how well the child may move in a zig-zag pathway. Because it is important in many sports to change directions quickly with the body, it is therefore more useful to measure children in tasks that require quick changes of direction while running, as well as in straight-ahead bursts of running speed (Fleishman, 1964). A more complete picture of how a child is likely to move in many games will be obtained than if a single measure of running speed is employed.

Balance.   Throughout childhood, youngsters continue to perform better and better on tests of both moving (dynamic) and static (posturing) balance. Technically, balance is not a skill but a rather important movement quality underlying the performance of a large group of skills. Among the tasks influenced by the degree of stability the child possesses are throwing, running, quick changes of direction, and

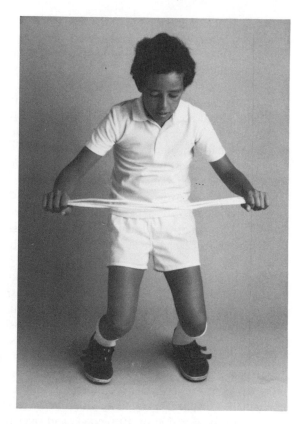

FIGURE 7.20
Among the stunt-type tests sometimes used to evaluate agility is a "cable-jump" to determine whether a child can jump over a hand-held cable or rope, as shown.

FIGURE 7.21 Mature running form and mechanics contribute to fast speeds in late childhood, as seen in this 10 year old boy.

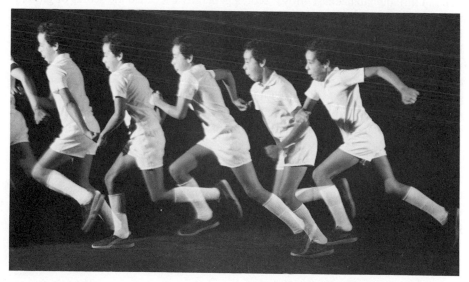

variations of locomotion, including hopping, skipping, and the like. Contemporary authors discussing balance in children are not in agreement as to how to classify it. Gallahue (1982) calls it a perceptual-motor skill, while Williams (1983) places it in a separate chapter that does not include gross motor skills.

It is possible that improvements in balance functions by middle and later childhood come about because of maturity of the motor system, since by that time visual attentional qualities, likely modifiers of early balance scores, are relatively mature. During the elementary school years neurologically sound children become able to walk narrow balance beams while posturing on one foot, sometimes with the eyes closed. However, useful comparisons of data from several studies are difficult. Small and ill-defined samples are often used, and such variables as height of the balance beam—and even practice—have been shown to exert significant influences on scores obtained in groups of youngsters (Wyrick, 1969). Clark and Watkins (1984), for example, found that body position, base of support, the use of vision, and foot preference had great influence on static balance in children from 6 to 9 years of age.

Stott has employed a number of balance tasks in his evaluation tool (1972). He contends that a child of 6 years, of either sex, should be able to posture for 15 seconds using one foot. A heel-to-toe walk is believed within the capabilities of 7-year-olds, using a 15-foot line. An interesting task for 8-year-olds combines the balance of objects with locomotion. The child must hold the bottom block, while balancing another on top, and at the same time walk a distance of 15 feet. At both 9 and 10 years, postures must be maintained using one foot placed on a block on the floor. By 13, it is expected that children of both sexes will be able successfully to maintain their balance on one foot, with the heel raised from the ground (on the ball of the foot) for a period of 10 seconds and over (Stott, 1972).

In our own research, we found rather steady improvement with age on variations of a static balance test. Boys' scores generally exceeded the scores of girls in this test from the ages of 6 to 8 years. After 8, however, the scores were almost identical. In contrast to many static balance tests that require a child to remain "as long as you can" in a one-foot stand, we required a demonstration of control in variations of a one-foot stand lasting from 4 to 6 seconds. By age 7 most children could maintain a one-foot stand with their eyes closed in a controlled and stable position for from 4 to 6 seconds. Eight-year-old boys could fold their arms while standing on one foot with eyes closed. By the age of 10, most children could hold a static one-foot stand on their nonpreferred foot with eyes closed (Cratty and Martin, 1970).

Static balance also improves with age. Seashore, for example, used a beam walking test and found steady improvement with age. Number of steps walked on the beam at each age were the scoring criteria (Seashore, 1949). For reasons that are not quite clear, however, Bachman (1961) found that static posturing on an unstable platform evidenced a decline with age during childhood and adolescence. The differences in the two tasks could have caused the contrasting findings.

Despite the presence of balance training in most programs intended to aid ba-

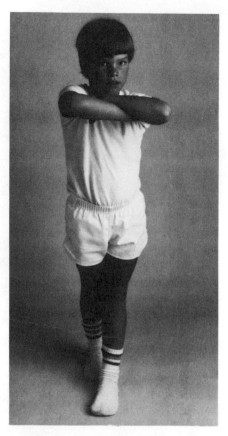

FIGURE 7.22
A more difficult static posture involves a heel toe stand, as shown, and is not accomplishable until middle childhood by most youngsters.

sic movement (and perceptual-motor) qualities, there is a dearth of evidence which indicates that training really helps. We found improvement in balance in a 1970 study (Cratty et al., 1975). And at the time, we were unsure whether we had improved balance as a basic quality or simply taught the children more effective work methods to use when attempting to posture on one foot. Cotton and Lowe (1974) used college-age students and found that improvement with training occurred on some balance tasks and not on others. Bordas, among numerous others, attempted to demonstrate improvement in balance among a group of children with developmental lags. Improvement with training did occur (Bordas, 1971), as was also seen in a similar study with a comparable population by Reeve (1976). Thus it appears that balance performance may improve with practice. What remains unclear, however, is whether balance training transfers positively to other movement tasks and to other types of perceptual-motor skills.

More work is needed with both normal and clumsy children to determine what subsystems contribute to and detract from balance tasks at various ages. For example, the relative role of vision, visual perceptual abilities, attention, and motor qualities might well be discovered if factor analytic methods were employed, assessing

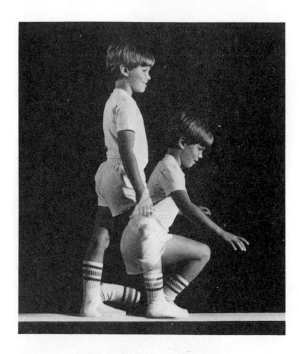

FIGURE 7.23
Older children can descend and arise
on a 4' balance beam, as shown.

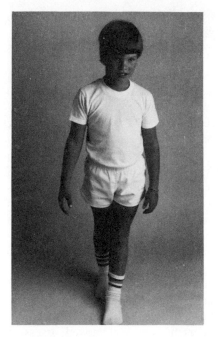

FIGURE 7.24
A heel-toe walk is sometimes included as a balance task
accomplishable by the 7th year.

just what qualities contribute to balance scores at various ages and/or during various stages of learning. This type of study has been conducted to explore contributors to motor learning tasks (Fleishman and Rich, 1963). Given our present state of knowledge, however, when assessing children's balance, a comprehensive look should be taken at visual as well as attentional contributors to the execution of an apparent motor task.

Ball Skills

Throwing.   Throwing continues to be an important group of skills to be acquired during childhood. Throwing is considered a collection of skills because of the increasingly larger number of missiles used by children and youth in the American culture. During the past week, for example, I witnessed several organized Frisbee football games in which the object to be thrown differs markedly from a ball, as does the wrist and arm action needed to give it impetus.

Over the decades, various ball-throwing skills have been researched. Efforts have been made to evaluate throwing mechanics, as well as accuracy and velocity (distance). In general, the throwing pattern of boys seems to mature more quickly than does that of girls (Cratty, Cortinas, and Kelly, 1973) for reasons that are not entirely clear. Additionally, as might be expected, older children can throw harder and farther than younger ones. In studies we have conducted, significant changes in throwing mechanics and accuracy were posted from the fifth to seventh year; a second improvement jump was found from the seventh to ninth year. After that time, in boys and girls no significant improvement was recorded (Cratty and Martin, 1970). In other studies, however, improvement in mean scores are seen at every age from 6 to 11 years (Keogh, 1965). Distance thrown may almost triple from the sixth to the eleventh year in both boys and girls. However, in late childhood the mean scores of girls are from 50 to 60 percent of the mean scores posted by boys (Keogh, 1965).

Several useful studies of throwing velocities have been conducted during the past several decades. Generally velocity evidences linear improvement with age in both boys and girls (Glassow and Kruse, 1960). Of most interest are results from a series of studies by Halverson and her colleagues extending from 1977 to 1982 in which the same children were studied in a longitudinal investigation (Halverson et al., 1966, 1982). Overall it was found that the children improved in velocity about 5–8 ft/sec each year in the case of boys; girls improved each year 2–4.5 ft/sec. Yearly shifts in the mean scores were obtained from kindergarten through second grade, and then again at seventh grade. Although the girls seemed to close the gap on the males in the study by the seventh grade, they were still five "developmental years" behind by the age of about 12 years, measured in velocity of throw. They also found, however, that girls' throwing velocities were more stable over time, based upon interyear comparisons of the throws of the same children.

Halverson and her helpers also sought information concerning what might have caused female-male differences in throwing speeds and interviewed their sub-

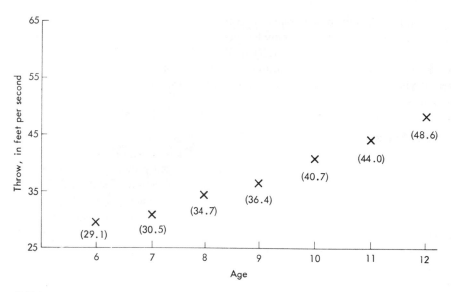

FIGURE 7.25 Throwing velocity changes in girls ages 6 to 11 years. From R. N. Glassow and P. Kruse, "Motor Performance of Girls Age 6–14 Years," *Res. Quart., 31* (1960), pp. 426–33.

jects concerning the amount of practice they engaged in each week at the age of 12. The boys reported more exposure to throwing than did the girls. Most of the boys (15 of 22) said that they threw hard from 3 to 5 times a week; only 5 of the 17 girls reported the same amount of experience and practice.

In several of the series by Halverson (1977, 1979), as well as in studies by others (Goldstein, 1983; Dusenberry, 1952; Dohrman, 1964; Toole et al., 1982), efforts have been made to evaluate the possible effects of training on throwing distance (velocity), as well as upon throwing mechanics. For the most part, the various investigators have not reported a great deal of success when studying training effects on throwing. As was pointed out in Chapter 6, Goldstein found that she could modify the immature throwing patterns of some girls of 5 to 6 years, while the throwing patterns of others seemed resistant to modification through training and demonstration. Dohrman (1964) similarly found that a special throwing training program did not show any particular improvement when contrasted to a regular physical education class. In two investigations, Halverson (1977, 1979) found that training did not improve the throwing velocities of boys and girls in the early elementary school years. It is possible that the training programs were not well structured, or did not afford the children enough time in which to evidence measurable improvement. Any changes that may occur in throwing seem to have to come with a great deal of practice, and with highly structured styles of teacher-centered teaching (Toole et al., 1982).

Moreover, training programs may have to overcome negative socio-cultural stereotypes and training that may curb the development of mature throwing patterns in some young children (East and Hensley, 1985).

Throwing mechanics continue to improve throughout childhood. But as Halverson found when surveying her subjects (1982), even by 12 years of age immature patterns continue to persist. However it also appears true that to change immature and/or inefficient throwing patterns in early or late childhood, a highly structured and prolonged program of instruction may be necessary. Throwing velocities, unlike some of the other physical qualities surveyed in this chapter, seem not to be greatly influenced by body build (Seils, 1951). Sustained exposure to correctly throwing peers probably has greater influence.

Throwing accuracy seems to improve with age. However, so great a range of target sizes and throwing distances have been used that solid data reflecting age changes are hard to come by. One investigator even varied the distance from target at which he placed children of various ages, making age comparisons somewhat difficult (Keogh, 1966).

Consistent sex differences favoring boys appear in all the available data, both in velocities attained, as well as in the maturity of the throwing patterns evidenced. Further work is needed, however, to untangle the possible influences of cultural expectations, social modeling and anatomical-physiological variables on the purported sex differences seen in throwing. It is likely that with newer trends in what constitutes appropriate physical activity for young girls, at least the correctness of the throwing pattern will not evidence the marked differences seen in earlier studies when the efforts of boys and girls are contrasted.

Catching. During childhood, patterns of catching continue to improve. Some of this improvement probably occurs because of improved motor abilities, particularly the ability to coordinate more than one action pattern at a time. Catching involves visually following the ball through an extended arc and moving the body some distance to intercept a ball. Important information-processing qualities are thus probably involved. Information processing as variable was evident in a study by Williams (1968) involving children from 5 to 12 years. In middle childhood, as the children watched the first part of a ball's arc, they were often quite late when trying to locate their bodies at the point of hypothesized final impact. However, in late childhood they left immediately to locate themselves where the ball would finally arrive. Moreover, the accuracy of these judgments improved markedly in early, middle, and late childhood. Seils, for example (1951), found that skeletal maturity, based upon carpal X-rays, correlated moderately with catching success in both boys and girls.

Often various apparently similar measures of ball interception and catching do not correlate. Two subsections of a test used in my test battery, for example, do not intercorrelate. One consists of asking the child to touch a ball on a string swinging in a plane parallel to the child's shoulders; the second task involves catching a ball bounced to the child 15 feet away. Apparently the ability to judge the position of a ball subject to the physics of a pendulum action is different from whatever judgments and/or movement qualities are needed to catch a ball bounced directly at the child.

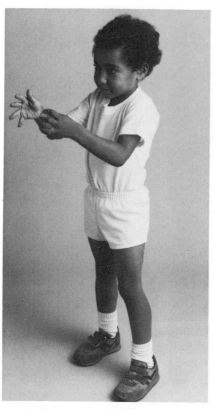 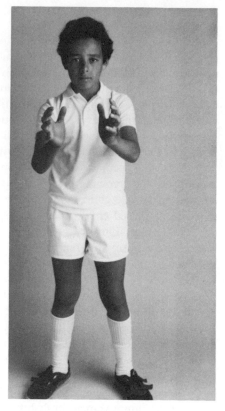

FIGURE 7.26
Not only do the abilities to track and catch balls change from early to later childhood, but the postures assumed preparatory to the catch may change. In (a) the boy of six awaits tensely, and may have to partly trap a ball against his body when it arrives. In contrast, the boy in (b) waits with his hands in a relaxed, extended position, and will usually catch a small ball using his hands only.

In general, most children at the ages of 6 and 7 are able to intercept a ball (8 inches in diameter, air-filled) when it is bounced once from a distance of 15 feet. However, the abilities necessary to catch small balls thrown from greater distances evidence marked individual differences through childhood and continue to show improvement with practice during this same period of time (Randt, 1985).

Differences in measured proficiency when testing younger children's catching behaviors may differ from task to task. For example, when the child has given impetus to the ball himself or herself, intercepting it is apparently easier than if it is projected in an unpredictable way by another. Stott (1972) suggests that 5-year-olds should be able to bounce a tennis ball on the ground and re-catch it using both hands by the age of 5. By 6, Stott believes that this same interception problem should be accomplishable with one hand, using the same small ball. However, Stott does not include the interception of a tennis ball thrown by another person in his test battery until tasks purportedly achievable by 9-year-olds are listed.

Randt as the result of her 1985 study indicates that not only should children of 7 and 8 be exposed to the catching of tennis-ball size missiles, but that using balls of this size will likely have beneficial training effects (Randt, 1985).

Additional improvement with practice during childhood is evident when children must move their total bodies in various ways to intercept balls. First, lateral movement is acquired when the ball is apparently coming to their left or right. Later more difficult forward and backward movement of the body is learned, as correct positions for ball interception are acquired in various sports. Special refinements are somehow acquired by, or must be taught to, children relative to ball interceptions accompanied by relocations of the body. For example, the child must somehow feel whether it is quicker and more efficient to take a sliding step to the side while facing the ball in order to intercept it, or whether it is better in a given situation to turn and run a short distance with the side of the body momentarily toward the direction of the incoming ball, before turning and facing it again in order to catch or stop it.

Kicking. A variety of actions that involve kicking a ball are needed in various sports and playground games. Soccer, increasingly popular in the United States, has during the past decade focused attention on this category of skill in young children. For the most part, a mature one-footed kick of a ball requires balance sufficient to permit the child to posture momentarily on one foot, and to take the stress of the pendulum and striking action of the other. Children with poor balance should not be permitted to participate in soccer because their kicking attempts may prove self-injurious. Additionally, some kicking tasks require the perceptual skills needed to catch well. The child must often predict where a moving ball will later be in relationship to his or her body.

Relatively little solid research has been done on kicking skills in children (Dohrman, 1964). The limited data available suggest that boys are superior to girls in kicking distance, while training children to kick better is not an easily accomplishable goal. Williams (1982) suggested that a child passes through three stages of kicking before the age of 5 years. These gradually involve more and more arm action, body lean, and greater ranges of motion in the kicking leg. However, it is believed to be more tenable that the three stages may or may not be completed during the preschool years. Many children may continue to move through these three stages well into the elementary school years. Furthermore, there are several more advanced stages in kicking behaviors involving the striking of a moving ball and the kicking of hand-released balls of various types.

The difficulty in kicking, just as is true with ball interception and striking skills of various types, depends in part upon whether or not the child releases the ball, or whether it is propelled in unpredictable ways by others.[2]

---

[2]Essentially all interception tasks involving striking, catching, or otherwise dealing with missiles may be what are termed *open* or *closed* skills. Open skills involve unpredictability; another person's actions and reactions influence the direction and velocity of the incoming missile. A closed skill, on the other hand, is one that is highly predictable because the interceptor has usually imparted initial impetus to the missile. A closed skill would thus include a single child bouncing and catching a ball; an open skill would include striking or catching a ball thrown or projected by another person.

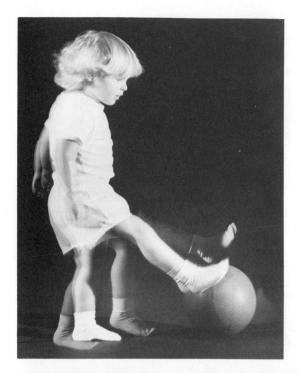

FIGURE 7.27
This girl of 2.4 years lacks the balance skills that permit a full range of motion by the kicking leg, but does pretty well in contacting the ball.

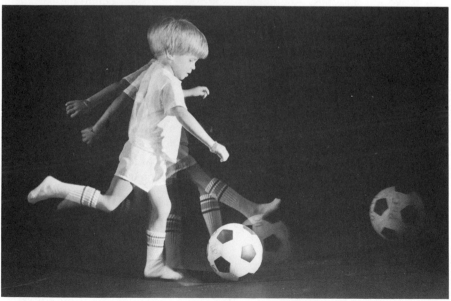

FIGURE 7.28   In contrast to the child in Figure 7.27, this older child demonstrates a more mature kicking action with appropriate weight shift forward, accompanied by appropriate arm actions.

One of the more advanced kicking problems now facing children in our culture are pictured below (Figure 7.29). Furthermore, kicking skills used in soccer come in an infinite variety, and often involve subtle guidance of the ball and a great deal of precision. Dribbling the ball, trapping it, passing it to a teammate are only some of the skills required. Thus in this specific game, improvement in these skills may be expected, with practice, throughout childhood. The role of maturation and so-called basic qualities, if the child is not neurologically impaired, are probably subordinated to the effects of learning, teaching, and practice.

Dribbling. A number of games, including basketball and team handball, require a child to dribble a ball. The task can prove a vexing one for the maturing child, particularly if it must be performed under the stress caused by social pressures in a competitive game. Little solid data are available on this skill, as differences in ball size and dribbling tasks would cause wide variations in scores obtained by children at various ages. Gallahue (1982) has identified three stages in dribbling that may appear at virtually any chronological age, depending on the youngster's experience with this complex serial task.

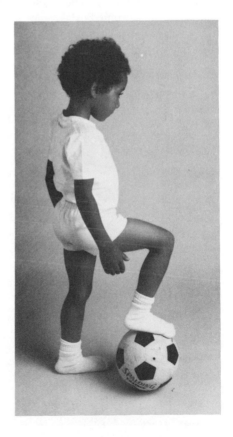

FIGURE 7.29
By six years many children can learn to execute a number of soccer (football) skills including dribbling and trapping the ball, as shown.

1. First the ball may be just held, dropped, and re-caught, with no attempt to move it continuously. Variations in the force of each downward throw (or drop) may be recorded. Variations in the height the ball bounces are also likely.
2. A second stage may involve one hand, with a pattern that is irregular and not completely successful. The ball may be slapped at instead of gently stroked, as during the last, more mature, stage. At times the child may lose control of the ball.
3. A final mature stage involves continuous and relaxed stroking motions of the hand. The hand "gives" as it touches the ball during its ascent and guides it downward without a slap.

Striking.   Striking missiles involves two possibilities. The hand or arms are striking the missile, or an extension of the body is used to strike a missile. Generally, movement patterns used in either of these two types of actions become more effective and mature as more and more body rotation precedes the hit, coupled with an increased amount of rotation by the shoulders and a weight shift of the body, usually forward. During an immature phase, the child will strike a ball or use an implement (racket, bat) with little weight shift, giving impetus primarily with arm action itself. During the later stage, forces are summated, beginning with those engendered by the hips, shoulders, and finally the arms. Williams (1983) has reported data in two of her unpublished studies which indicate that velocity improves from 4 to 8 years of age. The child is able to generate more force using both arms than if only one arm is used (Williams et al., 1971; Williams and Breihan, 1979).

Striking patterns may start using a stationary ball. Later the child, still using

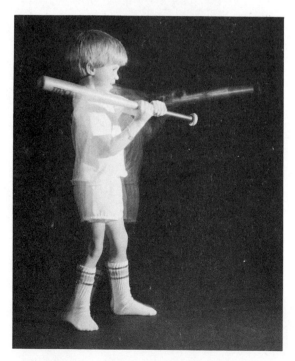

FIGURE 7.30
This boy of less than five years takes a somewhat restricted swing at the ball using a limited range of motion and body rotation.

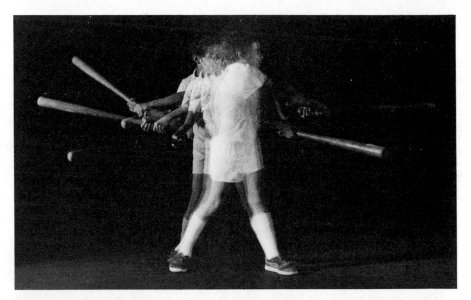

FIGURE 7.31 In contrast to Figure 7.30, this boy of 10 years takes a "full cut" at the ball, evidencing a complete range of motion, good body rotation, and a weight shift forward, which was barely evidenced in the 4.5 year old's swing.

the hand, may hold a playground ball with one hand and hit it with the other. This second act is relatively difficult if the child's neuromotor system is immature, as overflow (see Chapter 9) may make applying force with the striking arm-hand difficult while keeping the holding arm-hand in a relatively relaxed position.

Striking missiles with an extension of the body (bat, racket) presents even more difficulties for children younger than 7 or 8 years of age. The racket offers more linkages that need organizing than a simple hitting action of an empty arm-hand. The racket, for example, may be held at various distances from the body. In the case of tennis and racketball, the child must learn how far he or she must stand from the future position of a small ball to achieve a free swinging action of the racket or paddle. A reasonable amount of neuromotor maturity is thus needed before even beginning to learn such skills.

SUMMARY

Youngsters evidence marked improvement in a variety of skills during the elementary school years. Yearly improvement is measurable in strength, agility, balance, and in velocities reflected in running speed and in distances balls are thrown or hit. Coupled with measurable performance increases are improved body mechanics. Body parts become better integrated. The arms become more closely integrated with the legs as maturation takes place. Positive changes are measurable both in the product of the actions (distances balls are thrown), as well as in the quality of the actions produced by youngsters during these formative years.

In recent research delineating motor development changes during the elementary school, several useful trends are discernible. (1) Some longitudinal work is being carried out delineating changes at each year in children studied for a prolonged period of time. (2) Individual differences are being discovered in how, for example, children jump, rather than arbitrarily assigning specific mechanical methods to designated age groups, as has often been done in the past.

QUESTIONS FOR DISCUSSION

1. What seem more important to consider, sex differences or age differences, when formulating useful motor development programs for children from 5 to 10 years of age?
2. What trends are seen in children's balance scores, strength scores, agility measures, and ball skills from the ages of 5 to 7, 8 to 10?
3. What considerations should be kept in mind when trying to change the manner in which children throw, catch, and engage in body mechanics when jumping?
4. What compensations may be made when a child is physically awkward and is asked to play with more capable peers?
5. Why are comparisons of children's agility scores difficult, given the available literature?

STUDENT PROJECTS

1. With permission, observe a playground containing elementary school youngsters. Attempt to ascertain which ones may be physically awkward from observing their social behaviors. What youngsters seem physically superior? How do their verbal and social behaviors seem to stand out?
2. Prepare a checklist of gross motor skills probable in a 5-year-old child. With a parent's permission, evaluate a child of that age. How did your expected list correspond to the actual abilities seen in the child assessed?
3. Using information you gained from Chapter 6, contrast the skills you would expect in a child of 3 and a child of 7 years. Contact two children this age, with parental permission, and determine the correspondence between your expectations and their actual performances. In what tasks do these children tend to evidence similar behaviors? In what ways are they different?
4. Observe playground behaviors within schools in two parts of your city containing different ethnic groups. How do the behaviors contrast? In what ways are they similar? Can you account for the differences or similarities?

CHAPTER EIGHT
THE HANDS
The Development and Meanings of Manual Abilities in Infancy and Childhood

Humans evidence no more complex movement abilities than those exhibited by the hands. The human hand not only supplies a system through which the infant and child may manipulate the environment, but also stimulates and is a reflection of intellectual, social, and verbal and emotional behaviors. The hand grasps, hits, writes, communicates, feels, displays jewelry, and strikes blows. What the hands do is often the final result of numerous neurological-anatomical backup systems, including structures mediating speech, vision, hearing, and complex thought.

The human hand begins as a rudimentary "bud" within the first weeks after conception (Chapter 2). Its development continues through infancy at an accelerated rate. The products and outcomes of the hands provide an ever-changing pageant throughout life. Painting skills and intricate dexterities may, in some, continue to evolve into the eighth and ninth decades of life. Segovia in his eighties is currently giving guitar concerts. The paintings of Picasso, produced in his nineties, bring high prices.

Before the turn of the century, several studies were published describing drawing accuracy in youngsters (Bryant, 1892; Woodworth, 1899). During the first decades of this century, straightforward descriptions of manual abilities appeared in the literature. Some of these provided useful descriptions of the developmental stages seen in infants and children (Halverson, 1931). Other studies explored the ways in which factory workers use their hands (Gilbreath, 1917).

In the 1960s and particularly in the 1970s, studies about what youngsters do with their hands proliferated. More and more contemporary scholars have become interested in the ways in which the hands reflect other functions, primarily intellectual operations and stages in linguistic development. Bower, reacting to tenets of Piagetian theory dealing with object permanence, has produced numerous studies dealing with possible perceptual and cognitive bases for various actions of the hands (Bower, 1974). Goodson and Greenfield have looked for parallels in linguistic development by observing the manipulative play of children (Goodson and Greenfield, 1975). Still another author has described the rudimentary slashes and scribbles of children as motor manifestations of early attempts at speech (Alland, 1977).

Moreover, recent literature on the subject of manual skills has taken a more theoretical direction than was true among the descriptive studies of the past (Moss and Hogg, 1983). For example, it is becoming increasingly apparent that a simple stage-approach to the study of manual skill acquisition in infants and children is not a true picture of the complexity of the process and subprocesses involved.

Two other trends may be seen in the recent literature. One concentrates upon the sensory qualities of the hands. Studies have been carried out dealing with whether or not a youngster can perceive various parts of the hand and fingers when they are touched. Other sensory qualities explored deal with the information the child's hands are able to obtain when touching objects. The second trend emerged several decades ago from neurological clinics. This thrust has been toward the exploration of various sensory and motor deficits seen in both the young and the old. At times these investigations of problems in manual awareness and hand dexterity have afforded important insights into normal development. This type of data has also stimulated the formulation of useful testing devices.

The development of various abilities in which the hands are involved may be considered as numerous overlapping processes. Before birth, it is possible to elicit a grasping reflex. During the first weeks of life, an interaction of rhythmic stereotypes and reflex actions occurs similar to the processes involving the larger muscle groups described in Chapter 3. During these same early weeks and months, the infant begins to (a) pair vision with action in intricate and increasingly efficient ways; (b) discover new uses for the hand, and hands, including how both may be used together; and (c) gain more and more information from tactually exploring objects with increasing sophistication.

Cognitive qualities emerge as the infant becomes more and more curious about the nature of objects and realizes that hidden things may be rediscovered through manual efforts. As the middle of the first year of life is reached, infants begin to exploit objects in ever more creative ways. These exploitations tend to instigate social behaviors with others (Chapter 7). By the end of the first year, linguistic behaviors are stimulated as objects are not only picked up and held, but named. As the first year comes to an end, many youngsters, if appropriate objects are available, enter a general stage that both reflects and stimulates a great amount of intellectual behavior. Graphic efforts begin, branching into two major subdivisions by the second, third, and fourth years. One includes representations of thoughts using letters, words, and sentences in printed, manuscript, and later written form. Second, efforts are made to portray things, feelings, and thoughts by drawing and painting images and pictures.

EARLY REFLEXES, STEREOTYPIES, AND VISUAL–MANUAL SKILLS

At the sixth fetal month, a grasp response may be elicited. At birth the prehensile reflex appears in a rudimentary form that will undergo several transitions during the first year of life. Additionally, during these same early weeks a variety of rhythmic stereotypies emerge. These rhythmic flappings appear in the arms, hands, and fingers, and reach their zenith from the sixth to the twelfth month of age (Thelen, 1979). Other movements seen early consist of apparently inherent swiping patterns when the infant is confronted with an object. These three types of early movements (reflexes, stereotypies, and swiping patterns) during the middle of the first year of life, when the infant is able to sit and free the arms and hands, contribute to the acquisition of useful voluntary hand patterns and of hand-eye coordinations.

Phases of the Prehensile Reflex and Withdrawal Reaction

At birth the simple grasp reaction seen in the fetus begins to undergo several transitions (Twitchell, 1979). During the first eight weeks, for example, the reflex closing of the hand is most likely initiated if the arm is pulled away from the body. The flexion of the fingers in this case is accompanied by a parallel flexion at the elbow joint. This early appearance of the prehensile reflex is seemingly influenced by the tonic neck reflex. That is, when the tonic neck reflex appears, if the infant's arm on the skull side is pulled, the reflex is facilitated. However, if the arm is gently pulled on the face side (the arm toward which the face is looking in the tonic neck position), either a greatly diminished response is elicited, or no response at all.

During these same early weeks, this first component undergoes refinement and change, perhaps due to the maturation of supporting neural structures. If the infant's palm is pressed heavily, the same flexion of the limb may occur, accompanied by a closing of the thumb and index finger toward each other. Several other important changes in this reflex occur between the fourth and tenth months of age. During this period, if the palm is pressed the hand will close without a parallel flexion of the limb. Two final refinements of this reflex are both interesting and important: (a) The hand shows a tendency to orient toward the direction it is stroked. That is, if the thumb side is stroked, the hand will turn upward; if the little finger side is touched, the hand will turn in that direction (pronate). (b) A light touch to any part of the hand will elicit the closing of that part. This first appears in the index finger and later in other fingers that close when a moving or stationary touch is made.

Important changes during this last phase, at about the tenth and eleventh months, include (a) the eliciting of flexion reactions of parts of the hands to light touch rather than to the heavier touch that was previously required; (b) the closing of parts of the hand in appropriate ways to grasp objects with increased precision when the reflex is triggered. Also important is the fact that these refinements of the grasping reflex are not dependent on visual stimulation or control. They will occur often without the infant's visual inspection of the object being placed in the hand. These reactions are apparently triggered because of change in sensory information transmitted by the muscle, tendon, and joint receptors (proprioception).

In most infants there are also variations of a withdrawal reaction. This kind of response is elicited by light contact during the first month, and may consist of a spreading outward of the fingers and a flexion backward (dorsi-flexion) of the hand. As is true with the prehensile reaction, this reaction becomes more refined during successive months and may be seen later in avoidance by various parts of the hand, in various directions, when lightly stroked. These avoidance reactions, if too strong, may be indicative of neurological impairment, just as is true if the prehensile reflex does not become lighter and more refined later in the first year.

To elicit an increasingly mature grasp during the latter part of the first year, avoidance reactions and prehensile reactions must interweave in ways that permit the child to begin to reach, grasp, and finally to release objects that are first contacted, held, perhaps used, and then put aside. Indeed, releasing objects is a far more difficult task for the child than securing them. It is not until the twelfth to fourteenth month that the normal child is able easily to let go of an object. In some brain-damaged youngsters, a letting-go schema is often difficult or impossible to accomplish.

Rhythmic Actions, Stereotypies

It was suggested in Chapter 5 that various flappings and wavings of the limbs and trunk constitute important signs of early neurological training. Whether this is true or not remains to be seen. However, the existence of these actions and their placement in time seem strongly to suggest that they are in some way developmentally useful to the infant. These rhythmic stereotypies appear in several forms that involve the hands, arms, and fingers. Moreover, their appearance coincides with the appearance and refinement of the reflexes previously discussed, as well as with the onset of stages in early voluntary hand-eye coordinations of the young infant (Thelen, 1979).

Thelen has documented the appearance of several types of hand, finger, and arm movements in infancy. At times these movements were done with objects, and at other times the limb-hand was without a "load." These actions were divided into those involving objects and those without. Arm waving, for example, is seemingly divisible from arm banging, when the arm-hand contacts a surface at the end of the downward excursion. Arm banging can also include the use of an object to make a noise upon contact during the downward movement of the arm-hand. Other arm stereotypies seen in infancy include a rhythmic clapping together of the hands in a pat-a-cake movement, as well as a back and forth movement of the arm and rubbing an object against a surface; also scorable are arm actions involving a circular rubbing of the ear or hair near the ear.

During infancy, the hands normally are seen to make two kinds of rhythmic movements: (a) a rhythmic bending and extension of the wrist, and (b) a rotating action of the hand involving alternating pronation and supination.

Scorable and observable finger movements in infancy include: (a) a flexion response that may or may not include scratching a surface as the fingers (sometimes all four) come in contact with something, and a flexion response without any surface contact; and (b) a finger rotation that involves a turning outward of both the fingers and the hand. These actions are shown in Figure 8.1.

As can be seen in Figure 8.2, stereotypes reflecting manual abilities do appear, primarily during the second half of the first year. It is possible that this is true because the hands and arms become free from their support functions by that time; the infant need no longer rest upon hands and elbows when in a prone position. Or they appear in order to prepare the child for actions using the hands. It is also interesting to note that the distribution of finger actions occurs throughout the first year of life, without evidencing marked differences from the fourth to fifty-second week.

Further work should serve to define more precisely the functions of these interesting and ubiquitous actions. The manner in which they interact both with the reflex changes noted previously in the hands, as well as with voluntary grasp reactions, would be interesting and useful topics of further research. Additionally, patterns of stereotypies among neurologically impaired youngsters would be fruitful to contrast to the findings of Thelen, who used normal infants as subjects (Thelen, 1979).

Early Signs of Object Awareness and Contact

Infants begin rather early to detect the presence of objects and their movements. Additionally, various protective movement responses are often seen if an object is made to travel at moderate speed toward infants. The head will turn away, and the arms will seem to be attempting to ward off an impact with the object. Controversy exists, however, as to just how basic are tendencies for the infant to display early manual contacts with objects.

Bower (Bower et al., 1970), for example, seems to take an innate position. He and his colleagues found that infants within the first weeks of life would expect to contact objects with their hands. When the objects were projected holographic figures, their young subjects would evidence consternation, concern, and various physiological responses reflecting surprise and agitation. Not all researchers in the intervening years, however, have been able to replicate Bower's results (Franco and Muir, 1978). At the same time, if there *is* an apparent built-in hand-to-object expectation in youngsters, it seems to disappear and then reappear again in a more sophisticated and complicated form later in infancy.[1]

[1]This tendency of some behaviors to appear, disappear, and then reappear (discussed also when the stepping response was covered) is termed *decalage* by child development specialists.

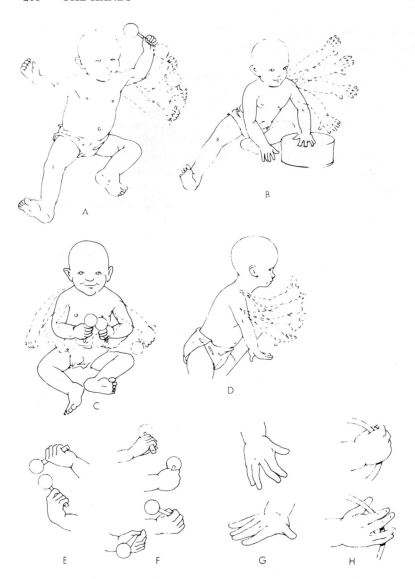

FIGURE 8.1 Rhythmic stereotypies of the arms, hands, and fingers. (a) Arm waving with object. (b) Arm banging against surface. (c) Banging both arms together with object. (d) Arm sway. (e) Hand flex. (f) Hand rotation. (g and h) Finger flex. From E. Thelen, "Rhythmic Stereotypes In Infants," *Animal Behavior,* 27 (1979) pp. 699–715. With the permission of the editors, Bailliere, Tindall, London.

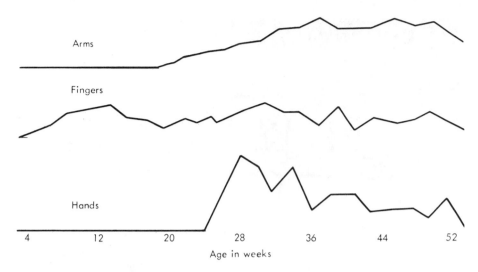

Arms

Fingers

Hands

| 4 | 12 | 20 | 28 | 36 | 44 | 52 |

Age in weeks

FIGURE 8.2 Frequency and distribution of rhythmic stereotypies during the first year. Frequencies have been expressed at each age as a percentage of the total "bouts" of that stereotypy group seen at that age. The vertical scale on the left is the same for each horizontal axis. From E. Thelen, "Rhythmic Stereotypes in Infants," *Animal Behavior*, 27 (1979), pp. 699–715. With the permission of the editors, Bailliere Tindal, London.

A more traditional and popular conception of the emergence of early object-hand behaviors in infants involves the gradual learning and unfolding of both visual-perceptual and motor behaviors. Initially, visual inspections of both moving and stable objects occur somewhat separately from movements of the hands and arms. Then gradually, in a number of steps, the two behaviors are put together.

The infant, it has been hypothesized, passes through several major stages in the acquisition of the hand-eye coordinations needed to contact objects. During the first two to three months, the infant spends a great deal of time visually inspecting the surroundings, including both static and moving objects. This inspection period also includes visual attraction to the infant's own hands (White and Held, 1967).

During these same first months, objects coming into view are likely to elicit what Bruner (1964) has called *athetoid responses*. These movements consist of spastic-like extensions and contractions of the limbs, without any apparent contact or purpose. At times, the appearance of objects during the first 90 days of life will elicit other changes in behavior. These can include modifications of heart rate and changes in the sucking response, as well as respiratory changes.

During this inspection period, a number of ingenious researchers have determined that the infant is able to perceive the three-dimensional characteristics of objects, despite possible changes in orientations relative to the child. A cube viewed head on is not seen simply as a square, but is viewed as the same object if rotated so that it assumes various shapes relative to the child (or imposes different retinal images) (Bower, 1966; Day and McKenzie, 1973; Caron et al., 1979). More accurate perceptions of the manner in which things of the same shape might appear under

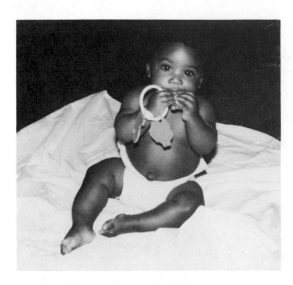

FIGURE 8.3
Mouthing is an important adjunct to
manual inspection of objects and adds
useful information.

various orientations seem to be enhanced by experience. That is, if the child has
once seen that an object can assume various apparent shapes, discrimination will be
facilitated if that object appears again (Ruff, 1980).

Another important motor response may also be seen during this early period.
The child frequently extends an arm when in the presence of a distant object. This
behavior was originally believed to mean that real reaching was being attempted,
with the infant evidencing poor depth perception. However, more recent hypotheses
have included the proposition that this apparent fruitless reaching reaction is a
method of somehow using the arm and hand to "measure" depth, and the properties
of visual space, by the immature infant (Bower, 1974).

Mouthing will also occur, along with visual inspection, during this period.
Objects placed in the hand will be brought immediately to the mouth (Uzgiris,
1967). Thus, rather early in life the mouth becomes an important prehensile tool
through which the infant gains information similar to that acquired through the
hands. Toward the termination of this first period, inspection of objects becomes
more precise, and less and less time is wasted on new objects, or on details previously assimilated in previously viewed objects.

SECOND, THIRD, AND FOURTH STAGES OF MANIPULATIVE
BEHAVIOR

Second Stage: Third to Tenth Month

This second stage is marked by an expansion of manipulative behaviors.
Swiping at objects becomes elaborated, refined, precise, and slowed down during
the middle and latter parts of this period. Objects may be in the hands while various

rhythmic stereotypes occur, and thus things are shaken, struck against surfaces, and even released in primitive throws.

During the third month, the hands often meet at the body's midline, initially to rub against each other and later to conduct simultaneous inspections of objects (White and Held, 1967). This midline grasp may be stimulated by early handling and visual enrichment of the infant. The action may also help to train the visual apparatus to converge at near-point, a quality later needed when reading and writing at close proximity to the body. At first both hands will hold objects or inspect them in similar ways. Within a month or two, however, the hands will evidence differentiated functions. One may hold the object (usually the nonpreferred one), while the second (the preferred) will engage in more precise manipulations of the object or of its parts. Hand preference may thus begin to emerge, in ways discussed in Chapter 9.

Even during these early weeks the infant may make manual contact with moving objects. Von Hofsten and Lindhagen (1979), for example, found that infants at about 18 weeks of age were able to "catch" objects moving at about 30 cm/sec. At this same time they were also successfully reaching for stationary objects. The early onset of these interception and reach behaviors suggested to these reseachers that the prediction of an object's future location when moving, and its interception through motor efforts, is innate (Von Hofsten, 1980), rather than being a carefully learned behavior composed of discretely acquired stages. Even experimental arrangements that made it difficult for infants to see their own hands when reaching did not seem greatly to disrupt reach and object contact responses at about this time of life (Lasky, 1977).

With practice, reaching reactions toward both moving and stable targets become more accurate and precise. Also, with maturation targets moving at increased speeds may be contacted (Von Hofsten, 1980). Finally, and most useful, the infant begins to slow down when reaching toward objects near the end of this period. The child is said to be displaying a "Piaget-like" reach. This consists of first carefully inspecting the object and slowly bringing the hand toward it, while glancing back and forth from hand to target until contact is made (White and Held, 1967).

This period of life is also marked by an increased tendency to exploit objects. The infant seems intent upon discovering what objects can do, what their properties seem to be. Among the types of exploitative behaviors seen at about this time are these: (a) Objects are struck on surfaces. (b) Objects are picked up, transported, and released. With practice, they are placed into smaller and smaller holes and containers. (c) Objects are dropped, and later crude throws are seen as objects swung through the air are pulled away from the hand because of the outward force that is exerted.

Objects are examined in ever more complex ways during this same time. Uzgiris, for example, has identified the emergence of what she terms an "examining" schema at about the sixth month that continues through the tenth month of age. This schema consists of poking at objects to ascertain rigidity, feeling surfaces and parts to obtain ideas about texture, and turning objects to gain information about shape. This tactile information is paired with visual information obtained as the infant watches the object in his or her hands.

Toward the end of this period, at about the tenth month, objects will be used increasingly to elicit social responses from others (Chapter 13). Things will be held out and shown to nearby adults and to adjacent children. If the parent or peer mistakenly takes the object offered, objections will usually be voiced by the apparently unselfish child. The purpose of this kind of showing schema is to initiate social contact and is at first not the unselfish offer to share a plaything with another (Uzgiris, 1967).

Third Stage: End of the First Year to the Middle of the Third Year

Toward the end of the first year and the beginning of the second, a number of shifts in manual activity will take place. A explosion of the graphic behaviors, beginning with scribbling, will emerge and gradually become refined during this period. This subphase is discussed later in the chapter. Additionally, as the second year begins and progresses, verbal behaviors will become more likely to be paired with manipulative efforts. For example, midway through the first year, Uzgiris has identified the appearance of what she terms a "naming" schema. The child will accompany the first efforts at naming things with simultaneous picking up of the object to be named. It is apparently useful to the child as first efforts are made to acquire nouns and other parts of speech. Experimental work with young children indicates that simultaneous handling of objects, together with naming them, enhances verbal retention (Uzgiris, 1967; Levin, 1978).

A final and most important trend is also noted toward the termination of this period, during the second and third years of life. More and more, a normal child will begin to substitute thought and simple visual inspections for direct contacts with objects. Previous matchings of tactual perceptions of shapes and of other qualities of objects with their names and functions enable the youngster more and more to cease handling everything, to confine efforts to the exploration of new and novel objects. Thus, as previous motor copies are contrasted cognitively and visually with contemporary objects and matches are made, only new motor copies need be acquired through handling.

Fourth Stage: Early and Middle Childhood

A fourth stage begins near the beginning of the fourth year. This is characterized by two main classifications of behavior, one of which involves translating sounds and thoughts into letters and words. The second main manual ability emerging in the 4-year-old involves the ability to begin to integrate and coordinate manual schemas with other behaviors (motor, perceptual, verbal) occurring simultaneously. Thus it is not unexpected that children of 4 and older will become able to run, to watch a ball, and at the same time to position hands and fingers in readiness to intercept the ball. Objects may be carried while walking and not forgotten or dropped, as might have happened a year or two earlier. Dinner-time conversation may be held while the youngster successfully manipulates knives and forks.

This final period, lasting from early to later childhood, is marked by increasing efforts on the part of children to explore their manipulative potentials as they relate to the arts. Musical instruments are played well by many children. Others expand their artistic abilities by gaining the capacities to represent thoughts, forms, and things with increasing sophistication during this same time of life (Kellogg, 1969). The skills needed in sculpturing, wood carving, and clay modeling are often developed during this period, given encouraging conditions.

Each of these four stages overlap in time. The infant and child will often progress and retrogress in the kinds of manual skills in evidence. At the same time, there are many subsequences of behaviors within each of the four stages described. In the following sections, a survey will be made of some of the more important parts of these developmental sequences.

LEARNING SEQUENCES WITHIN THE FIRST MONTHS

A number of scholars have proposed a sequence of learned acts that lead toward mature manipulative efforts (Trevarthen, 1979; Williams, 1983). Studies have been carried out to provide baseline normative data from which to study the effects of various enrichment programs on young infants (White and Held, 1967). These sequences, which reflect learning, contrast somewhat to models which suggest that many hand-eye coordinations are inherent, built in prior to birth (Bower, 1974).

The steps in this type of sequence are as follows:

1. During the first week of life, infants attempt to visually center their eyes on an object, and then extend the fingers of one or both hands in its direction. If objects are moved slowly, they are tracked through movement of the eyes, and sometimes by the torso, hands, and even feet (Trevarthen, 1979).

2. By the second week the infant may anticipate reaching objects by displaying grasping movements, and extending and withdrawing the arm. At times, movements of the mouth and tongue are seen in the presence of objects.

3. Also during these first two months, infants may be seen to make thrusting movements of the arms and hands toward objects. It has been suggested that these constitute a method of focusing attention, rather than signaling real attempts at manipulation (Hofsten, 1982).

4. As objects continue to be swiped at in the space field, the infant discovers body parts, including the hand. The fist is increasingly brought in front of the eyes, and by the third month, the fist may open and close while being inspected (White and Held, 1967).

5. At this same time, the first crude contacts with objects are made with ballistic throws of the arms that at first seem to contact objects by chance.

6. By 5 months, a more controlled form of reaching appears. Arm movements toward objects and head movements become coordinated (Trevarthen, 1979). A slowing down occurs that involves the Piaget-type reach described previously, as the hand is brought toward objects, with alternate glances being made from hand to object as con-

tact is made. At times the first attempts to touch objects will be accompanied by a closure of the eyes, as the infant seems to wish to concentrate more on kinesthetic cues emanating from arm and hand position.

7. The next step in object contact involves a crude palmar grasp reaction. The object rests against the palm, and the fingers close as a unit around the object, trapping it between fingers, palm, and thumb.

8. Following the sixth month, and as the tenth and twelfth month approach, infants exhibit more precise and delicate finger contact with objects. One or two fingers may contact an object and capture it between fingers and hand. The fingers may travel over objects to gain information about their (a) size, (b) rigidity, (c) weight, (d) location, (e) texture (smoothness versus roughness), (f) distance from the child.

9. Measurable differences may be seen between the quantity of manipulative activity engaged in by boys and girls. Moreover, full-term infants have been seen to manipulate more vigorously than pre-term infants (Kopp, 1976).

10. Finally, during this last half of the first year of life, qualities possessed by the objects may influence manipulative behaviors by infants. Objects differing in shape seem more interesting to children and encourage more handling than do those differing in color, for example (Ruff, 1982). Objects that permit modification seem more stimulating to the manually explorative infant than those that are rigid and unchangeable.

During the first year, when these manipulative actions become more refined, a number of other sequences intermesh with the ones just described. For example, various concepts about objects' weights and sizes serve to modify how an object will be gripped and otherwise dealt with muscularly. Furthermore, the two hands become more coordinated and act as a single examining unit. These and other sequences are described below.

For the most part, novel shapes elicit more exploration by infants. But as novelty wears off, there is lessened interest and thus diminished manual contact. This tendency has led to the formulation of a motor copy theory to explain the perceptual and conceptual underpinnings of manual behaviors in infants and children (Sokolov, 1960).

According to this model, orienting reactions of infants both manually-tactually and visually are alerted when in the presence of novel stimuli. As this information is acquired and stored neurologically, future stimuli are contrasted to already acquired images. If subsequent visual stimuli and/or objects are different, they are acquired and also stored. However, if successive objects (either seen or seen and touched) correspond to already stored impressions, inhibitory mechanisms in the nervous system tend to block additional visual and/or tactual inspection. Often an increase in manipulative variability is seen among infants of this age range (Moss and Hogg, 1983).

Age differences in the amount of tactual-manual activity may be explained using this model. The younger infant, and the child needing to establish a base of stored impressions, needs to engage in a vast amount of manual exploration, coupled with visual inspection. And indeed this is the case. However, as more and more impressions become stored with age and experience, there is a lessening of manual and visual-manual activity, except when confronted with new and novel information.

DIFFERENTIATION AND COORDINATION
OF THE TWO HANDS

Most manual activities confronting both children and adults require both hands. Often different parts of the task are assigned to each hand. This differentiation of hand function must be learned by the infant. At the same time, an opposite quality is necessary, the putting together of the two hands in various actions. Thus the infant and young child is faced with seeming paradoxical problems: (a) how to assign different functions to each hand, and (b) how to get the two hands to work in concert. These two contrasting qualities emerge early in infancy, and continue to mature and interact well into childhood. After the sixth month, many children can transfer a cube from hand to hand, for example (Noller and Ingrisano, 1984).

Initially the infant may accidentally discover that indeed two hands exist on the body by accidentally touching them together. During the third to fourth months, infants will continue this contact in front of the eyes, at the body's midline, and can be seen rubbing one hand with the other. In this way the initial perceptions needed for later bimanual controls are gained, together with some sensory information about both hands.

Often, by the sixth month children can evidence differentiated functions in either hand. One hand, usually the nonpreferred one, may hold a large object, while the other (usually the preferred) will examine a part of the object with more precision. It may be several years, however, before one hand is easily able to cross over into the space field in front of the opposite shoulder when manipulating objects. For the most part, this early bimanual manipulation of objects takes place directly in front of the youngster.

More and more, as two hands are employed, they may be differentiated as to force applied. By the end the first year and into the second, a vigorous movement may be made with one hand, while the other may remain relatively relaxed. As maturity occurs, less and less overflow will be seen from one hand-arm to the other, as one is being used vigorously (see Chapter 9). Differentiation of function matures well in neurologically intact children. By the fourth year, for example, it has been found that youngsters become able to make movements that cross the body midline with some ease (Schofield, 1976). Bilateral manual activity may take place within various space fields around the body as convenient, with further practice and maturation.

FINGER DIFFERENTIATION

Infants during the final half of their first year of life seemingly evidence a mature grip, and prehension of objects involves the finger pads, rather than the whole palm. As early as 18 months, for example, it has been found that some infants can grasp a grain of rice between their thumb and index finger, and by the third year this task is usually mastered (Noller and Ingrisano, 1984). It is a year or two later, however, before children are able to evidence precision in *individual finger movements*. Indeed, the ability to use each finger individually is often beyond the capacities of many brain-damaged youngsters, and they continue to use their hands as though they were encased in a fingerless mitten.

To evaluate finger differentiation, two primary types of tasks are employed. One is intended to determine how well a child is able to sense each finger. The hand may be hidden from view, and the child asked to respond either verbally or through a movement when individual fingers are lightly touched. The second type of test purports to discern how well the child can move each finger individually, and with what precision. This test of finger opposition is often used by pediatric neurologists to acertain possible neurological impairment, as well as by researchers exploring movement functions of the hands by children at various ages (Denckla, 1973; Grant, 1973; Holbrook, 1945). These and similar tests have been used to explore the possibility that some children lacking the ability to use individual fingers may also lack early mathematical skills because of the inability to use the fingers as efficient counters (Kinsbourne and Warrington, 1963; Neilson, 1938).

Early signs of finger differentiation appear within the first year of life. As has been mentioned, by the end of the sixth month children can be expected to oppose forefinger and thumb when picking up small objects (Kuhlman, 1939). Crude imitiation of finger-thumb opposition may be seen as early as the beginning of the third year in the presence of a visual demonstration of one action at a time (Kuhlman, 1939). However, while the motor abilities for this type of task seem to be present, perceptual discrimination of individual fingers seems to lag during early childhood. For example, only about 50 percent of the 3-year-olds in one study were able to touch each finger in order to the thumb, when the finger to be moved was touched by the examiner and not seen by the child. When the finger to be touched was indicated visually by pointing, there was only a slight improvement in performance.

In the 1970s several experimenters measured improvement in finger opposition, and related tasks, in children from 3 to middle childhood (Denckla, 1973, 1974; Lefford et al., 1974; Grant, 1973). Generally the task is scored under speed stress in either of two ways (a) number of cycles of finger opposition (forefinger to little finger, and back) within a given amount of time, or (b) the time to perform a single trip from first to little finger and return (Stott, 1966; Denckla, 1974). Touch errors are also scored when a finger is missed, in order to obtain an accuracy score.

Innumerable variations of finger opposition tasks have been employed. They have included repetitive touching of the forefinger to the thumb, finger opposition without the aid of vision, tactile cues as to which finger is to be touched to the thumb, nonvisual manipulation of various fingers to thumb in a sequence, and comparisons of finger opposition in the two hands under the various conditions outlined above (Denckla, 1973, 1974; Lefford et al., 1974). Regular improvement in this kind of finger differentiation task can be seen from the third to the eighth years. For the most part, girls are more likely to be superior to boys, but this does not always hold true. At times a plateau is reached at about the age of 5, but generally significant improvement is seen from the third to the fourth year, and from the

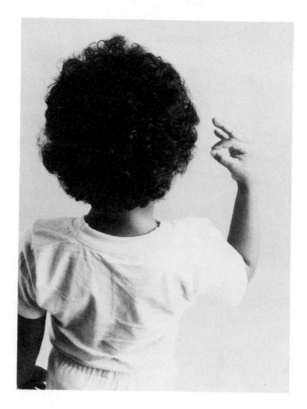

FIGURE 8.4
Finger opposition is a task frequently used to evaluate manual abilities and finger differentiation in children. Requiring a child to touch each finger in order to the thumb imposes a "target" problem for the placement of each finger.

fourth to the fifth year. Another significant jump in mean scores is usually recorded between the fifth and seventh years. Often the performance of children (particularly girls) at 8 years approximates that of adults.

Third year. At 3, the task, when demonstrated visually, is a difficult one for the majority of children. Only about 30 percent can be expected to complete a cycle of finger opposition under these conditions, and it is carried out slowly and with a great deal of visual inspection by the child. If more input is given to the child during the demonstration, more children will be successful at this age. For example, if the examiner touches each finger and guides it to the thumb in order, about 85 percent of 3-year-olds will be successful. However, if the movement sequence is attempted at this age without visual inspection as it is performed by the child, less than 30 percent will be successful.

Fourth year. Significant improvements are seen in the various ways this task may be performed by the middle of the fourth year, when contrasted with the scores of 3-year-olds. Over 30 percent will now be successful when the task is demonstrated visually, while with manual guidance almost all will be able to perform it reasonably well.

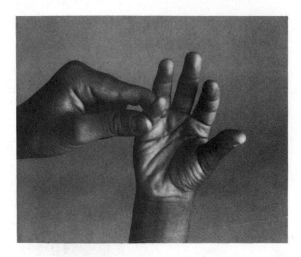

FIGURE 8.5
Children of three need their fingers manually guided in order that each reaches the thumb.

Fifth year.   Twice as many 5-year-olds can successfully execute a cycle of finger opposition than was true among 3-year-olds. Moreover, with less and less information during the demonstration phase of task administration, more 5-year-olds will be successful than was true among 4- and 3-year-olds. When the demonstration, for example, includes both manual guidance and visual inspection by the child, virtually all 5-year-olds can complete one successful cycle of finger opposition (Lefford et al., 1974).

Sixth to seventh years.   This kind of finger quality continues to improve during these two years. Cycles are made more rapidly and more accurately than was true among younger children (Denckla, 1974). Tasks involving finger opposition and those requiring children to touch a single finger repetitively to the thumb evidence improvement at 6 and 7 years.

Overall it is found that superiority in the preferred hand is seen more often in tasks requiring successive touches of the same finger, while sequential finger movements (finger opposition) are often performed equally well by both the left and right hands in right-handed children (Denckla, 1974). Right-handed superiority is also seen among children exposed to cutting circles with scissors (Zurif and Carson, 1970), as well as when engaging in precise placement of small objects (Rapin et al., 1966). Thus both hemispheres seem to contribute to repetitive and apparently purposeless actions, whereas when the actions involve sequencing and an obvious objective, it is possible that there is a greater contribution by the left hemisphere.

Precision of finger movement is an important quality in the childhood motor skills armament. This type of precision seems essential when the child begins to try to master shoelace tying, dressing, and using buttons and zippers, as well as holding writing implements. Failure to develop this quality is likely to lead to considerable frustration as the youngster begins to try to master the various everyday self-care skills demanded by parents during the formative years.

COGNITION AND MANIPULATION

Numerous parallels might be drawn between movements of the arms and hands and thought. Some of the more obvious are measures of object permanence discussed in Chapter 1 and the emerging abilities of a child to grasp and remove the cover of an unseen but desired object. This resolution of a problem through action constitutes an important concept called *equilibration* in Piagetian theory. This means that essential to learning is the child's resolution of apparently confusing and conflicting information. And in this resolution, positive change in mental growth takes place.

T. G. R. Bower has, in a now classic study, demonstrated how equilibration may be seen in the maturing infant and child as objects of different sizes and shapes are grasped and accommodated to with varying degrees of force. This sequence takes place from before the sixth month of age until the middle of the second year.

Prior to the age of 8 months, the infant grasps objects in a relatively unchanging way: Some infants habitually close the hand hard, while others have a more flaccid grip, but in general they are consistent within themselves. At this age, there is some accommodation to the varying weights of objects, but the accommodation is not anticipated; that is, the infant does not prepare the arm and shoulder muscles to support a large and/or heavier object by using only visual cues prior to its coming into the hand. Thus, when infants of this age are presented with an object, the arm may quickly drop as the object is grasped by the hand; the infant is not ready quickly enough to adjust it its weight (Figure 8.6).

During the following months further accommodations take place, and infants at times will adjust more quickly to falsifications in initial judgments of the weight of objects seen but not immediately handled. Bower suggests that this kind of adjustment to object-size-weight undergoes the following four changes during the first months of life:

Stage I   (prior to 6 months): No differentially produced arm-shoulder response to objects of different weight.

Stage II   (about 7–8 months and older): Differential response to objects of different weight after initial grasping has taken place.

Stage III (about 1 year): The response of the arm-shoulder musculature differs, but the child anticipates that the same object will weigh the same on repeated occasions.

Stage IV   (18 months): Response differs, or remains the same, based on two premises: (a) that the same object will weigh the same upon repeated presentations; and (b) that objects varying in length will correspondingly vary in weight.

By the ninth month, according to Bower, this seemingly inefficient behavior changes. That is, the infant, on the first trial, suffers a hand-arm drop due to unexpected weight changes as he or she grasps an object. But upon a second presentation, as shown in Figure 8.7, a kind of kinesthetic learning has begun to take place, and the arm does not drop as much. The arm-shoulder muscle receptors begin to

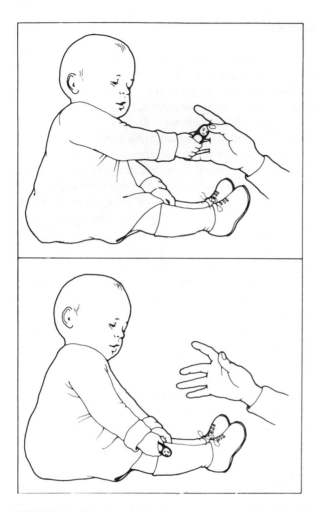

FIGURE 8.6 This picture shows two arm positions: (*top*) the position on taking the object, and (*bottom*) the position of the arm at the end of its first excursion. It clearly shows how the baby's arm falls as he or she takes the object. Drawn from photos in *Development in Infancy*, by T. G. R. Bower, San Francisco: W. H. Freeman and Company, copyright © 1974.

accommodate to the object weight upon subsequent presentations; in other words, the infant has begun to consciously or unconsciously correctly anticipate the weight of the approaching object when she or he has inspected it before. At this point, however, the adjustments are only for a specific object. When new objects are presented, the hand-arm quickly drops again, evidencing no ability to generalize shape-size-weight relationships and the adjustments in arm-shoulder musculature that are needed. As Bower suggests, a rule something like "the same objects weigh the same every time they are picked up" has been formulated. But newly perceived and handled objects still present problems of kinesthetic adjustment.

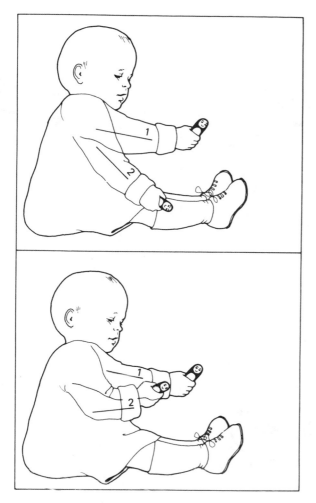

FIGURE 8.7 Each picture shows two arm positions superimposed: the position on taking the object, and the position of the arm at the end of its first excursion. On comparing the top and bottom pictures, it can be seen that the information about the weight of the object gained in the first presentation is applied immediately on the second presentation of the same object. Note the greatly diminished arm excursion. Drawn from photos in *Development in Infancy*, by T. G. R. Bower, San Francisco: W. H. Freeman and Company, copyright © 1974.

Midway through the second year of life, another modification occurs. Behavior appears which suggests that the child is anticipating the weights of objects to be presented. Thus, if the infant is given one object of a given weight and size, and then handed a second of the same size and shape, but heavier, the arm will suddenly "fly upward." As seen in Figure 8.8, the child overestimates the weight of the object because of some kind of prehandling response set. Such generalizations as "the longer an object will be, the heavier it will be" are established, leading toward more efficient kinesthetic adjustments, as revealed in behavior produced when the "rule" is violated by the clever experimenter.

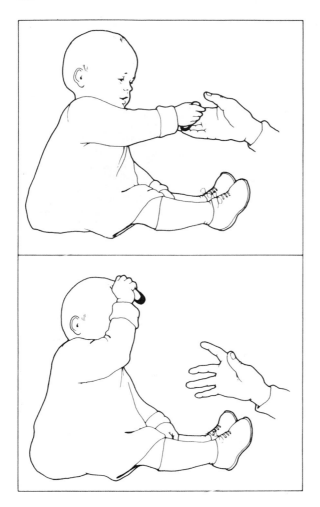

FIGURE 8.8 Here the baby has overestimated the weight of the object and her arm flies up. Drawn from photos in *Development in Infancy*, by T. C. R. Bower, San Francisco: W. H. Freemen and Company, copyright © 1974.

These first stages in the use of and judgments about objects represent rudimentary first steps in a process that continues throughout childhood and even in adulthood. As the child confronts more and more objects to be used as tools, continued adjustments must be made. The objects must be incorporated into the child's total body schema, and their uses refined with practice. These first calibrations documented by Bower and others are the first stages in a series of calibration and recalibration processes. The use of such tools as pencils, sticks, and the like continues to be refined long after these implements are merely grasped by the young child. First the hand is used as a tool, and then the hand uses tools that are relatively short and light in weight. Finally, heavier and longer tools come to be used by the child (Schwartz and Reilly, 1981).

As tools are used, two types of feedback systems are operative: (a) one involving the use of direct visual feedback obtained as an action is in progress, and (b) a second system involving the conceptual formulation of programs, and the comparison of results of tool use with expectations. More and more reseachers are beginning to explore skills that bridge the gap between the child's use of the hand and the use of extensions of the body in the form of tools of various kinds.

At least nine different types of grips have been identified when children and adults grasp an object, for example (Moss and Hogg, 1981). Thus analyses of grip must take into account not only precision and power, but just how the hand happens to rest on an object while manipulating it. Only when grip and tool use have been analyzed as a system can the manner in which children gain the ability to use tools be properly analyzed.

GRAPHIC ABILITIES: FROM SCRIBBLING TO WRITING

Scribbling has been described by more than one author as a type of kinesthetic or "motor" babbling similar to the primitive vocalizations commonly produced during infancy. As the child matures, scribbling and the forms that arise from early efforts take on momentous proportions. The inability to print and to write well may be labeled a *specific learning disability,* and greatly lessens chances of success in the first grades of school.

In a less serious vein, graphic representations of a child's emotions, visual impressions, and thoughts can be fun and creative. Several useful research programs have explored the esthetic qualities emerging in youngsters' desires to produce artistic renditions of their lives and feelings.

The stages through which children pass when scribbling and learning to draw and to write are generally as follows:

1. One child may simply attend to a writing implement by holding it; another child may use this implement to make marks on paper and on other surfaces.
2. Crude scribbling is engaged in and random marks are made seemingly without any plan and without producing any coherent designs.
3. The child reacts to some kinds of stimuli on the writing surfaces. He or she may draw lines and squares, and may balance out a figure on one side of a piece of paper with a spiral of scribbling on the other side.
4. Simple geometrical figures are drawn, usually consisting first of crude crosses and simple spirals.[2]
5. More exact geometrical figures are drawn; figures are placed in combinations of two and more; and pictures are colored with increasing accuracy.
6. More complex designs are made; drawings are made of people, of houses, and of other objects familiar to the child.

[2]In general it has been found that the higher primates (gorillas and chimpanzees) are able to accomplish steps 1, 2, and 3 and can often make simple crosses on a page, such as one short line crossing another short line.

7. Block printing and cursive writing are taught in school and are learned by the child.
8. With proper training and/or interest, pictures and figure drawings of three dimensions and involving increased complexity are drawn.

The Grips

As children begin to use writing implements, their technique undergoes predictable changes. Scribbling and early marking efforts are accomplished by a crude grasp, sometimes backhand, in which only the pencil touches the page. The arm and hand are in the air, unanchored. Later the elbow and little-finger side of the hand may come to rest on the page, and movements may be made with actions of the hand and figures moving as one unit. Finally, sometimes with instruction, the child will begin to evidence a more mature writing technique. The fingers and hand move separately. The hand anchors, while the fingers move together. This may occur sometimes between the fifth and seventh years. Children with problems perceiving their fingers may adopt other methods, including putting all fingers on the pencil. A hooked grip is sometimes used by left-handers, so that they will not cover the material just written. The adoption of a mature technique varies from culture to culture, depending on the emphasis upon graphic skills directed toward the young (Saida and Miyashita, 1979).

Scribbling

Although it does not often seem so, the scribbling behavior of the infant from 15 months to 2½ years and older proceeds within reasonably discernible stages.

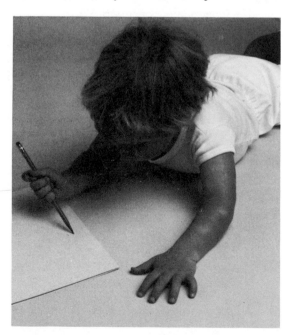

FIGURE 8.9
First attempts to handle a writing implement usually involve a crude grasp, using the fist, as shown.

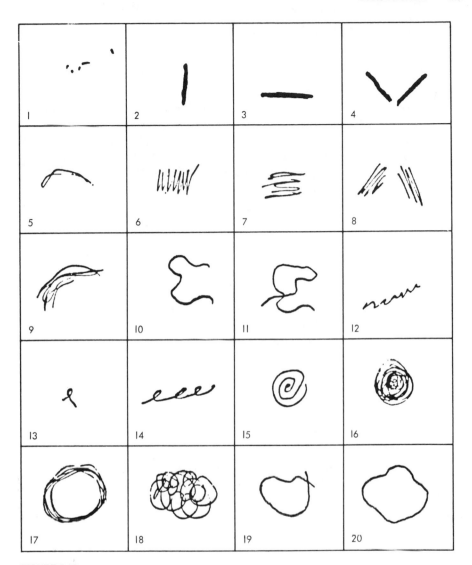

FIGURE 8.10

These sequences become apparent, however, if the efforts of a large number of children are analyzed and classified. One of the several scholars interested in this facet of a child's perceptual-motor behavior is Rhoda Kellogg, who during a period of twenty years collected and classified over 1 million drawings and paintings by infants and children (Kellogg, 1969).

Kellogg lists four steps in the acquisition of hand-eye control seen in drawing and writing. These include the scribbling stage; the combine stage, during which diagrams and combinations of two diagrams are drawn; the aggregate stage, during which three or more geometrical figures in combination are drawn; and the pictorial stage, during which pictures are made with increasing accuracy.

Within the initial scribbling stage, about twenty substeps are identified by Kellogg (Figure 8.10). Despite these classification systems, it is difficult to obtain exact developmental norms for the acquisition of various degrees of drawing and scribbling competence because of the influence of a number of variables on children's efforts. It is obvious that a child who observes others writing and drawing within the home and who has pencils and other implements available will acquire competence before a child who has no opportunities to observe and to practice drawing skills. The reader should keep in mind, therefore, that perhaps more than other skills, scribbling, drawing, and writing are shaped to a large degree by conditions within the home environment.[3]

Random and Repetitive Actions

The initial stages of scribbling may emerge by accident as a child makes a mark on one object with another object. The visual cue becomes reinforcing, and other marks are made. The first marks are usually done hesitatingly, and with practice these marks become bolder and more repetitive.

As can be seen in Figure 8.10, the majority are circular in shape (5, 9, 15, 16, 18, 19, 20). The next most frequent are alternating lines (11, 12, 13, 14), while there are only two each that are vertical (2, 6), horizontal (3, 7), and diagonal (4, 8). Kellogg *does not* believe that these appear in any regular order. However, combinations of these designs may be used to construct most letters, numbers, and a variety of representative pictures of people, structures, and the like. Thus these scribbles, like the primitive babblings of infants, seem to provide basic data that is later molded into a variety of realistic graphic representations important in art and in the classroom, just as primitive speech particles are combined and modified into words important in a culture.

The first scribblings seem stimulated by the joy children find in the movements themselves, as well as in the marks made. However, during the second and third years, youngsters may begin reacting to visual characteristics of what else may appear on a writing surface (Goodenough, 1926). Some of these reactions involve responses to visual forms seen on a page. Moreover, children from different cultures are likely to respond differently, even at this young age. Japanese children have been found to fill a page with repetitive but intricate designs, while children from other cultures may place a single figure in the middle of a page, or from a central figure tend to work outward (Alland, 1983). Young children from artistically rather bland environments, even at these early ages, may not produce as great a quantity of simple figures—nor will the figures evidence the variety seen in the drawings of youngsters living in more artistically rich cultures.

---

[3]Kellogg's amazingly detailed text contains an important chapter entitled "Children's Art as a Mental Test," in which the author poses important questions for those attempting to evaluate mental and emotional attributes through children's efforts at drawing geometrical designs and representational figures—i.e., the human figure. I believe her evaluation of these tests is among the most lucid I have encountered, and I recommend it to the readers of this book.

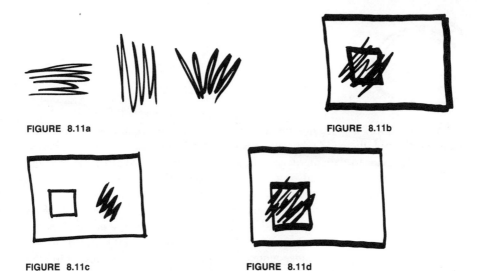

FIGURE 8.11a

FIGURE 8.11b

FIGURE 8.11c

FIGURE 8.11d

Children from all cultures will begin to react to stimuli confronting them. For example, if a form is on a page, they may obliterate it by marking over it (Figure 8.11b). On the other hand, children may try to "balance" a form on a page with efforts on the opposite side (Figure 8.11c). If the form is large, children may begin to evidence a desire to stay within its boundaries (Figure 8.11d).

Enclosing Space

As more control is gained, children will slow down their movements and begin to attempt to guide them with the eyes (during the early and middle parts of the second year). The first efforts within this second phase seem to evidence a need to enclose space (Figure 8.12). These lines may rove and contain a loop or two (Figure 8.13). They may be made by children as young as 2.5 years.

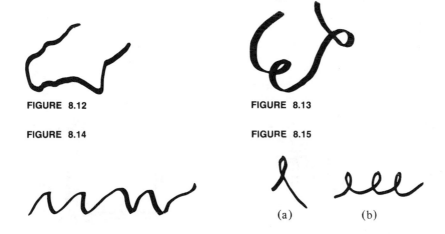

FIGURE 8.12

FIGURE 8.13

FIGURE 8.14

FIGURE 8.15

(a)

(b)

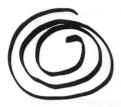

FIGURE 8.16

Waving lines, usually horizontal but at times either vertical or lateral, may appear shortly after the child begins to enclose space in a restricted area on the page (Figure 8.14). Prior to the emergence of the often seen ''curly-haired'' loop is the single loop, which is followed by a repetitious loop (Figure 8.15).

After children find that they can travel with the repetitive loops, they discover that they may make a spiral within a smaller amount of space (Figure 8.16). With practice, they may produce an overlaid circle, and then gradually a circle that contains multiple circumferences with a clear center will emerge (Figure 8.17). As the circular movement is placed under more strict control, the child begins within the third or fourth years to make imperfect circles consisting of a single circumference (Figure 8.18).

At about the same time that children's scribblings evolve to the ability to make a crude circle, children's efforts may also lead them toward the drawing of rudimentary squares. First attempts at replicating geometrical configurations usually take the form of simple crosses, and with practice they make repetitive crosses with both horizontal and vertical lines (Figure 8.19). Thus by 3 years, children begin to attend to characteristics of visual models they may try to copy. By the time children

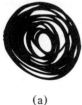
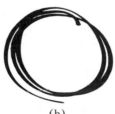
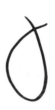

(a)   (b)

FIGURE 8.17 (a) Overlaid circle. (b) Circle with several   **FIGURE 8.18**
circumferences.

FIGURE 8.19 (a) Simple cross. (b) Crossing-bar configurations.   **FIGURE 8.20**

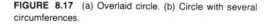
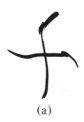
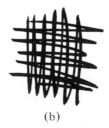

(a)   (b)

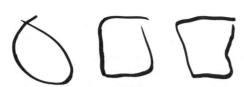 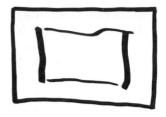

FIGURE 8.21   **FIGURE 8.22**

reach the middle of the third year, they may begin to enter what has been described as the diagram phase. Squares may begin to emerge in several ways. Children may begin to leave spaces within repetitive vertical and horizontal lines (Figure 8.20).

At other times, they may begin to "square off" circles (Figure 8.21). Another child may copy squares by following the sides of the paper with straight lines (Figure 8.22). By age 4, more and more angles are seen in children's drawings.

The Diagram Phase

Numerous investigators have produced studies describing the qualities seen as children from 4 to 12 years reproduce various geometric figures. Often it is assumed that early success in these endeavors will be predictive of letter printing, and thus of first-grade success. Indeed, some data support this contention. Vane (1968), among others, has found moderate relationships between early figure drawing accuracy and success in the first grades of school.

Conceivably, however, the skills needed to draw geometric figures (alone or in combinations) involve different neural processes (and different hemispheric participation) than does the reproduction of letter forms containing verbal-cognitive meanings. It is thus sometimes found that children who may "fail" figure drawing tests, even as young as 5 years, will be able to produce legible letters. These qualities are seen in the figure drawings of children of various ages.

Five years.   The 5-year-old shows considerable improvement, particularly in the production of angular figures, when compared to the more rounded figures seen in the 4-year-old's drawings. By 5, in most cultures, clear differences will be seen between drawings of circles and squares if the child is provided with visual models of each to copy (Noller and Ingrisano, 1984). A 5-year-old will make a clear and accurate cross with lines, while the 4-year-old may still have difficulty with this task. More than one-third of all 5-year-olds will be able to produce a recognizable triangle (Birch and Lefford, 1967) containing properly proportioned sides and in a correct orientation. Lines will become straighter and angles of figures more sharp by the sixth year. Five-year-olds may tend to draw figures, and their first letters, larger than will be the case a year later.

Six years.   At 6, angular figures improve, and they are more likely to be drawn in a continuous motion, moving from side to side, than was true a year earlier. The child may be anchoring arm and hand more, and thus produce difficult figures such as the triangle and diamond in smaller size than was true a year earlier. Maximal change may be seen in children's diagrams between the fifth and sixth years, according to some investigators (Birch and Lefford, 1967). Diamonds continue to plague the 6-year-old, and they are not drawn well until about the eighth year by both boys and girls. Most if not all 6-year-olds will draw triangles in a proper upright position, without any rotations. Moreover, shapes are drawn with lines that are considerably straighter during the sixth year than was true a birthday earlier (Ilg and Ames, 1965).

Seventh to the ninth years.   More and more children can execute freehand drawings of common geometric figures during these years, including the previously difficult diamond. Variability of performance decreases during these ages, and normal children more and more tend to resemble one another in the rendition of geometric figures. The use of line grids, drawn to scale, seems to facilitate geometric figures at these ages, as the children seem to be able to grasp the notion of scale (Birch and Lefford, 1967).

Diamonds are drawn in correct spatial orientation by most children at these ages, while the quality of the lines forming figures continues to improve. As children grow older, they tend to become consistent in directional behaviors. That is, figures tend to be drawn in ways that begin at the upper-most angle and proceed downward, and they begin at the left of the figure more often than to the right (if the children are right-handed) (Bernbaum et al., 1974; Cratty and Martin, 1970). We have found in our investigations that right-handed children usually begin in the upper left-hand corner of figures and proceed in a counterclockwise direction until the figure is complete. Left-handers usually start in the upper right-hand corner and proceed clockwise.

Combines and Aggregates

The combine and aggregate stages are developmental levels labeled by Kellogg and occur during the years in which children draw single geometrical figures. The combine stage is marked by the attempt of a child to combine more than one figure at a time into a pattern (Figure 8.23). The aggregate stage involves the inclusion of three or more figures into various designs (Figure 8.24). The

FIGURE 8.23   **FIGURE 8.24**

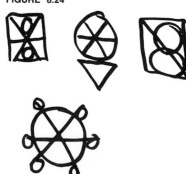

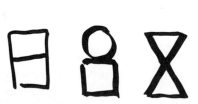

mandala-shaped aggregate in the lower part of Figure 8.24 is seen, according to Kellogg, in many cultures of the world (Kellogg, 1969).

Pictorial Stage

Around the age of 5, children begin also to draw pictures of things within their environment. Their first efforts are often unrecognizable, but in the next several years more accurate pictures will be drawn. Often the first *thing* to be drawn will be the tadpole man, a circle with line-like legs extending directly from it (Gardner, 1973). This is considered a pivotal point in the development of graphic behaviors by children. Moreover, as pictures continue to emerge from children, two major types of "artists" have been identified.

One type has been referred to as a *patterner*. This child tries for accuracy in drawings, producing draftsmanlike representations to the limits of his or her ability (Gardner, 1973). A second type has been labeled a *dramatist*. This child makes up elaborate, often romantic descriptions for what are often ill-formed figures. As Arnheim has stated, such children draw equivalents of seen objects, and then employ verbal symbolism to enhance the drawing when asked about it (Arnheim, 1964).

Goodnow (1977) has identified several stages through which children pass reflecting general ways their drawings evolve:

1. At first they are extremely thrifty with their uses of forms and units. They experiment with a basic vocabulary of movement strokes. A circle containing random dots may stand for a human.
2. Next, parts are related to each other in line with specific principles. In the case of the human figure, arms and legs are added to a circular face.
3. Parts are related in sequence. Children begin and end drawings using a regular pattern. The order in which they add parts to a human figure, for example, is consistent and predictable.
4. Finally, at the most mature level, children draw things which indicate that their graphic thinking approximates that of most adults.

As children begin to reproduce simple forms in space, it is infrequently found that these take the forms of objects within their world. Circles are labeled "suns" and "faces," and triangles and squares are sometimes called "houses."

Some of the more important objects within the environment are the other people with whom children associate; thus it is not surprising to find that they begin to attempt to reproduce the human form.

As in the case of the aggregates previously discussed, the various forms of the draw-a-person test are utilized to assess a wide range of subtle and obvious attributes in children including emotional stability, intelligence, and social competency. In addition, the accuracy with which a child draws the human figure has been employed by many researchers to assess body image, intelligence, and social adjustment. Ilg and Ames utilize a test in which an incomplete figure is presented and the child is asked to complete the drawing (Figure 8.25).

Several researchers have traced the manner in which skill in drawing the hu-

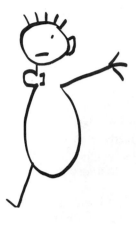

FIGURE 8.25

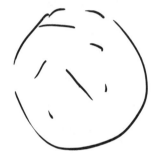

FIGURE 8.26

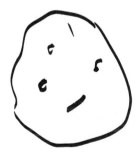

FIGURE 8.27

man figure evolves in the maturing child. In general, the following sequential steps emerge. Circles with marks in or around them are seen first (Figure 8.26). The circles begin to contain marks that represent facial features (Figure 8.27).

The round face begins to evidence "stick" arms and then legs projecting directly from the circumference (Figure 8.28). The tadpole man shown has been found in many cultures, but may be delayed in appearance in some ethnic groups relatively devoid of artistic stimulation for their young (Alland, 1983).

The figure gradually becomes more refined. The figure may be drawn with a continuous outline, but at the same time more and more parts are discernible (Figure 8.29). Finally, the limbs assume two dimensions, or width, as shown in Figure 8.30.

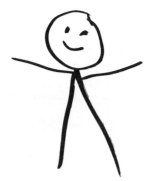

FIGURE 8.28

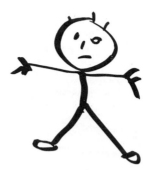

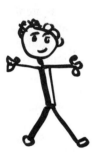

FIGURE 8.29

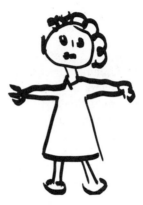

FIGURE 8.30

Printing Letters and Numbers

Paralleling efforts at drawing various figures, houses, and the like are attempts on the parts of 4-, 5-, and 6-year-olds to print letters and numbers. When printing letters, the 4-year-old is likely to scatter them on the page; he or she has no stable base line for the efforts. Lettters may be placed on their sides and may be slanted to varying degrees.

Many 5-year-old children are able to print their first names. And by the age of 6, most children can print the alphabet, their first and last names, and the numbers from one to ten. According to research by Stennet and his colleagues, lowercase letters are somewhat more difficult to copy than uppercase letters. Even at the end of the third grade, there remains difficulty in reproducing the lowercase letters. Letters with horizontal and vertical strokes (H, I, T) are easier for the young child to replicate than letters with slanted lines, or those combining curved and slanted lines (D, Z, G, N) (Stennet, 1972).

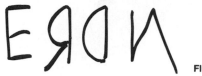

FIGURE 8.32

By the sixth and seventh years, the letters are aligned horizontally, as are the numbers. As children mature, the sizes of their efforts change. The 5-year-old child is likely to make letters and numbers from .5 to 1 inch in height; some even utilize 2 inches for their productions. By the age of 7 years, however, children utilize only about .25 inch for each number and letter they attempt.

The 5-, 6-, and 7-year-old children are likely to have difficulty arranging their figures in an even manner. Uniform spacing of letters and numbers is not achieved until about the age of 9. Richards and his colleagues (Richards, 1975) formulated a "name printing" test with which to assess developing maturity in children 5 and 6 years of age. Over 2,000 children were used in the experiment, which produced good interrater reliability and positive correlations between name-printing accuracy and the teacher's appraisals of the children's general classroom performance.

Each child has a unique way of writing numbers and letters during the formative years. The 7, 8, and 9 are often executed in two parts using two separate strokes, and the 3, the 4, and the 5 are often written in a continuous manner (Figure 8.31). Children of 5 and 6 years may reverse numbers and letters in a variety of ways. Individual letters and numbers may be reversed (Figure 8.32).

At times, two-digit numbers may be reversed: 10 may be written as 01, and 20 may be written as 02. A lack of rhythm may be seen as children reverse the order in which they write two-digit numbers; yet the number will appear in its final form in the correct order. For example, the child may write the 5 before writing the 1, but the number 15 will appear correctly. According to Ilg and Ames, about 60 percent of all the 5 ½-year-old children reversed letters and numbers, and 52 percent of the 6-year-old boys and 64 percent of the 6-year-old girls reversed their numbers. By the age of 7 years, however, only about 12 percent of the children surveyed evidenced reversals of numbers and letters (Ilg and Ames, 1965).

FIGURE 8.33
(a) Cylinder, (b) Face-on cube, (c) Point-on cube.

Three-Dimensional Representations in Drawing

Ilg and Ames tested the ability of children between the ages of 5 and 10 to copy correctly various three-dimensional forms. This kind of task proved considerably more difficult than copying the two-dimensional figures discussed previously. Three forms were utilized in their evaluation of this interesting task: a cylinder, a face-on cube, and a point-on cube (Figure 8.33).

The 5-year-old child is likely to represent the cylinder with a single circle and will often state that it represents either the bottom or the top of the figure. Until the age of 8 years, the child will draw a rectangle in response to the cylinder and state that it is the front of the figure. By the age of 7 years, only about 22 percent of the boys and about 32 percent of the girls were able to make a fair replication of the cylinder, but the base was likely to be drawn straight rather than curved. By the age of 8 years, about 22 percent of the boys and 28 percent of the girls drew a curved base line to their cylinder. By the age of 10 years, about 40 percent of the boys and 64 percent of the girls drew a reasonably accurate replication of the cylinder.

Drawing both the point-on and the face-on cubes proved equally difficult for the children tested by Ilg and Ames. Usually between the ages of 5 and 7 years, the children gave little indication that they were aware of the three-dimensional characteristics of the two figures, and they often drew single squares or diamonds in response to the stimulus figures. Even at 10 years of age, most of the children surveyed evidenced difficulty in putting together all the surfaces of the two cubes in the correct perspectives. By the age of 10 years, the boys were slightly superior to the girls in the drawing of both figures, and the point-on cube proved easier to replicate than did the face-on cube. About 34 percent of the girls and 46 percent of the boys drew a correct point-on cube by the age of 10 years, but only 2 percent of the girls and 20 percent of the boys could correctly draw the face-on cube at the same age. The researchers note that this is one of the few figure-drawing tasks surveyed in which the performances of boys were superior to those of girls.

By middle and late childhood, many youngsters will become able to depict a third dimension within two-dimensional drawings of people, places, and things. With proper instruction in artistic principles that imply depth, relatively mature landscapes and portraits may emerge from the paintboxes of many children by the ages of 8, 9, and 10.

THE PERFORMANCE OF FINE MOTOR TASKS
IN CHILDHOOD

A variety of other tasks have been and are employed to evaluate the dexterity of children. Often these tasks are scored with the child under some kind of speed stress. The object may be to drop as many pennies as possible into a small slot within 30 seconds, for example. At other times the tasks involve an integration of the left and right hand in an alternating manner, or the task performance is scored for each hand separately, and the results compared.

A two-handed task involving the winding of string around a spool has been used (Holbrook, 1945). Marble dropping tasks are often employed (Stott, 1972), as are tasks requiring the child to construct things from two or more objects. Stott uses several such tasks in his test at the 5-year-old level. A bilateral aiming task is also found in the Stott battery at the 7-year-old level, requiring a child to push a pencil into holes on a board held by the other hand. This task, like many similar measures, is timed.

Bilateral placement of two matchsticks, moved simultaneously, was used on the different versions of the Oseretzky and has survived in various modified forms today. Threading beads has also been used (Keogh, 1968).

Most of these tasks require precise grasp by forefinger and thumb, transport of an object, and placing it with precision into a small hole. However, other tasks to which children have been exposed involve more macroscopic hand-eye coordinations. Williams, for example, reports the results of an investigation sampling what she terms "dynamic eye-hand coordination." She used a pursuit rotor to determine how well children from 5 to 12 years of age could keep the tip of a stylus in contact with a spot on a rotating disc in the shape of a phonograph record (Williams, 1983).

The measure used was time on target, and overall there was a linear improvement with age. Children at 12 could contact the moving target about three times longer than was possible by 5-year-olds. Boys were slightly superior to girls in later childhood and continued to improve after the age of 10 and 11. Girls' mean scores, on the other hand, plateaued in late childhood.

In a variety of manual skills, particularly when scored under conditions which require that the child work accurately and rapidly, youngsters continue to improve during childhood. As children gain experience attacking such problems and formulating strategies that work better and better, performance increments will usually be recorded. It is difficult to determine, particularly after middle childhood, how much improvement may be attributed to (a) changes in neuromotor maturity, in contrast to (b) experience in formulating useful work methods and attending to other cognitive and perceptual components of the problems confronting them in such situations.

SUMMARY

The development of the human hand, and its ability to move with precision, parallels other emerging qualities in children, including language and cognitive behaviors. The first movements made by the infant's hand involve the intricate interweaving of variations of the prehensile reflex, coupled with subtle avoidance responses of hands and fingers. Objects when first seen by the infant are reacted to in a spastic-like manner, with no real contact taking place. It is only with maturation and experience that the child becomes able slowly to reach an object, grasp it, and examine it in any kind of organized manner.

Although controversy exists as to whether hand-to-object contact is learned or innate, most agree that the abilities are acquired in discrete phases. These include moving from crude swiping responses to more delicate examining actions, often involving both hands.

By the ages of 3 and 4, a variety of manual abilities may be assessed in children. These include fine finger dexterity, usually measured in finger opposition tests; simple graphic behaviors, assessed with simple drawing tasks; as well as manipulative activities involving self-care skills such as dressing, washing, and the like.

Distinct changes in the sophistication of movements of the hands, as well as in drawing behaviors, are recorded when children of 5, 7, and 9 are contrasted. Letter size is reduced, while letter accuracy improves dramatically from ages 5 to 7, and later. Likewise, the sophistication of artistic renditions also changes markedly from early to middle childhood.

QUESTIONS FOR DISCUSSION

1. Relate the material found in the next chapter (9) dealing with handedness to the facts given in this chapter reflecting early manual behaviors.
2. With what kind of daily living tasks needed in childhood might measures taken from various forms of a finger opposition test correlate?
3. What graphic and manual behaviors might be used on checklist (pass-fail) used to measure these qualities in a 3-year-old? a 7-year-old?
4. What kinds of drawing behaviors are seen in many cultures? What kinds of drawing behaviors and associated abilities seem molded by cultural influences?
5. How do cognition and hand-arm adjustments seem to relate in the example given of equilibration in the chapter? What stages are involved in this example?
6. Can you give another example of equilibration involving manual dexterities not specifically described in the chapter?

7. What does the motor copy theory mean relative to the presence or absence of play objects in a given cultural setting? What behaviors might you expect from children from a bland versus an enriched culture when various objects are present? What qualities in objects seem to elicit the most and least manual inspection by maturing children?

8. What kinds of tasks are used to assess manual dexterity of children in middle and late childhood? What role does the concept of speed stress have in these evaluations?

9. What sex differences are seen in various manipulative and graphic behaviors displayed by maturing children?

10. How do language and manipulative behaviors interact? Can you give specific examples?

STUDENT PROJECTS

1. Evaluate children of 3, 4, 5, and 7 in tests of finger opposition. What kinds of variations in administration are necessary to permit children of various ages to do this task? What kinds of self-care skills are dependent upon this kind of quality?

2. Observe an infant from 1 to 3 months of age. Do you notice, or can you record, any hand-arm stereotypes? What kinds of grasp and avoidance reflexes are you able to elicit? Can you relate the nature and strength of these to the infant's age?

3. Collect the drawings of children from 5 to 7 years. What differences do you notice in quality, quantity, accuracy, and/or sophistication? Can you relate these to possible opportunities the various children have had to practice with writing implements?

4. Using a manual task, such as placing pennies for speed into a small opening, study the influence of speech stress upon the accuracy of performance of children from 8 to 10 years of age. When you require faster speed, what accuracy decrements do you notice?

5. Study how difference in direction may alter the kind of human figure drawn by a child of 7 to 8 years of age. Vary your directions: draw a person; draw a child like you; draw a child as accurately as you can (and press for more details); or draw your family.

CHAPTER NINE
QUALITATIVE CHANGES
IN MOVEMENT BEHAVIORS

Some dimensions of infants' and children's emerging physical qualities are easy to identify. Obvious changes such as jumping heights and distances, running speeds, and how far a ball is thrown are among the more traditional measures of interest for those who have studied motor development. However, a number of more subtle qualities and capacities that interact in important ways with children's movements have not been given a great deal of attention by scholars. Some of these represent qualitative changes reflecting how well the child is able to demonstrate increasing efficiency when calling up and exhibiting efficient neuromotor programs. Other qualities contribute to, or detract from, the movement capacities the child and youth may exhibit once the motor program has been formulated.

Some of these qualities have been measured for over a century by experimental psychologists. These include reaction time and handedness. Other qualities have been given attention by clinical neurologists studying what happens when the brain undergoes trauma. These latter, more subtle molders of movement characteristics include the ability to plan a series of movements, as well as the degree to which the child can focus movement in select body parts, rather than exhibiting extraneous overflow of actions in body parts not directly involved in the task at hand. Often important lessons about how normal movement qualities develop in the maturing child may thus be learned by observing how actions appear when the nervous system has been traumatized.

It is believed that only by considering some of these parameters can we gain real insight into how children and youth mature motorically. Therefore, in this chapter we survey five of these qualitative dimensions of movement activity: (a) The laterality of the body, including the symmetry and asymmetry with which the body seems to function. (b) Reaction time, usually defined as the time taken for the individual to begin to react to some kind of situation or stimuli. (c) Overflow, or the appearance and disappearance of tensions and movements in body parts not directly involved in the task at hand, (d) Motor planning, sometimes referred to as praxic behavior, reflecting the degree to which the youngster is able to produce a reasonably complex movement series in response to commands, demonstrations, or thoughts. (e) Rhythm.

These qualities are not neatly divisible, and they often interact. Reaction times that are prolonged may reflect problems in effective motor planning. Additionally scientists and developmental specialists have not distributed their efforts evenly throughout these categories. Overflow has been paid only cursory attention by measurement specialists, while recently laterality and cerebral dominance have enjoyed a resurgence of effort of remarkable proportions, reflected in literally hundreds of articles, coupled with several survey texts (Springer and Deutsch, 1981; Corballis, 1983; Bryden, 1982; Bradshaw and Nettleton, 1983).

A chapter about these qualities was included in this text for several reasons. First, previous surveys of motor development either ignored these dimensions or passed over them in a cursory manner. Second, it is believed that understanding the contributions of these more subtle parameters of developmental movement provides insights into the processes underlying the acquisition of action capabilities by the maturing child and youth. Third, evaluative efforts will become more sophisticated to the degree to which these less obvious motor qualities are understood. Finally, it is hoped that some readers, becoming intrigued by this material, will begin to explore in more depth and with more precise measuring tools qualities that have been afforded only cursory attention at this point.

LATERALITY: MOTOR FUNCTIONS

Humans have long been intrigued by the fact that maturing children prefer to use one hand or the other in intricate tasks. Special attention has been paid throughout the ages to those perplexing individuals who seem to prefer their left to their right hands. No less a personage than Charles Darwin wrote in 1877 about the changing handedness of his son (Corballis, 1983), believing that the hand switching he noted during the first months of the child's life was due to qualities inherited from his relatives. More recent research has documented this same tendency in the early acquisition of handedness, but has given reasons for it not in line with Darwin's contention.

Other kinds of movement asymmetries have been scrutinized in recent and past investigations. These include head-turning responses and food preferences, as well as functional asymmetries associated with motor functions, including ear and eye preferences.

Contemporary interest in handedness and functional asymmetries of other kinds, as well as in possible associations with cerebral specialization and the lateralization of speech functions, has exploded in the form of hundreds of investigations since the late 1970s and in several review texts.[1] Accompanying this increase in interest are numerous controversial issues surrounding the development of lateralization in the child, and how hemispheric specialization of functions may be reflected in, or influenced by, one-sided preferences in hearing and eye use, as well as biases in hand and foot use.

The collection of more and more data has resulted in the formulation of several basic questions, including: (a) Whether asymmetries in hemispheric functions are caused mainly by innate biological tendencies inherited from parents, or are influenced by environmental stresses and experiences; (b) how relationships between preferred hand use and other neurological and behavioral asymmetries reflect either normal deviations from the "average" or pathological problems worthy of concern.

The focus in this section is upon motor functions and their asymmetries. A thorough consideration of even this one type of preference is made difficult because of (a) the different ways in which foot and hand preferences are measured, and (b) the often weak relationships between hand preference, eye preference, foot preference, and other asymmetries. Furthermore, it should be pointed out that despite the protestations of some to the contrary, there is only a weak relationship between preferences in motor function (hand usage for example) and hemispheric specialization. Most left *and* right-handers, for example, control speech functions in their left hemispheres, while spatial abilities are for the most part localized in the right hemispheres of both (Satz, Achenbach, and Fennell, 1967).

Early Motor Asymmetries

One of the first clear-cut asymmetries seen in the motor patterns of the infant is an unequal manifestation of the tonic neck reflex (Chapter 3). Like later handedness, there is a moderate but clear-cut bias of human infants to turn their heads to the right when evidencing this reflex (Leiderman and Kinsbourne, 1980; Michel, 1981; Turkewitz, Gordon, and Birch, 1965). Furthermore, several researchers have found that the side toward which an infant usually displays this "fencer's response" is moderately predictable of later hand use (Gesell and Ames, 1947; Michel 1981). Michel (1981), for example, in studying 20 infants with either left or right preferences when displaying this reflex, found a significant relationship between the directions the infant turned and hand preferences within the first year of life.

---

[1]Bryden (1982), Bradshaw and Nettleton (1983), Corballis (1983), and Springer and Deutsch (1981).

This relationship between reflex tendencies and hand use is far from a perfect one, however. It is unclear, for example, if the hand-turning preference to the right is a reflection of similar biases in right head-turning orientations seen when infants are presented with both aversive and nonaversive stimuli (Leiderman and Kinsbourne, 1980), or whether the bias in the tonic neck reflex is independent of other head-turning biases researched.

Despite some early indications of right preferences in both head-turning responses and in the tonic neck reflex, the assumption of clear-cut hand preference is not always apparent during the first months of life. When carefully measured, for example, both reaching and grasping responses are seen to shift from those predominantly of the right hand and then of the left hand during these formative weeks (Gesell and Ames, 1947). The infant's motor patterns seem to indicate an uncertainty as to which will later be the preferred hand. One hypothesis attempting to explain what is taking place suggests that as the brain hemispheres mature in uneven ways, first one and then the other may assume control over hand preference. Thus the infant may manifest this shifting of hand preference as first the right and then the left hemisphere matures throughout the first year of life.

The reasons presented for the fact that most human infants begin to manifest right hand use by the end of the first year are plentiful and varied. For example, some have suggested that the right hand is freer in the womb, resting against the yielding abdomen of the mother; while the left hand prior to birth is in a restricted position against the mother's back. Therefore some believe that the right hand has received more prenatal exercise than has the left. Others have explained that the right-turning tendency in the tonic neck reflex simply permits the infant to view the right hand more than the left, and thus right-handedness later predominates (Harris, 1980). Still others have postulated complicated neurological explanations for right hand preferences seen in most infants. These hypotheses are often combined with genetic explanations for hand preference tendencies toward the right in humans.

According to recent work the infant's cerebral hemispheres may be specialized for somewhat separate functions within the first weeks of life (Molfese, Freeman, and Palermo, 1975). Heart-rate changes (Glanville et al., 1977), as well as tremors in the arms and legs, have evidenced differences depending upon the types of auditory stimulation reaching either hemisphere of the newborn. This evidence in turn has prompted some to suggest that early hand usage similarly reflects early hemispheric specialization. Drawing conclusions between early hand usage and lateralization and maturation of the cerebral hemispheres, however, is fraught with peril. Most authorities suggest that hand usage is only a superficial manifestation of cerebral hemisphere maturation and function (Corballis, 1983).

At the same time, however, the findings from several interesting studies have indicated possible relationships between the localization of speech-language functions and hand usage. Kinsbourne and McMurray (1975) found, for example, that speaking interfered more with right-hand finger tapping than with left-hand finger tapping. This suggested to them that the overflow from speech centers usually located in the left hemisphere interfered more with right-hand functions controlled by the same hemisphere than was true when the left hand was moving. Ingram produced similar findings linking hand usage with speech functions in children from 3 to 5 years of age (Ingram, 1975).

Kimura (1976), after analyzing data reflecting speech-language functions, has formulated an interesting contemporary hypothesis linking right hand use with the verbal communicative functions usually controlled by the left hemisphere. Her theory may explain why most infants, children, and adults are right-handed, and the relationship between left hemisphere speech-language properties and right hand use in humans. She suggests that right hand use in gestural communication by primitive humans is carried over into later written communication with the same hand. Right hand use coupled with left hemisphere specialization for speech-language thus became linked early in our evolutionary development and persists today. Evidence that even now right-handed people gesture more with the right hand when speaking further supports Kimura's interesting idea.

In addition to hand use, infants evidence a striking right preference consistency in the stepping reflex at birth. According to several researchers (Peters and Petrie, 1979; Melekian, 1981), the foot that leads in this reflex is likely to be the right. The apparent inability of the environment to alter this right-stepping tendency has led to the speculation that this kind of foot preference may be a more valid indicator of cerebral specialization than are early biases in head turning or in reaching responses.

The findings of studies surveying hand usage in both infants and children have produced more questions than answers. For example, it is clear that among children, just as is true among adults, degrees of handedness exist. While most people are found to be predominantly right-handed, there exists a sizable percentage who use their left hands in many tasks. Many left-handers, as evaluated by preference for writing, use their right hands in other tasks. Some of this confusion is also created by the lack of correspondence often found when scores from various measures of hand preference, foot use, and/or eye and ear preference are contrasted. Traditional measures of hand use include performance preferences, level of dexterity, as well as questionnaire self-reports. Often it is found that both children and adults are largely oblivious to what hands they use in many daily tasks. In any case, in the following section some information concerning how hand usage develops in children is surveyed. These data should be helpful to those attempting to teach motor skills to youngsters during middle childhood (Benton, Meyers, and Polder, 1962; Satz, Achenbach, and Fennell, 1967).

The Acquisition of Handedness

Although it has been pointed out that hand usage often fluctuates in early infancy, there is a gradual acquisition of preferred and stable hand usage that seems to become ingrained by early to middle childhood (Gesell and Ames, 1947). The criteria for one-hand usage seem to play a part in determining when a preferred hand has been "settled" on by the child. Ramsey (1980), evaluating handedness by noting what hands made contact with various toys, found no evidence for a right-hand bias at the fifth month. However, two months later a right-handed bias was recorded in the subjects. It was not until the first year of life, however, that Ramsey and his colleagues (Ramsey, Campos, and Fenson, 1979) found what he termed "differentiated hand use." That is, the supportive role of the left hand and the more active role of the right hand when engaged in complex two-handed manipulations and explorations seem to emerge later than does simply one-hand preference in direct reaching, contact, and manipulation tasks.

The data from several studies comparing the strength and apparent endurance of the grip of infants place hand preference at an age earlier than the fifth month. Tests given as early as the first and second months of life often indicate an advantage in strength and in duration of grasp by the right hand by the majority of infants tested (Petri and Peters, 1980; Hawn and Harris, 1979; Caplan and Kinsbourne, 1976). However, hand preference becomes quite apparent between the twelfth and twenty-fourth month (Rice et al., 1984).

Handedness appears to become more ingrained throughout childhood, and to develop just as does the child's perceptual and cognitive abilities. Coren (1981) and others have documented the increased tendency for right hand use by large populations measured from the nursery school years through adulthood. More and more innate, inherent, and genetic explanations are being used to explain the acquisition of handedness in infants, children, and adults. For example, most surveys of relationships between the hand use of parents and that of their offspring dating from the 1920s (Chamberlain, 1928) to contemporary investigations (Annett, 1973; Bryden, 1979) indicate that right-handed parents tend more to have right-handed children than do parents who are both left-handed. Moreover, it is more usual to find a left-handed mother producing a left-handed child than is true if only the father is left-handed. However, despite these tendencies a relatively substantial percentage of left-handed parents produce right-handed children (50 percent). So simple theories involving inheritance are being augmented by other explanations, often including the influence of environmental factors and social pressures.[2] The apparent innate nature of both neurological and functional asymmetries is further substantiated by the increased kinds of structural differences discovered when the right and left sides of the brain are surveyed (Geschwind and Levitsky, 1968).

A number of researchers have attempted to determine whether or not there are identifiable and significant differences in motor abilities when left- and right-handers are compared. The authors of these studies have differed as to the skills studied, as well as to how they have measured handedness and mixed preferences, so the findings are often difficult to evaluate and to compare (Vogel, 1935; Irwin, 1938; Horine, 1968). However, overall the data indicate that when a large, undiffer-

---

[2]A detailed survey of these models is impossible within the space available here. The enterprising reader might consult a survey by Bradshaw and Nettleton (1983), or more specific models proposed by Blau (1946), Annett (1964 and 1972), as well as by Levy and Nagylaki (1972) and Corballis and Morgan (1978). Recent data from 272 infants finding no parental relationships between hand preferences of their offspring also brings into question a simple inheritance theory.

entiated group of left-handers are compared to right-handers, little or no differences are seen in their abilities to perform physical skills.

Typical is the investigation by Horine (1968), who contrasted the motor abilities of four groups: (a) pure (or homolateral) right-sided, consisting of 35 percent of the sample; (b) predominantly right-sided (three of four laterality components being right, 45 percent of the subjects); (c) mixed laterality (13.6 percent of his subjects); and finally (d) pure left and predominantly left (6.4 percent of the subjects). Using measures of explosive strength, balance, agility, and motor educability, no significant differences were found when the groups were contrasted. Horine did, however, find slightly higher scores among those who were completely right-handed, and thus suggests that further studies be carried out.

In contrast was a study by Way (1956), who found that the subjects she tested exhibiting mixed preferences were superior in motor abilities stressing accuracy of movements and throwing to fixed targets, than were children who were predominantly right- or left-handed. It is possible that youths whose preferences appear to be mixed when life's daily activities are surveyed are those who can best adapt to sport skills requiring mixed preferences, as is the case for the switch-hitting batter in American baseball or the soccer-football player who may use both feet equally well. However, hard data supporting this assumption seem at present to be lacking.

Roth (1942) explored the possibility that dissimilar eye and hand preference may reflect problems in motor control and coordination. However, he found no differences between those whose eye preferences were similar to their hand preferences and those of mixed preferences, whose eye preferences were unlike the hand they preferred to use, when various scores of motor ability were contrasted.

Overall, these studies have not differentiated well among the groups evidencing various preference tendencies. In particular, they have not discriminated between left-handers who evidence a familial history of left-handedness and those who do not. It is possible that some left-handers who may have been forced to use their left hand because of a cerebral insult of some kind may evidence problems in some tasks requiring accuracy and/or control. However, data verifying this assumption are presently lacking.

Leg Preference

Many important skills in childhood involve single leg use. As was pointed out, leg preference seems to be one of the strongest and earliest indices of functional motor asymmetry seen in infants when the stepping reflex is elicited. Hand preference for the right side seems stronger in humans, ranging from 85 to 90 percent; however, foot preference is a close second, and 80 percent of all children seem to evidence right foot preference. However, as with handedness, foot preference is not a simple nor single quality, and its identification may depend upon the test. Vanden Abelle (1980) suggests a difference in the concepts of footedness and leggedness, and suggests that measures of this quality be considered separately and consist of (a) posture: what limb is preferred for load bearing when standing or kneeling; (b) operant behavior: leg used when kicking, stamping, or doing some complex motor task; and finally (c) locomotion: what leg is used when stepping forward.

Leg and hand preference tend to correlate, but the relationship is not a perfect one (Porac et al., 1980; Porac and Coren, 1979). Correlations also seem to be found when foot and hand *performance measures* are obtained (Peters and Durding, 1978). However, it is usual and normal to find both adults and children who may prefer the hand opposite to their preferred leg. Right-handers may tend to kick with their left foot (Annett and Turner, 1974). In addition, it is often desirable to teach a child to use both feet well in such sports as soccer or football. The child who may best be able to accommodate to teaching that encourages ambidexterity is one whose hand and foot preferences tend to be mixed, rather than one who does most things with either the left or the right foot. Indeed, some theoreticians believe that simple right-handedness or left-handedness is not inherited, but rather the strength or asymmetrical function may be what is inherited from one's parents. Thus the child whose parents are relatively ambidexterous may be the same child who may quickly accommodate to sports that similarly demand the use of both arms and/or both legs (Coren and Porac, 1980; Corballis and Morgan, 1978).

It is probable that a child's tendency to use a consistent leg becomes more marked with age, just as is true with hand use. However, at this point I am unaware of substantiating data on this subject. Overall, however, it is apparent that the human sensory processing systems and motor subsystems reflect a variety of asymmetrical functions and processes. Often these functions are poorly correlated. Expecting or demanding that a child will kick or throw with similar-side limbs is not in line with current findings.

Sex Differences

There seem to be marked differences in the manner in which cerebral functions localize themselves in females, in contrast to males (Buffery and Gray, 1972). Some have speculated that feminine superiority in some tasks may be due to the fact that general neurological maturation proceeds faster in girls than in boys. Overall, however, it is also apparent that there are more left-handers among populations of boys than among girls, and similarly left-handers tend to be less strongly lateralized (Loo and Schneider, 1979; Thompson and Marsh, 1976). Still, consistent data tell us that there are more boys among neurologically suspect populations. Thus there is a moderate but consistent relationship between sex, neurological problems, neurological maturity, and handedness.

Girls, consistent with the previous information, tend to be less likely to be ambidextrous than boys. However, some have speculated that females, sometimes more submissive to testers, may report handedness differently on questionnaires (Bradshaw and Nettleton, 1983). In any case, girls tend more to be right-handers, and in a paradox, tend to be more strongly handed (left or right) than boys, despite the fact that speech and spatial functions are more generally and broadly represented in the hemispheres of females than in males. That is, speech seems mediated to various degrees in both hemispheres of females, making women less likely to suffer speech losses when they incur cerebral strokes later in life. Studies dating back over a hundred years (McGlone, 1980) indicate that anatomical measures are more likely to be symmetrical in females than in males (Wada, Clarke, and Hamm, 1975).

The Puzzling Left-Hander

Sorting out the developmental meanings of handedness, sensory asymmetries, and hemispheric specialization is difficult enough if everyone is right-handed. However, the presence of left-handers in our midst makes theoretical and practical speculations even more tenuous. Just as is true among contemporary neurologists, left-handedness was a topic of intense speculation among the ancients. Scientific and pseudoscientific speculations attempting to explain why some of us are different in this way range from the bizarre to the sublime.[3]

Genetic theories are confronted with the fact that in many monozygotic twins one is a left-hander and one a right-hander (Boklage, 1980). Left-handed parents more often produce right-handed offspring. Most tenable are models that propose several types of left-handers—those who have somehow inherited the tendency, and others for whom left-handedness is some kind of neurological compensation, perhaps caused by some kind of insult or injury early in development to the left hemisphere of the brain. Still a third explanation is that left-handedness is acquired by some infants whose right hemisphere matures earlier than does the left (Annett, 1973; Zurif and Bryden, 1969).

Substantiation for a theory coupling brain pathology with left-handedness is found in numerous studies of clinically abnormal populations in which a disproportionate number of left-handers are often found (Springer and Searleman, 1980). Moreover, left-handedness is more often found in larger babies, as well as in other populations likely to undergo higher risk of birth trauma, including those born first or born later to older parents (Bakan, Dibb, and Reed, 1973).

However, a useful explanation for left-handers is that they may stem from several types of populations (Bradshaw and Nettleton, 1983). These include (a) those from an environment that has traumatized them, such as a difficult birth (the environmental pathological), (b) those inheriting the tendency from within a pathological population (the genetic pathological), and finally (c) a group who have normally inherited handedness (the genetic left-hander). Thus the simple presence of left-handedness in a youngster should not be taken as an indication that something is wrong, for indeed such a child may simply need to be taught differently—to hold the pencil in a way that permits observation of the writing without undue tension or strain. Moreover, left-handers in many sports contexts are desired and provide useful skills, as is true among first basemen in American baseball, as well as in the boxing ring. Indeed, some researchers contend that left-handers may be more crea-

---

[3]An interesting historical survey of the left-hander (the sinister sinistrial) may be found in the review by Springer and Deutsch (1981).

tive than right-handers because of the balanced involvement of both hemispheres in the formulation and execution of various tasks. In support of this contention is the fact that Leonardo da Vinci and Benjamin Franklin were both left-handed.

Overview

While much remains puzzling about handedness, cerebral function, and hemispheric specialization, current and past research has made several points clear. (a) Hemispheric specialization for speech and spatial functions bears only a slight relationship to hand preference in children. (b) Left-handedness and mixed preferences in both children and adults are often normal conditions and should not in themselves be a cause of concern. (c) Hand preferences and foot preferences appear rather early during the first year of life and continue to mature as development continues. (d) There are only moderate correlations between the various functional as well as sensory asymmetries, and thus it is not either unusual or pathological to find a child who kicks with one foot while writing with the opposite hand. Likewise, a child who prefers to use one eye in a sighting task will often prefer to write with the opposing hand. Finally, accommodation to left-handedness or mixed preferences have important implications for teaching and learning intricate one-handed skills deemed important by a culture, both in sport and in other aspects of life. (e) Hand preference, as well as mixed preferences, are not likely to be predictive of motor abilities or of levels of motor coordination and control.

MOTOR PLANNING

Even the casual observer of the newborn is struck with the often rigid and imprecise movement patterns that emerge. Bruner (1968) has characterized this time of abrupt, erratic, and seemingly purposeless movements the athetoid phase. By this term he refers to the similarity of these early poorly planned and executed movement patterns to those seen in some individuals who evidence the athetoid type of cerebral palsy.

Relatively soon, however, the infant's movement patterns smooth out, and actions of increased complexity are acquired. Most important, during the next months and years infants and later children are able to copy actions demonstrated by more mature and able brothers, sisters, friends, and parents. Later youngsters become able to perform actions when simply given the verbal command to do so, or when an object such as a hammer obviously requires that some kind of physical task be executed. In essence, therefore, the infant and later the child are able to perceive and to plan actions of increasing complexity with maturation.

This acquisition of motor planning abilities, however, does not proceed in the same way in all children. Some seem unable to chain together a series of actions into an integrated whole in the same efficient way that others can. Some children evidence confusion when given a simple demonstration of a daily task, such as shoe tying, while others not only effortlessly acquire essential self-care activities but rather quickly begin to learn a number of sport skills and to display artistic drawing abilities.[4]

Motor planning qualities in people were first studied by neurologists during the second half of the last century. Hughlings Jackson (1866) and others (Steinthal, 1871) began to notice that many who evidenced various forms of brain damage and the disruption of other behaviors, notably speech, also were apparently unable to perform simple voluntary actions of the hands and limbs and movements of the mouth and tongue. Later case studies of atypical adults revealed that this kind of deficit in motor planning was often independent of the individual's ability to understand what was required. Further work made it clear that motor planning problems (apraxic behaviors) were conditions separate from simple muscular weaknesses, and reflected instead problems within the central nervous system.

Motor planning problems, or apraxic behaviors, continue to be studied within various handicapped groups today, including the learning-disabled and brain-damaged child, as well as adult victims of cerebral strokes (Haaland, Porch, and Delaney, 1980; Wyke, 1971). Research of this nature has afforded important insights into the relationships between motor behaviors, speech-language functions, and cognitive-intellectual qualities (Kimura, 1982). Several writers are engaged in important searches for a theoretical rationale underlying motor planning deficits.[5]

More recently, researchers have noted that deficits in motor planning appear in some children who otherwise may be free of traditional and obvious neurological impairments (Gubbay, 1975). However, it was not until the late 1970s and 1980s that efforts were made to quantify motor planning capacities expected in normal children (Cratty, 1978; Cratty and Samoy, 1984; DeRenzi et al., 1980; Kools and Tweedie, 1975; Cratty and Gibson, 1984). Generally these contemporary efforts have focused upon (a) establishing general averages expected by children at various ages, and (b) attempting to analyze what subabilities may be required to execute various groups of tasks successfully. This research has also helped to begin the development of various tests needed to identify motor planning problems that may exist among children who are otherwise free of more obvious sensory, motor, and/or conceptual problems.

Developmentally, it appears that if children are presented with various actions normally seen in their culture, and whose complexity is not great, reasonable success will be seen by the age of 6 years. Children of 6 in one study responded accurately to such requests as "Pretend you are drinking a glass of water," "Clap your hands," "Pretend you are shaking hands with someone" (Kools and Tweedie,

---

[4]Some (Gubbay, 1978) equate overall motor coordination and physical awkwardness with motor planning problems.

[5]Those interested in exploring the theoretical underpinnings proposed recently might consult the work by Heilman et al. (1982), Heilman (1973), Roy (1978), Kelso and Tuller (1981). Motor planning problems are usually classified into several basic groups, including *ideational apraxia,* reflected in a lack of understanding of the movement itself; *ideomotor apraxia,* indicating an improper sequencing of a serial act; *limb kinetic apraxia,* involving an improper execution of a submovement; and *construction apraxia,* assessed when the child is unable to employ an object or objects properly and in proper sequence.

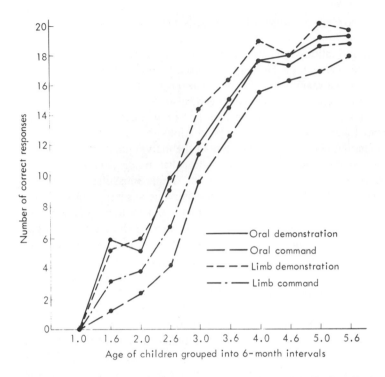

FIGURE 9.1 Changes in different types of praxic behaviors early in life. From Kools and Tweedie (1975), with permission.

1975). Easier for the younger children is to respond correctly when presented with a visual demonstration of the same movements. Kools and Tweedie (1975) divided their tasks into those involving the hands and arms and those involving the face and tongue ("Click your tongue and sound like a horse running"). Additional subdivision used tasks elicited by a verbal command and those triggered by a visual demonstration (see Figure 9.1).

This kind of division of the tasks has elicited the finding that in normal children, responding to visual demonstrations of both hand-limb movements, tongue and facial movements are of equal difficulty. This similarity occurs despite the fact that children can seldom see their own face-tongue actions, while those of the hands and limb are often easy to observe. More difficult for children are complex responses to verbal commands without an accompanying visual demonstration. Overall, it is becoming apparent that tests of motor planning in children should consist of several kinds of tasks, as often the correlations between these various measures are nonexistent or low (Cratty and Samoy, 1984; Kools and Tweedie, 1975; Conrad, Cermak, and Drake, 1983; DeRenzi et al., 1980). These tests should include:

1. Those involving the hands and fingers which require an imitation of a visual demonstration.

2. The imitation of limb movements, visually demonstrated.
3. Actions that replicate daily activities found in life. These may be demonstrated or commanded orally.
4. "Nonsymbolic" or nonsense actions not previously practiced by the child.
5. A series of actions involving the total body.
6. Actions required to be performed with objects, usually duplicating those used in daily activities.

Care must be taken to present such tests visually through a demonstration as well as orally on command. Often how the tasks are presented is more important than the part of the body involved (Kools and Tweedie, 1975).

The presentation of nonsense actions may reveal the maturity and facility of the child's right hemisphere. The duplications of actions that make sense and that can conceivably be translated into a verbal formula, on the other hand, may involve the maturation and health of the child's left hemisphere (Kimura and Archibald, 1974). However, hard evidence for this clear-cut division of functions of the two hemispheres is hard to come by. Indeed, a better case could be made that in normal children the left hemisphere is likely to mediate most motor planning functions.[6]

It appears that by the age of 6 or 8 imitation of both simple and complex gestures (both those that are life-related and nonsense movements) is able to be duplicated by most children. It appears, however, that the ability to engage in increasingly complex motor planning actions continues to mature after those ages (Kools and Tweedie, 1975; Cratty, 1984). In a series of studies we have carried out since the middle 1970s we explored motor planning tasks of several kinds. These included (a) the ability of children to duplicate from 1 to 7 hand movements in a series, (b) the duplication of from 1 to 7 limb positions in a series, (c) the ability to duplicate a series of from 1 to 7 positions jumped to on a mat marked in one-foot squares, and finally (d) the ability to duplicate the drawing of a figure containing 7 strokes of a pencil, with from 1 to 7 strokes presented at a time. These tasks were selected to represent a variety of motor planning qualities, including manual praxia (the hands test), limb praxia (limb positioning), trunk praxia (jumped positions of the total body), and finally the planning needed as geometric figures are drawn by the child. Additionally, other measures were contrasted to other task scores by children of various ages. These included measures of impulsivity (Cratty and Gibson, 1984), teachers' ratings of proficiency at small and larger muscle activity, self-control, and printing proficiency (Cratty and Samoy, 1984; Cratty, 1984).

Only the tasks evaluating the planning of a series of limb positions and hand positions correlated, and the correlations were small. Otherwise it seems more ap-

---

[6]This may not be true in some handicapped groups, however. In a recent study, we found that motor planning abilities in profoundly deaf children were equal to or superior to those of hearing populations tested, despite the probability that the deaf children did not have internal speech to describe the movements presented. Thus either the movements were amenable to right hemispheric processing by the deaf, or the deaf children possessed unusual visual memory, superior to that of the hearing children tested, because the former had had to depend upon visual memory when learning to sign (Cratty, Cornell and Omata, 1986).

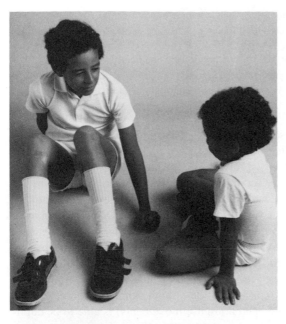

FIGURE 9.2 One kind of motor planning task requires the child to copy from 1 to 7 positions of the hand, demonstrated one a second.

FIGURE 9.3 Another kind of motor planning task we have used requires the replication of a series of arm-positions, from 1–7.

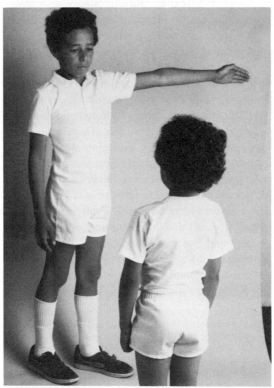

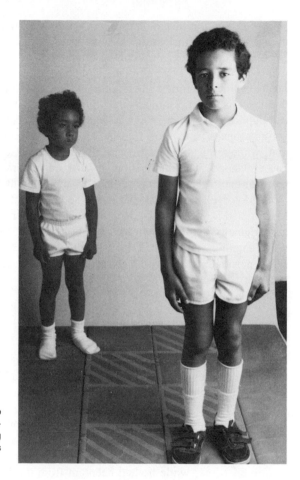

FIGURE 9.4 Motor planning can also involve the replication of a series of positions of the total body, remembering into what squares a previous child has jumped, for example.

propriate when discussing motor planning abilities (or disabilities) of children to specify just what kind of ability seems to be adequate or deficient. Conrad, Cermak, and Drake (1983) have also found that motor planning abilities should be described with specific reference to the type of test applied.

In contrast to our research, which was based primarily on tasks involving nonsymbolic (or nonsense) movements, Conrad and his colleagues used both symbolic and nonsymbolic tasks. These included symbolic motor planning involving the use of common objects (a comb, for example). Two other types employed included tests assessing what they term "optic-spatial" planning involving the imitation of nonsense positions and gestures, and (c) "dynamic qualities" evaluated by studying movements of the arms and hands, one of which resembled the test of hand praxis we have used in our research. They also found that at least two separate motor planning qualities were evaluated by the tests and in their discussion urge precision of evaluation of motor planning disabilities and abilities in both normal children and those with learning disabilities.[7]

Generally in our data children improved with age when given up to 7 movements to duplicate. For example, children of 5.5 years duplicated from 3 to 4 movements or limb positions when presented one a second; while children a year older duplicated about 5.5 movements on the average. By late childhood many children can duplicate 7 movements in a sequence. In a recent study, over 50 percent of the young subjects from 8 to 11 years of age could duplicate 7 positions jumped to on a mat, while replicating positions of the arms was also carried out with some ease by late childhood. The duplication of hand movements in the same children proved more difficult. They averaged under 6 positions at these same ages.

Motor planning tasks evidence few sex differences (Cratty, 1985; Manni, Martin, and Sewell, 1977). Moreover, for younger children the Gestures Imitation test originally devised by Berges and Lezine (1965) seems adequate. Tests that involve common implements, as well as those that contain up to 7 in a series of nonsense movements or positions, seem best when evaluating children older than 6 years of age.

OVERVIEW

Motor planning skills, if deficient, may represent a huge obstacle in the life of a child or adolescent. A few years ago we evaluated a 17-year-old boy about to graduate from high school. Although otherwise intact neurologically, academically, and intellectually, he was plagued by the inability to chain together useful series of movements necessary within three critical areas of his life. He had recently been fired from a part-time job because of his inability to make hamburgers successfully! His social life had been dampened because of his inability to learn dances important among his peers, while he had been cut from the basketball team because he had been unable to manage the complex drills and floor patterns essential in the sport.

Earlier in life, the maturing child evidencing planning deficits may find it difficult to dress or undress, to manage a fork and spoon, as well as to master important playground skills. Success in the first grades often rests on the child's ability successfully to plan and execute the formulation of letters (both written and printed), as well as the chaining together of letters into readable words.

Children who cannot process and then replicate a series of more than three subactions by the age of 6 should be exposed to extremely patient teaching, instruction that carefully confronts such youngsters with demonstrations of simple kinds

[7]In the study by Conrad, Cermak, and Drake (1983), as is invariably true in studies of motor planning, children labeled neurologically impaired and/or learning disabled are likely to post scores beneath those of children who function normally in classrooms and in other tests of motor coordination (DeRenzi et al., 1980).

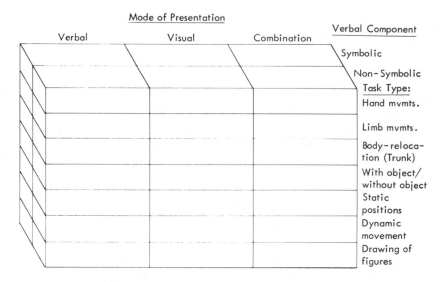

Mode of Presentation

Verbal   Visual   Combination

Verbal Component

Symbolic

Non-Symbolic

Task Type:
Hand mvmts.

Limb mvmts.

Body-reloca-
tion (Trunk)

With object/
without object

Static
positions

Dynamic
movement

Drawing of
figures

FIGURE 9.5 A model for the study of motor planning behaviors.

and of short durations. In contrast, children who may appear precocious when confronted with tests of motor planning, and who may, for example, be able to duplicate a series of five or more acts chained together by the age of 6 or 7 years might be considered apt candidates for higher-level skills training.

Finally, it is clear that motor planning is not a unitary quality but a collection of subabilities that in older children are not likely to be highly related (Kools and Tweedie, 1975; Cratty and Samoy, 1984; Conrad, Cermak, and Drake, 1983). This differentiation of motor planning into several subabilities appears to be more marked in older children than in younger ones. Below the age of 3 years, for example, correlations between various tests of motor planning based upon responses given to both oral commands and visual demonstrations are likely to be related (Kools and Tweedie, 1975). However, by the age of 5 or 6, it is more useful to select (or formulate) tests of motor planning that rather exactly correspond to specific kinds or types of serial motor skills whose execution it is desired to explore. Figure 9.5 portrays some of the dimensions of motor planning.

Three dimensions of motor planning evaluation are shown. These include how the task is demonstrated or requested (mode of presentation), whether the task is one involved in daily living that can be described in words (symbolic), or whether it is a nonsense movement (nonsymbolic). A fourth important dimension, not pictured, is a subject dimension. Results from these studies will be influenced by the age of the subject, as well as by the presence of possible pathological conditions, such as left or right hemisphere lesion. Moreover, the verbal abilities of the subject may make a difference.

RHYTHM

Rhythm permeates both the psyche and the physiology of humans. The beat of the heart, the regularity of breathing, cyclic fluctuations of mood and energy, as well as the presence of music and dance within all cultures of the world attest to the truth that rhythm is indeed an essence of life itself. The term *rhythm,* however, may mean different things to various observers of movement and motor performance. Movement therapists see rhythm as an indispensable tool when working with the emotionally disturbed, particularly the severely withdrawn (Richman, 1976). Dance specialists perceive rhythmic variations as important in the construction of performance presentations. Those obtaining relatively hard data about rhythm, while in the minority, attempt to dissect various measurable qualities within rhythmic experiences, including the influence of various stimuli upon regular movement, as well as qualities and quantities in the actions themselves.

Child development specialists have begun to take a closer look at various rhythmical qualities in the actions of children and infants. Thelen's important work, reviewed in Chapter 3, may have begun to unveil only one part of this most important quality embedded within the unfolding movement personalities of youngsters (Thelen, 1979). Numerous other problems await other energetic researchers in the years ahead.

The first studies of motor rhythm in children surveyed the accuracy with which a youngster could match movements to sound cues given regularly or irregularly and with increasing difficulty (Seashore, 1926). More recently, rhythm expressed in movement has been measured by assessing not only the simple accuracy of the movement response, but also the accuracy of the space through which a movement occurs (Smoll, 1973).

When measures of both response accuracy and amplitude of movement are employed, regular improvement is noted from the age of 5 to 10 and 11 years (Smoll, 1974). A plateau effect is noted in such studies at about the age of 10 years, and sex differences are not usually found. Age seems a more important modifier of response accuracy than does the speed with which the auditory cues are given. Occasionally, however, racial differences in rhythmic movement responses have been obtained. Van Alstyne and Osborn (1948) found black children to be more accurate in their responses to sound cues given rhythmically than were their young white subjects.

Rhythmical qualities and movement are combined in various ways. The infant, to give one example, seems to be born with the tendency to make regular responses with many parts of the body, within a predictable schedule, during the first year of life (Thelen, 1979). These important responses seem to be triggered by an internal drummer and are not in reaction to obvious external stimulation. It is not until months later that the child is apparently stimulated by external cues when making regular actions of the body. Thus two basic classifications of rhythmic movements are those that are the apparent product of interal programs, in contrast to actions that are the result of sounds or sights outside the body.

Other dimensions of rhythmic movement consist of (a) a consideration of various preferences for rhythmic movement speed and quality if, for example, a child is simply asked to move rhythmically; (b) preferences for various kinds of stimuli to which to move, such as auditory cues and visual stimulations (both demonstrations by another human, as well as light cues); (c) ethnic variations in rhythmic qualities and abilities; and (d) formulation of a difficulty scale depicting the order in which movements of various complexities are engaged in rhythmically by children of various ages. Unfortunately, only cursory attention has been paid to the questions apparent within these various categories of problems. Most books purporting to cover the topic of motor development either ignore the subject of rhythm entirely or pay only superficial heed to this most important quality embedded in the unfolding movement behavior of children.

Periodic attempts have been made over the years to ascertain whether the accurate response to a rhythmic beat reflects athletic ability and/or experience in dance or music (Huff, 1972; Bond, 1959; Annett, 1932; Thomas and Moon, 1976). Generally there seem to be some differences in younger children who have had experiences in music and dance at earlier ages (Annett, 1932). However, when the rhythmic abilities of older adolescents are contrasted, differences between those with experiences in athletics and dance and those without these backgrounds are not always apparent (Huff, 1972).

Developmentally, most children are first attracted by and tend to move rhythmically to sounds rather than to simple visual cues (Smith, 1970). However, it is a common observation that when the visual cue to rhythmic movement is an adult engaged in a dance movement important within a culture, nearby infants, even though to young to stand, will often pick up the beat with their bodies and limbs. As children grow older, they become better able to replicate a regular beat with bodily movements. Indeed, Marie Montessori declared years ago that until children can relate to and replicate a rhythmic action in response to sound cues, they are not otherwise ready for an education (Montessori, 1914). Also, as children mature, they become capable of more complex and different rhythmic movements (Cratty, 1981). For example, first seen are actions that simply replicate a relatively slow and regular sound cue. Next to be acquired are variations in the timing of movements in response to an irregular beat. Force changes seem next to be acquired, when the sound cue is made to differ in intensity.

Movements in a horizontal plane are acquired before those that involve up and down movements of the arms. Walking movements are among the easier rhythmic responses to be seen in children of 2 and 3 years of age. Indeed, locomotion itself takes on more and more regular rhythmicity during the second year of life. Finally, circular and lateral movements are seen in children. Moving an arm from a raised position over the same shoulder to a low position next to the opposite foot seems more difficult to replicate, perhaps because of the difficulty children have in acquiring the ability to cross the body's midline with movements (Ayres, 1969; Williams et al., 1971).

The assumptions of rhythmic beats by various of the extremities, either alone

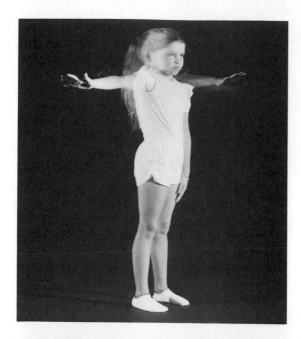

FIGURE 9.6 Movements in horizontal plane are often easier.

FIGURE 9.7 Vertical movements are next in difficulty.

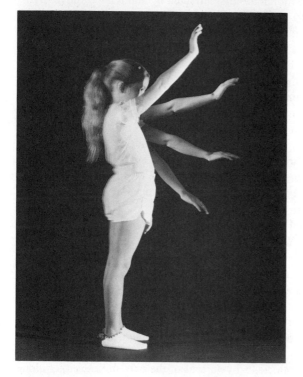

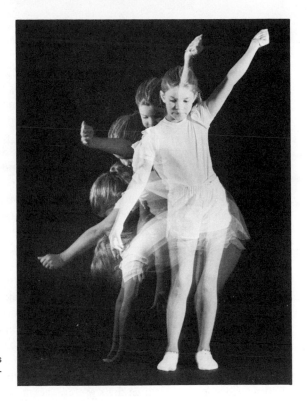

FIGURE 9.8 Lateral movements tend to be harder to make, rhythmically.

or in combination, may correspond to the order in which control is gained over various movements (DeOreo, 1978; Gesell, 1946; Seefeldt, 1972). As the infant and child matures, the following movements are seen to occur in the lower limbs: (a) Bilateral and simultaneous movements of the legs, with the child in a lying position; (b) bilateral and alternating movements of the legs, again in a lying position; (c) bilateral and simultaneous movements of both legs, either while being held upright or in a lying position against gravity; and (d) single rhythmic movements of a single leg.

Upper limb control also seems to follow predictable patterns that would seem to predict the types of rhythmic patterns the infant and child is able to assume, and the order in which they might appear. Control of the arms usually occurs before control of the hand, and hand movements occur before precise finger movements. Thus one upper limb sequence involves progression from large arm movements to precise finger actions. A second sequence of upper limb control involves (a) one arm-hand actions independent of the other hand-arm; (b) bilateral movements involving the simultaneous use of both arms; and finally (c) alternating movements of both arms in which one arm-hand may assume an action different from the other. One arm-hand may assist while the other beats a drum, for example.

Rhythmic transfers of patterns from one side of the body to the other also show changes in children from 5 to 8 years of age. The emerging ability to, for example, engage in an alternate hopping pattern of two hops on one foot, and then two on the other, may be due to the maturation of the corpus callosum, the structure forming the bridge between the two cerebral hemispheres (Keogh, 1968). The sex differences favoring the girls in this type of task may be due to the acknowledged neurological precocity of females during early and middle childhood. Essentially the data indicate that approximately 50 percent of girls tested can accomplish this task at 6 years of age, and by age 8, 90 percent of all girls tested can successfully accomplish this rhythmic task. In contrast, boys at 6 years are not likely to do this successfully, but by 8 and 9 years of age, most of them can also hop alternately. By 8 years of age girls can also hop from foot to foot in a 3-2 rhythm. Again, boys are as a group not as proficient at this kind of task until a year or two later.

One of the more interesting rhythmic qualities in both children and adults involves the preferences they show for tempo when asked to move rhythmically in various ways. Marked individual preferences are shown when adult and child subjects are asked, for example, to tap their hand rhythmically, or to exhibit rhythmic hopping or foot tapping. Generally the available data indicate that in the same kind of task, people are markedly consistent over time (Rimoldi, 1951). That is, from year to year a child is likely to tap at the same tempo when given a drum to beat. However, in contrast, personal rhythms in various parts of the body are not likely to correspond very closely. A child who may prefer to hop rapidly when asked to do so rhythmically may be slower when asked to tap rhythmically. Asking people to vary rhythms slower or faster than their preferences has unusual effects upon time perception, and may require real practice and learning (Dinner et al., 1963). Moreover, those teaching children dance rhythmics that may contain tempos different from the child's preferences may have a more difficult time than if the child's speed preferences correspond to those required by the music and/or teacher. That is, the teacher may be faced with encouraging the child to break out of preferences for rhythms that may be rather deeply ingrained within the youngster's movement personality.

Testers attempting to obtain valid measures of such qualities as accuracy of rhythmic hopping face similar problems. The examiner's personal tempo preference when demonstrating actions, when not in congruence with the child's preferences, may result in scores that are more a reflection of the individual differences in personal tempos between tester and child than in the true qualities possessed by the youngster. Also, more than one researcher attempting to assess rhythmic responses has had the data modified by what may be a child's personal rhythm preferences (Smoll, 1974). If a high score in such tasks is obtained when a rhythmic movement is demonstrated by a tester, it may be caused by a similarity between the child's preference for rhythmic speed and that of the tester. A low score may, in contrast, merely indicate a lack of congruence between the personal speed and tempo preferences of child and tester.

Rhythm appears in many types of movement tasks other than those obviously requiring this quality. Most sport skills contain rhythmic elements. Cooper (1982) reported a technique of teaching sport skills based upon their rhythmicity. He first recorded the rhythms within skills exhibited by outstanding athletes. Using these rhythmic patterns, he then taught beginners the same skills, accompanying the teaching with drumbeats corresponding to accents within the tasks. He reported that novices performed and learned better using this approach.

Rhythmicity also appears in academic tasks such as reading and writing. However, when children evidence both a learning deficit and a problem in rhythmic motor behaviors, improving sequenced action patterns will not necessarily modify academic learning.[8] Exposing children to rhythmic tasks, particularly those involving the duplication of regular and irregular beats, may heighten auditory discrimination and improve attention in general. Indeed, it is probable that improvement in the duplication of an auditory or visual cue with rhythmic actions may be due more to improved attention and maturation of the nervous system rather than to changes in movement abilities themselves (Thomas and Stratton, 1977).

OVERFLOW: ASSOCIATED MOVEMENTS

When younger children perform movement tasks, they often seem to be "cuter." When running, for example, their wrists may curl upward. Their first attempts to use a pencil are often accompanied by the appearance of the tongue moving slowly back and forth outside their mouths. These and similar movements are referred to as *associated movements* and represent some kind of neuromotor overflow that results in the involvement of actions in body parts not directly involved in the task. This kind of residual tension is often seen in the action patterns of preschool children.

However, by the seventh and eighth year of age, the action patterns of normal children become more precise and biomechanically correct. Persistence of these extraneous actions are signs to the pediatric neurologist that some kind of neuromotor immaturity is present. A moderate or minimal neurological problem may often be diagnosed using various tests of the presence of these actions. For example, if associated movements occur more in one side of the body than in the other, a lateralization syndrome may be present. That is, the child may not be completely lateralized relative to one-sided function, and/or the child may be afflicted with a mild form of one-sided cerebral palsy (hemiplegia).

Several tests have been devised by observers of this phenemonon during the past two decades (Abercrombie et al., 1964; Connolly and Stratton, 1968; Fog and Fog, 1963; Zazzo, 1960; Touwen and Prechtl, 1970). Generally these evaluations seek to determine the precision with which a task is carried out, unaccompanied by tensions and/or movements in body parts not involved. Often the hands are used in such tasks. The child may be asked to spread the fingers on one hand while an observation is made of finger spreading on the opposite hand of which the child may

---

[8]Lack of the ability to duplicate a rhythmic foot tapping while seated is used, with other similar tests, to assess possible neurological impairment in children.

be unaware. Finger opposition is required in one hand to determine if only that hand and not the other is involved in the task. The lower limbs may be required to display a strong extension pattern, as the child is asked to walk on the heels, for example. While this is attempted, observations of flexions of the hands and wrists, as well as extensions of the arms at the shoulders, may occur in the upper limbs. Clinical neurologists refer to this overflow as "mirror movements." Still another test consists of asking the child to smile and to squint the eyes, while observing whether or not the fingers spread apart at the same time. The tendency for these associated movements to spill over from the hands to the face and vice versa is probably due to the proximity of the areas that mediate these two types of functions within the sensory-motor cortex.

While clinical tests of this phenomenon abound in the literature, exact scores from these measures when applied to various age groups and the establishment of norms are relatively scarce. Most authorities agree that it is "normal" for children of 2 and 3 years to exhibit these extraneous patterns of movements, while by the age of 7 and 8 they are largely believed to be almost absent (Touwen and Prechtl, 1970). However, more precise assessments await further research. Furthermore, it is apparent that the appearance of associated movements may be specific to various combinations of body parts and segments. Complicating the picture further is the fact that various factors or conditions may contribute to their appearance, in addition to neuromotor maturity. These conditions include (a) the order with which tasks are presented in an evaluation, (b) the complexity of the movement involved, (c) whether or not the preferred hand is being used, and (d) the intensity with which an action is undertaken. With reference to the intensity of the task, a considerable amount of this kind of overflow is likely to occur in most adults if the strength effort exerted is forceful. With progressively increased resistance, for example, an increased amount of overflow is to be expected in normal adults and children (Waterland and Hellenbrandt, 1964).

Despite the lack of precision with which this quality may be assessed, its presence in children's movement patterns to an inordinate degree is likely to cause several problems.

1. Extraneous actions appear unesthetic to playmates. Peculiar writhings of the mouth or limbs are likely to be seen as somehow different by a child's peers, and may result in derision directed toward the offending youngster.

2. The presence of these associated actions, particularly during high-intensity efforts, are likely to disrupt or interfere with correct and efficient production of a movement or a movement sequence. A child who, for example, evidences extreme flexions in the upper limbs when extending the lower limbs in a jumping pattern is not as likely to rise as high as one whose arms and legs reflect a synchronized and mature pattern of jumping. In this same movement the flexion, and thus the lifting of the arms in an inappropriate manner, will also make the child more unstable, as the center of mass is lifted at the same time.

3. Extraneous associated movements may also produce quicker fatigue than if the child is directing force and energy only in the body parts appropriate to the task.

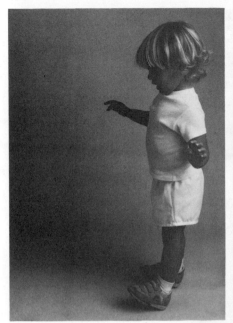
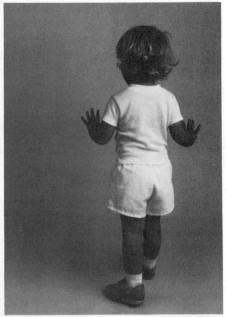

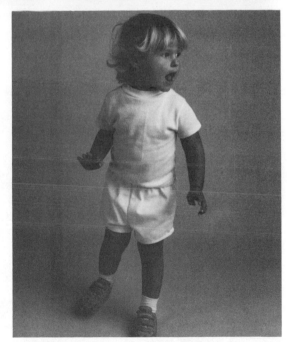

FIGURE 9.9 Heel walking causes a normal amount of overflow in the mouth and hands in this boy of 2+ years.

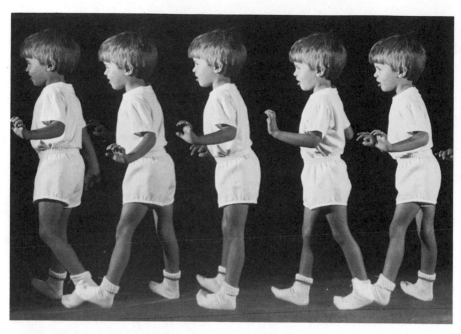

FIGURE 9.10 Heel walking, placing tension in the lower limbs, causes overflow in this boy of 4.5 years, both in the upper limbs and in the mouth region.

FIGURE 9.11 When a seven year old girl is asked to "heel walk" however, little or no overflow in other parts of the body are apparent.

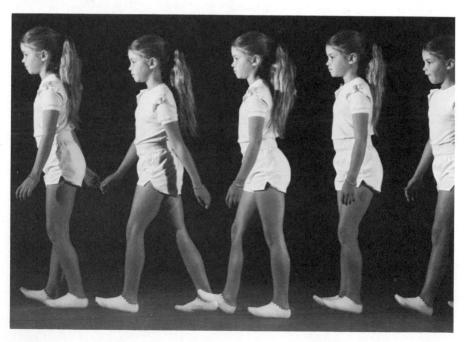

Reduction of these actions in children evidencing some kind of neurological deficit is often a difficult task. In our clinical program, we often feel successful when working with a youngster, only to have the unusual flexions suddenly appear when the child is placed under stress and/or becomes excited. Among the general approaches to reducing associated movements are relaxation training of various kinds and encouraging the child to reduce the actions by bringing them to his or her conscious attention.

Associated movements interact with the other qualities discussed in this chapter. As was pointed out, laterality problems may be reflected in an asymmetrical display of these actions. The inability of a child correctly to integrate body parts may be partially due to the presence of these undesirable actions interfering with appropriate task performance. It is not unusual to find that a child having an inordinate amount of overflow present in action patterns also has problems drawing lateral lines. The nonwriting hand-arm seems to be subtly fighting the hand used in drawing the line, thus making it difficult for the child to form the capital letter *A,* or to draw a triangle.

Movement educators, and those attempting to evaluate movement qualities in children and youth, should be cognizant of several principles and guidelines when encountering these interesting types of movement qualities:

1. The presence of these associated movements may be a signal of subtle neurological problems needing the advice and assessment of a medical doctor.
2. The reduction of these qualities may be a useful way to aid the child to move more efficiently. Furthermore, their reduction or control is likely to make the child more pleasing to look at while performing various playground skills, and thus more socially pleasing to peers.
3. The persistence of these extra actions in middle childhood may signal the presence of motor awkwardness that needs attention.
4. Subjective assessment of these qualities during a motor development evaluation adds depth to the assessment. Descriptive paragraphs or categorical scoring methods may be used to identify properly the presence, strength, and location of associated movements.

Overall, it appears that in early childhood the nervous system is not able to act with precision in the production of precise movement qualities. One way in which this imprecision is seen is in the presence of these associated movements. With normal development and maturation, however, the neuromotor structures begin to display less irritation and thus perform with increased accuracy, an improvement that is seen in the reduction and elimination of associated movements in normal children under moderate degrees of tension and stress. The assessment of these associated movements should be made while considering the amount of tension imposed in the task and the maturity of the child, as well as the complexity of the actions required.

REACTION TIME

An important quality accompanying efficient motor performance by children is the speed with which they react. Although sports writers refer to the reaction time of athletes to mean the speed with which a performer moves, technically *reaction time* involves no movement at all. Rather, it refers to the time taken to formulate an action and is timed from the appearance of something the child may be required to (or wish to) react to, and the time the resultant movement takes place.

Reaction time is therefore time during which at least four events are happening: (a) Time taken to assimilate the stimuli to be reacted to, such as the appearance of an incoming ball; (b) time taken to formulate the resultant action; combined with (c) any kinds of judgments the child may be making; and finally (d) the time taken for the program formulated usually within the central nervous system to reach the muscles. Most of the time involves phases (b) and (c); indeed, these two parts are often difficult to separate. That is, the child who may be slow to react may actually be slowly contemplating appropriate reactions rather than simply taking a great deal of time to instigate the program decided upon.

Numerous studies have been carried out on the reaction time of adults. Generally, the results indicated that a number of factors either speed up or slow down reaction time. For example, adults usually react faster if they know a simple response has to be made to some light or sound cue than if the light or sound is to be followed by a complex response. To a point, the more intense the stimulus (the louder the sound), the more quickly the action will be initiated. However, if the sound is made too loudly, reaction time may be slowed down. Similarly, if there is some kind of forewarning that a stimulus to be reacted to is to appear, the subsequent reaction will be quicker than if no warning is given to the subject.

Reaction times in various parts of the body (the hands) have been found to be more rapid than in other parts (the legs). In general, adult humans react more quickly to a sound than to a light cue. The dominant hand will usually react quicker than the nondominant hand, and practice in a reaction time situation will usually elicit only slight improvement on the part of the subject (about 10 percent in many studies, depending on the complexity of the response to be made).

Developmental trends in reaction time have been studied for many years. Even before the turn of the century, J.A. Gilbert found that reaction time in children decreases with age, while choice reaction time (reaction to one of more than one possible stimuli) decreases faster than does simple reaction time. Gilbert, like numerous researchers to follow, also found that the variability of children's responses will diminish as they get older (Gilbert, 1984).

Reaction time seems fastest at about 20 years of age (Pierson, 1959). At that age, times are significantly better than they are at the age of 12, or at 48 (Mendryk, 1960). Moreover, as age increases, correlations between reaction time and movement speed tend to decrease and become almost absent by adulthood (Pierson, 1959).

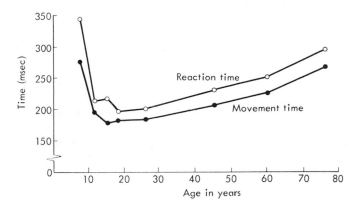

FIGURE 9.12 Reaction time and movement time as a function of age. From Hodgkins, 1962.

After the age of 8, as can be seen in Figure 9.12, reaction times markedly decrease until about the age of 18. Gradual increases in reaction time are recorded between the ages of 20 and 40 years, with more marked increases seen in averages after the age of 60. Movement time, while paralleling reaction time when mean times at each age are contrasted, does not correlate with reaction times for the most part. That is, knowing how quickly a youngster may *begin* a movement tells us little about how *fast* the movement may then be executed.

The measurement of reaction time in young children has not been studied in a large range of tasks. The information that is available indicates that in simple problems, the reaction time of 5-year-olds is twice as long as is found at adulthood. At the same time, there is a marked improvement of about 43 percent from the ages of 3 to 5 years. These findings indicate that a large amount of the motor ineptitude apparent in young children may be caused by inability rapidly to start a movement itself. For example, as Whiting points out, if a 5-year-old is expected to catch a ball traveling only 15 feet per second from a distance of 10 feet, he must initiate his response as soon as the ball has left the thrower's hand. Thus, in some measure ineptitude in this type of task might be attributable to slow reaction time rather than to the inability correctly to place the body and hands when catching the ball (Whiting, 1969).

The study of ball interception by children of various ages, discussed in Chapter 6, contains data that indicate the interesting relationships between judgment time, reaction time, and maturation. Children who were younger when attempting accurately to predict the final destination of a ball, when able to see only the initial part of its trajectory, reacted rapidly and inaccurately. Thus children of 5 to 6 years of age were apparently unaware of the complicated nature of the problem facing them. In contrast, youngsters in middle childhood took their time and, while posting a longer reaction time, actually evidenced a longer judgment interval as they apparently realized how difficult it was to solve the task. Finally, children in late childhood had seen balls traveling at them for some years, and thus apparently had prepared programs available to them. They reacted both rapidly and accurately at the ages of 10 to 12 to the same judgment of trajectory problem.

Reaction time aids and plagues the movement efforts of children in a variety of tasks as they mature. The shortening of this preparation interval as maturity occurs is probably a combination of several factors, including: (a) maturation of the nervous system, particularly the central structures involved in the formulation and storage of motor programs; (b) learning and experience the child acquires with a variety of situations that require similar or the same response patterns; (c) the development of analytic-cognitive skills enabling the child to more quickly size up situations that occur.

Several theories have been proposed over the years to explain how reaction time decreases in children who are older. Luria, for example (1932), suggested that reaction time is slower in younger children because when a stimulus appears, the youngster becomes generally excited, and this agitated state involves not only the motor system in general but other parts of the brain. The response or responses that then occur are therefore often not specific or appropriate. The previous section discussing overflow contains evidence that substantiates Luria's contentions. Luria further proposes that as children grow older, this diffused, general state of excitation becomes more focused and specific, resulting in more efficient and quicker responses to various stimuli.

Other theorists borrow from information theory. Elliot, for example (1964), suggests that attentional qualities as they mature produce more sustained and qualitative attention in older children than in younger ones. With increased attention, quicker reaction time is the result. Surwillo also proposed that the faster processing time possible in a mature brain results in an improvement in reaction time. He found that he could artificially modify reaction time in children by speeding up or slowing down selected brain waves using changes in visual stimulation (Surwillo, 1974, 1971).

SUMMARY

A number of qualitative aspects of movement have been discussed in this chapter, including laterality-asymmetry, overflow, rhythm, reaction time, and motor planning. Some of these qualities have been more thoroughly researched than others. The identification of some of these variables arose from the laboratories of the clinical neurologist, rather than from experiments with normal youngsters.

Hand and foot preferences are seen rather early, even as reflexes are triggered near birth. The stepping response, for example, evidences a right bias, as does the asymmetrical tonic neck reflex. Within the first half year of life, most human infants evidence some degree of right-handedness that sometimes seems to go and to return. Hand and foot preferences seem inherited, with some modification occurring later due to cultural factors.

Children also evidence regular improvement in the ability to observe and to replicate movement series of various types and complexities. Infants may imitate simple actions requiring one or two parts. By age 5, a three-part action will be repeated accurately; by middle childhood, youngsters can replicate a series of from five to seven actions. Individual differences in various components of motor planning abilities are likely predictors of later educability in a variety of self-care and sport skills.

Maturation also brings with it the ability of children to direct and make specific the force and accuracy of their movements. Less and less, as middle childhood approaches, are youngsters likely to evidence overflow of actions into body parts not directly involved in tasks. Children delayed neurologically may persist in evidencing these extraneous actions, resulting in problems at play, acceptance by peers, and inefficient mechanics in a variety of motor tasks.

Reaction time also improves in a linear fashion with age. As maturation takes place, there are likely to be fewer and fewer correlations between reaction time and movement speed measures. Maturation of the nervous system, freedom from diffused motor patterns, as well as positive changes in attention have all been proposed as reasons for improved reaction times among older youngsters.

QUESTIONS FOR DISCUSSION

1. How does the concept of hand preference differ from the idea of hemispheric specialization? Is there a correspondence or correlation between the two ideas?
2. How do foot and hand preference manifest themselves during the early months of life? To what have fluctuations in these preferences been attributed?
3. What changes are seen in hand preferences as children mature?
4. What does the idea of degree of handedness mean? How might you evaluate this degree in a 5-year-old child?
5. How can you define motor planning? What components of motor planning tests seem important to administer?
6. How do correlations between motor planning scores differ among younger versus older children?
7. Can you pair specific types of motor planning subtests with various skills needed in the home, at work, and at play?
8. What does overflow mean, and how might it inhibit the actions of a 7-year-old child?
9. How might overflow be evaluated? How might a 3-year-old versus a 7-year-old differ in the expression of this quality in movement?
10. What variables influence the amount of overflow seen in a child?
11. How is reaction time defined and measured?
12. What are some subcomponents of reaction time and movement speed (response time)?

13. What stages may be seen in the rhythmic behaviors of youngsters?
14. What factors might influence the quality of rhythmic behaviors seen in a youngster?

STUDENT PROJECTS

1. Ascertain the probable hand preference relative to beginning printing of a 5-year old boy by asking him to execute a number of relatively difficult (for him) one-handed movements. Would you have to score him (or her) over a period of time, or would one testing be enough?

2. Survey your friends to see how they execute various one-handed tasks. Are they consistent in hand use? Might you find differences between their reported hand use and their actual hand use?

3. Observe dance classes of children from 2 to 10 years of age or older. What differences do you see in the movement and rhythmic qualities they evidence? What conditions and/or variables in the classes seem to cause individual differences in the rhythmic competencies seen in the children?

4. Ask a child of 3 or 4 to walk slowly on his or her heels. Observe any extraneous overflow in the upper limbs. Contrast this overflow to that seen when a child of 7 or 8 is asked to heel walk.

5. Using reaction timers available in your laboratory, assess reaction times (simple and complex) in children of various ages. What differences are you likely to obtain, and in what measures?

6. Give a simple test of motor planning to a child of 5 and another of 8 years of age, asking them to replicate a series of from 1 to 5 movements. What differences did you notice? What might be the reasons for these differences?

7. Assess children's foot preferences in several ways and contrast these to their hand preferences in throwing and other tasks. What conclusions can you draw from the results of your survey?

CHAPTER TEN
ACQUIRING SKILL
Developmental Perspectives

During the first months and years of life, infants and children acquire an amazing number of physical, linguistic, and cognitive skills. During the early decades of this century, those interested in the abilities of youngsters seem to have concentrated on the identification of these emerging skills and on placing them at various age levels. While these efforts have formed a useful baseline of norms for the unfolding of physical skills, little attempt was made to unravel *how* children learned and acquired various movement capacities from birth to childhood.

During the past fifteen years, however, more and more behavioral scientists interested in children have begun to focus their attention upon processes that underlie the performance of various physical tasks, rather than simply recording outcomes. Some of these contemporary researchers seem to have been stimulated by the work of Piaget, and have extended and elaborated upon his ideas within experimental contexts more disciplined than that used by the Swiss epistemologist. Ideas surrounding the computer revolution may have also prompted others to describe memory, learning, and even physical skills in the jargon of the hardware and software salesperson. Whatever stimulated these recent efforts at explanation, contemporary research has begun to outline how children and infants seem to acquire skills.

Understanding motor learning processes as they are seen in children of various ages is a demanding undertaking. Finding out how infants and children learn skills is made difficult for the following reasons. Physical skills and the manipulation of objects in the environment seldom occur without the accompaniment of subtle and difficult to see cognitive processes. Expressive as well as internal language is often closely intertwined with actions children are performing and learning. Different social contexts are likely to influence, in various ways, how and why a youngster acquires a physical skill. Children evidence a wide variety of individual differences in the quality of skill they evidence, their rate of motor learning, and what motivates them to move and to learn. Finally, the terms used by contemporary writers are sometimes more confusing than enlightening. The term *schema,* for example, employed earlier by Piaget, has been bent into various molds by contemporary writers.

Despite these difficulties, however, it is important to try to understand what *is* presently known about processes underlying motor learning in infants and children. Illuminating these processes, even if with imprecise and broad strokes, should (1) lead to understanding how normal youngsters mature as reflected in their action patterns, and (2) aid in the better understanding of youngsters who evidence either developmental lags or developmental superiority when exposed to physical skill situations. These understandings in turn should lead to more effective programming and facility and equipment development, as well as to more sensitive teaching of all youngsters attempting to improve their abilities.

The following discussion does not, however, contain exact cookbook formulas for how children learn, and thus must be taught. The behaviors of children during their formative years bring up many paradoxical questions. Emerging action patterns rest upon little-understood inherent tendencies, and are formed by a multitude of intricately interwoven cultural expectations and experiences. It is thus proposed in this chapter to outline general principles rather than exact rules that precisely delineate developmental aspects of motor learning.

Broadly conceived, skill acquisition in the young may be considered through the inspection of three sets of phenemona. These include basic tendencies or inherent characteristics that seem to underlie most of what humans and many animals seem to do. On a second level are the observable behaviors themselves, what the child does when faced with a situation, person, or thought which impels physical interaction, interactions which may be refined through use. Finally, the outcomes or results of the child's actions and skills form another important dimension to consider. These outcomes often afford important insights into why the child persists, and why improvement and change occur in the child's action patterns with repeated exposure over time.

Basic tendencies, behavior, and the results of that behavior intertwine in intricate ways. Moreover, cognitive activity may operate at several levels as actions are acquired. A child may be moving, and at the same time be thinking about what to do next and/or about the results of the action taking place. As a youngster performs, various levels of behavior form a number of simultaneously operative feedback systems. Thus the consideration of motor behavior and learning at one level is at times superficial.

For purposes of clarity and organization, the following discussion has been sectioned as follows. Initially, basic tendencies are discussed. These are qualities that underlie the behaviors of humans in a variety of contexts and the behaviors of some animals. Next, various qualitative dimensions of motor learning are considered within a developmental framework. The roles of thinking and speech as they relate to motor skill acquisition are discussed next. The chapter concludes with guidelines for planning motor skills programs.

BASIC TENDENCIES

Information Seeking

Most observers of both animal and human behavior agree that organisms display strong urges to obtain information. Even the casual observer of the newborn cannot help but be struck by the vast amount of time devoted to looking at the environment. This complex behavior has been documented frequently within the past two decades, both in the work of Fantz (1961) as well as in that of Haith (1980).

Information seeking in infants may occur within a specific sensory modality— looking and listening, for example. With maturation, it is more likely to occur as two or even three sensory modes are combined. That is, rather early in life the infant will seek to touch and look at an object at the same time. If the target object makes a noise, it may be simultaneously shaken also.

Information seeking is invariably accompanied by two complementary processes. These include (a) storage into memory, and (b) comparison with what has already been stored during previous contacts with the world. These latter processes have the effect of modifying the amount and quality of an infant's and child's exploratory information-seeking movement behaviors. These behaviors tend to change from those that seem random and even impulsive in nature to actions that are increasingly refined and selective. Past experiences and the impressions obtained and stored are not repeated endlessly in normal youngsters. With maturation and experience, children will usually spend less time with the familiar and instead seek novel objects and experiences to deal with.

Capacity Utilization

Organisms invariably display strong needs to exercise and thus expand their capacities. In the human infant and child, capacities for action, speech, and thought will be employed and seemingly utilized for the sheer joy of exercise. Some students of human motivation have espoused the concept of the capacity primacy theory of motivation. This model is based on the premise that much of what humans engage in is simply an attempt to employ inherent sensory and motor capacities. In the animal world, this same model suggests that birds fly because they can, while lions roar because it is within their capabilities to do so.

In the human infant, seemingly imperative acts like sucking are played with and modified simply because it is fun to do so. Apparently inherent and simple visual looking and fixating responses quickly become modified in the same manner, and perhaps for the same reason. Grasping, initially a reflex, also becomes fun to play with and a capacity to expand for its own sake (Hogg & Moss, 1983). In a similar way, infants and children seem motivated to move, and thus begin to move vigorously because they have the capacity to do so. Moreover, as movement capacities expand, more frequent movements are engaged in.

Novelty Seeking

Human infants and children, and most members of the animal kingdom, seem to detest being bored. Children seek novelty both in play and in play materials and companions. Several theoreticians have argued that a primary reason children engage in play is to seek an optimum level of stimulation and to prevent boredom. Playful movement experiences may not serve any purpose other than to give the participant pleasure, prevent boredom, and arouse or calm the child to levels the youngster feels comfortable with. Berlyne, several decades ago, presented evidence that novelty seeking is a strong and seemingly inherent drive among animals, as well as among young humans (Berlyne, 1960).

Thus it seems that basic tendencies to seek information and novelty, and to exercise capacities, form an important foundation for the expansion and learning of action patterns in infants. However, as maturation occurs, a number of other trends emerge. Older children begin to think more, to move selectively, and to copy others. Additionally they begin to play games with strict rules formulated by others and to interact in ways not possible in infancy. In this next section, some of these dimensions of motor learning in childhood are explored.

DIMENSIONS OF MOTOR LEARNING IN CHILDHOOD

With maturation, a number of factors begin to mold how children acquire skills over the base of inherent tendencies to acquire information, seek novelty, and exercise capacities. Older children begin to mix language with skill acquisition and to think about how they are learning a skill, and even about what skills to acquire (Gachound et al., 1983).

Improved abilities to store information and to process quantities of information accompanying motor acts changes how motor learning occurs in early and middle childhood. As language capacities expand, children begin to employ internal speech in the form of ever more efficient self-instructions. By late childhood many youngsters begin to think about thinking itself, and to formulate elaborate plans about how they may acquire skills of a number of kinds—cognitive and linguistic, as well as perceptual and motor (Flavell, 1972). Among the trends seen by contemporary theoreticians that may influence motor skill acquisition are the following.

The Formulation and Use of Movement Rules

With maturation, children begin to acquire and to use more and more useful rules about movements and about movement learning. Contemporary students of linguistic learning in children (Chomsky, 1980) have suggested that unique word usage and sentence formations that have not been uttered previously are possible because youngsters learn and use language-speech rules. In this way children construct sentences and thoughts of increasing sophistication.

It is probable that movement rules are also formulated by youngsters as they confront more situations suggesting action. Initially these rules may consist of rather simple associations between effort and outcome. The infant in the crib, for example, soon learns that activation may produce results—or more simply put, "When I get excited in my crib, I may contact those interesting objects overhead." Later, two things occur: Not only is a single rule made more useful and refined, but an additional number of rules are formulated. Thus the initial rule about contact may be refined to become: "If I move slowly, and watch my departing hand carefully, my chances for contact are increased." At the same time, the infant learns more rules about social-motor interactions: "When I move my mouth in a certain way, the human hovering over my crib also moves her mouth in the same way and seems pleased with me." Or perhaps: "When I kick my legs just right I can uncover them and thus freely express my needs to kick vigorously" (Bruner, 1973).

As maturation proceeds, more and more rules are learned about how to produce efficient and vigorous action, about how to instigate social relationships, and about how to deal with balls. In infancy, these rules may be self-formulated. Later they may come from others and include formal instructions such as "See, put one foot in front of the other." In this manner, self-instructions often intermingle with the formal lessons offered by others in later childhood and adolescence.

These processes of rule making proceed in two general ways: (a) On the one hand, more and more rules make confrontations with movement situations easier. (b) Single rules becomes generalized to more and more ways in which actions are applied and performed by the child. Additionally, the manner in which children and youth think about rules in formal games undergoes evolution. In early infancy rules for games are nonexistent. The infant plays informally and in situations containing few formal restrictions. In early and middle childhood, rules for games are discovered and adhered to strictly. Finally, in late childhood and adolescence youngsters realize that rules may be made up and applied in various ways. Modifications of game rules are tried out, and in general a flexible attitude toward strict game rules may be adopted (Piaget, 1952).

Perception and Motor Learning

A number of perceptual tendencies change as children mature and attempt to acquire motor skills. In infancy, visual perception and movement seem often to operate independently. During the first months of life, the eyes may search and scan in ways that are seemingly independent of the action patterns engaged in. Infant stereotypies (Chapter 3) seemingly exist on their own, while the infant is apparently occupied elsewhere visually and auditorially (Anshel, 1979).

During the middle of the first year, the infant shows a tendency to begin to work hard to integrate visual input with movement capacities. Random and ballistic swipings slow down, and reaching begins to be accompanied by close and interested visual inspection. Visual-motor impressions of manipulations of the child's own body are replaced by the formation of visual-motor impressions of the numerous qualities possessed by objects contacted. Thus an object's texture, shape, size, weight, and articulations are explored in an integrated way by both eyes and hands. In a similar way, progress in locomotion is accompanied by close attention to the progress of the alternating feet, as well as to features of the footpath which may either disrupt or aid the child's initial attempts to locomotion.

Finally, during the second year and later, the child again begins to work selectively with various components of the perceptual and motor system. Now well-learned actions are taken without the apparent need for close visual attention, while the child may be occupied either with another skill or simply with internal thoughts. Most important, the child may choose simply to gaze quickly at some object or occurrence and then to shift attention elsewhere. The child has learned that (a) it is highly inefficient to visually *and* manually inspect all familiar features of the environment, and (b) that one may simply compare current and familar visual experiences and objects with those which are similar and which have been previously stored. Thus (c) one may confine one's attention to objects, events, and situations which are novel, unexpected, and/or interesting or threatening, and deal with these using both movement and vision, rather than waste time on the familiar and usual (Thomas, 1980; Kerr, 1982).

Thus a sequence is operative which includes an early phase that might be termed visual and motor, a second visual-motor integration phase, and finally a phase which is selectively visual, motor, or visual-motor, depending upon the characteristics of the situation and the interest and needs of the child. It is important to note, however, that these phases do not occur at any exact and predictable times of life, and at the same time these subsequences frequently overlap in time. Their occurrence may thus be specific for various kinds of situations. That is, the child may be functioning at a visual-motor level when dealing with one kind of situation, while when confronted with other types of situations and events may be operating at the higher level at which vision, thought, and movement are combined or kept separate as the occasion demands. Children who are labeled hyperactive are thought by some to be somehow stuck at the more immature middle part in this sequence, needing constantly and continually to visually and motorically inspect objects, people, and situations at ages older than is true of their more adequately functioning peers.

Variability and Precision

Another fascinating type of paradoxical problem in the acquisition of skill is the infant's and child's apparent need to engage in opposite processes. On the one hand the infant needs to explore, to create variability and complexity with movement, to evidence a variety of actions within a given classification of actions. That is, after learning to bring the food-filled spoon to the mouth, the infant may evidence different ways of accomplishing (or almost accomplishing) the same task. The spoon may be turned over before entering the mouth. Other unique and creative actions are invented to deal with the spoon, including using it as a missile, a hammer, or perhaps a weapon. Contemporary researchers have concluded that this seeking of variability is a useful undertaking, creating a variety of transfer possibilities to an ever-increasing number of skills (Kelso and Norman, 1977).

Moss and Hogg (1983), for example, in studying the acquisition of manipulative skills in children, found that with learning the children evidenced more variability and less consistency in the ways they handled objects. These researchers attributed this tendency for variability to several possibilities, including the fact that the children became bored and could easily modify their patterns without disturbing their task performance. Moreover, these researchers speculated, this tendency toward variability probably facilitated the transfer of one skill to another, and more additional learning, than if the child held strictly to a prescribed manner of manipulating an object.

One of the reasons it is hypothesized that children are so motivated to play with another child or adult, rather than to confine their efforts to solitary play with objects, is that people are more likely to give off a greater variety of responses and results than are objects. Indeed, in recent studies it has been found that objects and devices contrived to be interesting and complex to the extreme will hold normal children's attention for only a brief period, as compared to an adult or child playing in the same situation. People not only are able to emit more types of responses than do toys or objects, but are more unpredictable than a toy. This very unpredictability adds greater interest to the child's encounters with people than will be experienced when an object is manipulated in various ways. Thus play with others enhances the variations in responses made toward the child and that in turn the youngster is likely to make.

On the other hand, the child also seeks to refine specific skills. 'A decrease in variability in many skills is both desired by the culture and seemingly striven for by the child. Great amounts of visual attention are expended by infants as they try to make their first precise contact with objects; later, skills of eating, dressing, and playing certain games possess rather exact requirements which in the normal child are met with successful attempts at decreased variability of response.

As maturity occurs, the child encounters various cultural sanctions and encouragements for either type of behavior, variable or confined and precise. Movement educators dote on the child's ability to modify responses in accordance with various rather broad and nonspecific demands. Dance teachers and the child's art instructors similarly try to induce variations in responses. On the other hand, the child encounters specific sports skills and coaches of these skills for the first time, events which encourage the *only* or *best* ways of performing specific skills for maximum performance advantage. Thus, in natural ways the initial months of a child's life are occupied with both variability and efforts for precision of response, while later childhood years are also occupied with this same dichotomy of exactitude and creative variability of physical action.

Interesting individual differences in how this variability of response may be manifested have appeared in recent research. For example, when manipulating blocks and clay, some investigators have found that children may be classified into two types. On the one hand are those who use this kind of material to form ever-increasing patterns, arranging blocks in different designs or forming balls of clay into patterns that are unique. In contrast, one is able to identify those whose efforts are to assign ever-increasing functions to clay, blocks, and the like. These latter children are not concerned about the shape of blocks, or how they may form clay, but instead are quite interested in how many things they may make a block, or a group of blocks, do or stand for. At one point the block may become an imaginary truck; at another point, a building. These individual differences in how children create variation, and what kinds of variability they consistently evidence, has important implications for the types of mental processes they will later engage in well, and even perhaps in the types of occupations they may later succeed in.

Arguments persist among and between movement educators and those advocating specific skill teaching among children as to which approach is best, whereas in truth by the child's very efforts, tendencies, and actions, it is probable that both kinds of movement demands have their place in the motor development of the child. Both types may be encouraged concurrently within the same or separate formal programs. This paradoxical contrast in children to explore variability and at

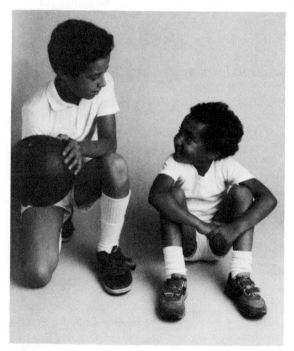

FIGURE 10.1 With maturity children are required to acquire specific skills valued by older peers.

the same time to achieve precision is a most interesting pair of goals in the movement behavior patterns of children. It is a dichotomy that presents a challenge to movement educators as well as to maturing youngsters themselves.

Children's response capacities become refined over time. Extraneous movements, or overflow, occur less in older children than in younger ones. Children acquire the ability to watch complex demonstrations longer as they become older, while their ability to respond quicker also improves with age. Thus a child's *ability* to emit a precise response improves in childhood. At the same time, if encouraged or unhampered, the child's *wishes* to continue to experiment with a variety and diversity of movement responses also may continue to be manifested during the same periods in middle and late childhood.

Wholes or Parts?

Developmentally, children's motor skills undergo modification partly as a function of their attention to a part or to the whole of the situations confronting them. Early in life, infants often become somehow locked in to a part of an action event with which they are confronted. They often have difficulty breaking away from a single component of the situation and focusing upon the broad context. Many young children single-mindedly follow a ball rolling into the street rather than observing oncoming cars.

Ball games in early childhood are often difficult if they are made too complicated. Young children seem to have a limited amount of perceptual energy in such situations, and thus deal mostly with objects and people singularly and in close proximity (Hogan and Hogan, 1975). When children enter school, another step in this whole-part pattern of attention is seen. They may then begin to attend to too many things at the same time. In contrast to infants, they often fail to select out important parts of a situation to attend to. Failure in ball games may occur when the child apparently becomes transfixed with the actions of too many things and people occurring at the same time (Chi, 1976). Finally, during middle and late childhood, a further sorting out process is seen. At this point youngsters begin to become able selectively to switch from either the broad or the narrow context. In games they may quickly transfer their attention from a moving ball to patterns of action seen in a number of moving people. The perceptually mature child in late childhood may, for example, accommodate to the need to focus upon the basket when shooting, and at the same time be aware of the location of players in the game (Thomas, 1980).

These three phases thus consist of (a) selectively and narrowly concentrating upon a single central part of a situation; (b) a broadly based attentional pattern, often excluding central stimuli; and (c) effectively switching from a central focus to a more broadly based attentional orientation. Children do not move neatly and predictably from one of these stages to another. Often a child may be perceptually immature in one situation, while in a more familiar one, more mature perceptual functioning may be seen.

Wholes and Parts

Another important part of the infant's and child's response tendencies, when confronted with need to manifest skill, includes tendencies for responses initially to consist of pieces and then later to become parts of larger and larger wholes. Often the infant is seen to emit even partial responses, which Piaget termed signifiers. These become full responses, which later become parts of still larger skills. Thus, following the acquisition of a single skill over time is not as useful as determining how well a child builds up various parts into a whole.

One example would consist of an outfielder in a childhood game who is able to watch a ball, judging its trajectory and termination, and at the same time move laterally, preparing the hands to make an interception, terminating with watching the ball. This total or global response of the 12-year-old outfielder is made up of at least four or five different subskills, including tracking the ball visually, moving laterally, stopping the body in preparation for interception, preparing the hands for interception, and finally making the catch. This response, fully elaborated, also includes decisions and actions that propel the ball to the appropriate place or base.

This gradual buildup and elaboration of responses into increasingly complex action patterns is characteristic of children's motor learning at all ages. Left to their own devices, this building up and elaboration process will usually be engaged in by normal youngsters under reasonably motivating conditions. Movement development educators need to be sensitive to how rapidly this buildup may occur in various skills and at what ages, and under what kinds of instructional conditions. In infancy, the neonate builds upon a simple sucking response while learning to mold to the mother's body and to grasp the bottle, just as the older child learns to field a ball in the outfield.

With maturity, the infant and child learn to do more than one thing at a time. This quality involves improved attentional abilities and is dependent upon the automatization of a single skill, so that attentional energy is not required, permitting attention to be given to another subskill, or to a component of the external environment. A new and difficult skill requires close attention, as when the child first tries to reach for an object with one hand; later the child learns to hold an object in one hand and manipulate a part of it with the other, as discussed in Chapter 8.

As attentional and skill capacities improve with age, the child may also attend to more than one skill, or selectively attend to a subskill while moving the body. This is a useful type of skill modification. Walking need not be closely attended to after the middle of the first year, permitting children to engage visually and motorically in other skills while walking, or even running (Thomas, 1980).

This same buildup is illustrated quite well when a child learns the complexities of typing. First single letter responses are acquired, and then word responses, which may be executed without thinking about a single letter. Finally, phrases are acquired. In a similar way, the child learns partial skills, and then increasingly larger wholes as he or she acquires the ability to tie shoes, dress, play an instrument, play basketball, and finally drive a car. The movement development teacher must learn just how rapidly to encourage the child to attempt the next level or chunk of a skill, or skill family, without overloading the child's response capabilities and perceptual abilities. Children progress at different rates, and what might be a partial skill to one child is a difficult whole to another. Thus individual differences in response capacities must be carefully dealt with during the formative years of childhood by instructors in physical skills.

HOW CHILDREN LEARN SKILLS: MODELS AND INSTRUCTION TYPES

A variety of reasons have been postulated as to why a child continues to be impelled to practice a skill, and why the child attempts a skill in the first place. These reasons include intrinsic interest in the task itself and feedback from the child's own efforts. Other reasons include the influence of various models—others who may be performing the skill and who may be copied. Still other reasons for the child's acquiring skill include instruction. This can be formal instruction emanating from others, as well as formal or incidental self-instruction the child may give to himself or herself. It has also been postulated that the child may learn accidentally, as some random event occurs and is paired with the child's physical efforts.

A survey of the literature makes it apparent that under various conditions and circumstances, and at various ages, several of these factors may be operative. Indeed, in a given situation two or more of these conditions may be influential in skill acquisition. In simple chronological order, the importance of the various methods might be as follows:

1. During the early months, feedback from the infant's own variable efforts seems to afford maximum inducement to move further. Piaget has named these *primarily circular reactions*. This feedback consists first of satisfying modifications of the child's own body, sucking responses, and hand to body and mouth, and later the reactions of the environment, as objects are randomly and then intentionally contacted (Piaget, 1952).

2. Rather soon in infancy, various models for movement may prove to be powerful inducements. Models, both at this age and later, exert both specific and general influences. That is, the mother or caretaker, both by expression and example, affords the infant a general model for action. They show the infant that the exertion of effort and action are generally desirable. In addition, the model both then and later will begin to exhibit specific skills the child may copy. An early initial skill might include a smile emanating from the mother. Later the mother might model the grasping of a spoon or of a rattle.

3. Also during this early period, intrinsic interest in the task itself proves motivating and sustains present actions while promoting further ones. Rhoda Kellogg, who studied the scribbling behavior of infants and children in great detail, believes quite strongly that early attempts at scribbling are sustained because of the results of the child's efforts themselves, rather than because of any attempt formally to teach the child, or because of the child's attention to objects and events external to the situation. This is, the early scribbler is satisfied, happy, and motivated by the sight of his or her own scribbles, and does not consciously try to copy the people, flowers, or houses that may be sug-

gested by these early efforts. This intrinsic task interest, or the motivation to move for its own sake, has been alluded to in numerous studies of movement qualities in children. Furthermore, this kind of motive may be blunted and corrupted if an inordinate number of extrinsic rewards are afforded the child in an indiscriminate way for exhibiting proficiency in general movement tasks or in movement skills (Yarrow et al., 1983; Kellogg, 1969).

4. Later the child may be susceptible to instruction from two sources. At first the child may in subtle ways begin to instruct himself or herself. By the age of 5, it has been found that children will realize that larger tasks are more difficult than smaller ones. By the age of 7 or 8 more sophisticated kinds of self-instruction will enhance both cognitive as well as motor tasks.

5. Overlapping self-instruction in time will be formal instructional programs emanating from others. This kind of formal instruction may have various effects upon the child's movement capacities ranging from traumatization to improvement. Often those engaging in formal instruction do not realize that the younger child is also trying to instruct himself or herself at the same time. Thus the making available of formal instruction to younger children, children who may have limited information capacity systems, should be done with care. A child who is being given formal instruction is usually also attempting to handle information from a variety of other sources, including feedback from the task itself, information the child is telling himself or herself, and information that may be given by other child models in the situation (Anshel, 1979).

INTENTIONAL AND ACCIDENTAL LEARNING

In a number of ways, the learning that accompanies the acquisition of motor skills may be either intentional or accidental. The random actions, the striving for variability, often result in action-outcome pairings which are accidental, but which at the same time are useful and/or satisfying and which result in the actions being repeated intentionally. Numerous examples of this occurring in the newborn are to be found in the writings of Piaget. Any parent carefully observing a child at play can attest to the occurrences of accidental learning that take place both in infancy and in childhood. An object held in the hand, while the arm inscribes a rapid arc in the air, may be pulled from the infant's grip, resulting in an initial crude throwing response. Objects struck against a surface as the infant attempts to make noises may also leave satisfying marks, and thus result in the first primitive scribbling responses, responses which are further elaborated upon in successive days and attempts. With maturation, the incidence of these accidental happenings may tend to decrease. Nonetheless, their occurrence at all stages in the child's career forms an important part of motor skills acquisition. These accidental happenings may be encouraged by the sensitive parent, who may "accidentally on purpose" place materials or arrange conditions so that the child's seekings for novelty are rewarded by new and happy outcomes. As these instances occur, the intelligent child not only seeks to repeat the more satisfying ones, but also adds to his or her list of rules that govern the interactions of actions and objects.

Modeling may also be accidental or intentional. A formal lesson may take place into which a planned model is inserted. On the other hand, the accidental presence of models within the child's world, consisting of brothers, sisters, and play-mates, offer other models to copy and emulate as skills are acquired. Learning itself may be thought of as accidental, acquired through random play, or the result of planned teaching-learning experiences. It is likely that the vast majority of the child's attempts to gain skills during the first months and years of life occur because of accidental and informal, rather than intentional and formal learning experiences. However, the attentive, sensitive, and creative parent may be able to create a great number of accidental learning experiences through their attitudes toward apparently random exploration, as well as through the judicious placement of objects and the affording of useful opportunities for the child to "accidentally discover" the useful-ness of a new skill.

MOTOR PLANNING: WHY IT CHANGES WITH AGE

In Chapter 9 a brief survey was made of quantitative changes in motor planning behaviors in children of various ages. However, simply measuring improvement in planning qualities is easier than finding out *why* more mature children are able to evidence more proficiency in putting together larger series of movement patterns. Proficiency in motor planning may be due to (a) the ability to attend to a prolonged demonstration of a movement; (b) the ability visually to organize and to remember what is demonstrated; (c) the maturation of integrative processes deep within the nervous system; and/or (d) the ability to execute a series of movements correctly (Cratty and Samoy, 1984).

It is likely that for many children, all these processes, involving organization of input, integration of input and output, as well as quality of output, combine col-lectively to improve execution as increased neuromotor maturity is achieved. Motor planning, according to our work, is not a simple and singular entity. The ability of children to observe and to execute hand movements is not highly correlated to the observation and execution of movements involving the limbs and the total body. So when it is decided that the child is either good or bad at motor planning, an addi-tional and more precise decision has to be made concerning just what kind of motor task(s) constitute the planned act to which one is referring. Measures of motor plan-ning thus represent a synthesis of a number of qualities that are likely to change positively as children mature. Attention span increases, enabling the taking in of longer demonstrations. Improvement in medium- and short-term memory also con-tributes to retention of parts of movement series demonstrated. Finally, with neuromotor maturation the ability to execute movements of increasing complexity is enhanced.

The further application and refinement of motor planning measures should give movement educators, and others interested in formal skill development, guidelines for determining just how much visual-motor-auditory information nor-mal children at various ages may process, integrate, and otherwise deal with. More-over, the elaboration of these measures will also provide helpful tools with which to evaluate children whose coordination may be less than adequate.

THINKING, TALKING, AND MOTOR LEARNING

Penetrating looks at motor skill acquisition as a function of age require analyses of just how various conceptual and linguistic elements reside within the evolving intricacies of physical actions. Cognitive elements underlie and influence infants' early experimentation, as well as their assessments of both intentional and accidental outcomes of actions undertaken at various ages. Moreover, verbal elements, words emanating from others and from the child himself or herself, invariably interact with efforts to move better as youngsters strive to interact with their world.

It is possible to project a rather neat sequence of events pairing verbal to motor behavior as a function of age. At the same time, however, which comes first, the chicken or the egg, or in this case the words or the actions, seems to depend on the situation and behaviors studied. For example, actions probably precede the child's first understanding of words emanating from the caretaking mother. The child acts, and then learns that Stop! has a distinct and often painful meaning. A number of acts may be tried and then the mother's words monitored before the child begins to lessen certain efforts when admonished verbally.

Rather soon, however, the infant learns that words may precede actions. The mother or father makes a statement—"Come here," or perhaps "What is it?" or maybe "Give it to me"—and then the child begins to experiment with actions that seem to somehow please the caretaker after these phrases are uttered. Next, the infant may initiate actions that elicit words from parents and siblings. When objects are shown, it is discovered, many times the parents name the extended object. During the first eighteen months of life, the child continues to play with movement and word combinations of various kinds, but for the most part the words played with emanate from others, as expressive speech is still to be acquired by the child. During the middle of the second year, however, a dramatic change may be seen both in the linguistic ability of the child and in the ways in which movements and words may be combined. The child begins to utter recognizable words, words that he or she soon learns may be used as adjuncts to the planning, describing, and executing of motor skills.

The first ways in which these words and later phrases are employed are in obvious and overt utterances. The child states out loud what he or she is about to do, and then often accompanies the subsequent action with a similar phrase. The termination of the action often triggers a similar phrase, reflecting what has just been done. Before the child rolls a ball, he or she might say: "Johnny is going to roll the ball." As the ball is pushed, the phrase is heard again: "Johnny is rolling the ball." Finally, after the ball has stopped its journey, the child might state: "Johnny rolled the ball." Thus words and later phrases are used as adjuncts to planning, as controls when an act is taking place, and then later as a kind of reflection, assessment, or reward statement after the termination of an action.

During the second and third years, these expressive phrases may be modified, shortened, whispered, or even left out entirely when an action has been well assimilated. A moderately well learned act may be accompanied later by subvocal internal speech; when further acquisition has taken place, the physical skill may be unaccompanied by any kind of speech-language, internal or external. At the same time, both children and adults are likely to again turn to expressive language (either external or internal) when confronted with new, complex, and/or difficult tasks. All of us, children included, seem to realize that an important aid to our thoughts and our actions are the phrases we may utter that describe how we are thinking or acting.

Virtually inseparable, except perhaps to the sophisticated linguist, are thoughtful phrases and cognitive behavior itself. It is thus possible to hypothesize that thoughts act in much the same ways as the thoughtful phrases noted above. Early attempts at motor skills acquisition, or the acquisition of difficult skills, require a great deal of thought by infants and children. Later stages of learning, or the confrontation of an easy motor skill, do not call for as much cognitive energy. At the same time, cognition and motor skill acquisition may be paired in several other ways. These combinations will be surveyed briefly, as a thorough and comprehensive discussion of cognitive development is beyond the scope of this text. It is likely that with increased cognitive sophistication, the processes and combinations described will translate into superior motor skill learning and execution in children of increasing ages. Briefly, thought and skill may be combined in the following ways:

1. Early stages of motor skill acquisition have often been described as the *discovery phase*, a period of time during which the learner tries to determine the similarity of the present skill with past skills acquired, and then tries to develop effective work methods for the task facing him or her. It is likely that as cognitive maturity is gained, the child will more quickly perceive similarities between a contemporary skill and one or several skills learned in the past. Moreover, the intellectually more able child will then more quickly adopt effective work methods when beginning the initial stages of the new skill. Research is quite clear that a mentally retarded youth will have more difficulty during this phase, and that if given special help in conceptualizing what the new skill is all about, will often equal a normal child when executing a skill.

2. One important type of cognitive ability is memory. Memory processes, coupled with retrieval, undoubtedly contribute to mature motor skill acquisition. In older children, improved memory, memory storage capacity, and retrieval from memory enable them to (a) store more templates representing an increasing variety of physical skills, (b) retrieve skills from storage when appropriate, and (c) apply skills to new situations in useful ways (Chi, 1976; Carson and Weigand, 1979).

3. Another cognitive dimension important in the understanding of motor learning is how action and thought blend together during the formative years. It has been found that how the child instructs himself or herself undergoes interesting modifications in early childhood and later.

At still another and more sophisticated level, children also become able and are more inclined to *think about thinking itself* as they progress from early to middle and to late childhood. Thus the child improves at two levels relative to the selection and application of a given skill or group of skills to situations encountered: (a) They engage in better planning strategies, and (b) they pay increasing attention and expend more intellectual resources to planning their planning. This second level of thinking about thinking is sometimes referred to as *metacognitive behavior*. Programs to help children acquire better skills at planning their thinking usually pay off in better performances of motor tasks and academic operations, but they also reflect increased general abilities to exercise better self-control (Flavell, 1972).

Among the kinds of evidence seen to support this important thread within the child's overall intellectual personality is the observation that when a 5-year-old is told that he must remember a group of objects (those present in the room), he or she may spend more time visually inspecting its contents before leaving. However, a child of 7 or 8 may be seen to recite the list of the room's contents aloud before being required to repeat what has been inspected.

Contemporary scholars often link metacognition with internal self-talk. They postulate that what the child says to himself or herself is an important reflection of the nature of the child's thoughts, and thoughts about thoughts (metacognition.). Additionally, contemporary students of metacognition have attempted to change how children behave by attempting to adjust the child's internal vocalizations. Much of the time these attempts at adjustment of self-talk, and the behavior they apparently control, have involved the use of motor tasks. A child, for example, may be given a relatively complicated drawing task. In an effort to reduce the child's tendencies to move through the task impulsively, the clinician might have the child recite careful planning statements aloud—for example, "I should first find out just what I must do in this task." Self-talk is also encouraged during the execution of the task—"There, I must hold the paper with one hand while drawing with the other." Additionally, phrases are required at the termination of the task: "I did pretty well that time, but still did not always stay between the lines." This final kind of self-talk may involve phrases that act as self-rewards, as well as self-evaluation of previous efforts—for example: "Not bad for the first time," and "I did not always hold the pencil correctly, however." In these examples, the clinicians often are employing physical tasks, only as means to get at improvements in thought strategies in a variety of school operations, including reading and mathematics. At the same time, these same kinds of self-talk, or metacognitive efforts, may to varying degrees be present as a child plans, executes, and reflects back upon motor skills themselves, skills used both in self-care tasks (shoelace tying) and in sports (throwing and serving a tennis ball) (Cratty, 1985).

It is logical to hypothesize that the more mature child, perhaps more intellectually capable, is likely to utter more effective types of internalized speech (self-talk) than is the less mature. Improvement in various aspects of motor skill acquisition thus is due not only to such subtleties as the maturation of the neuromotor system and changes in perceptual qualities, but also to the manner in which the child thinks about the applications of actions to situations.

Examples of how mature thought is likely to aid children's acquisition and application of skill include these:

1. The child who is intellectually able learns with experience to select out from the memory storage an exactly appropriate subskill to meet the precise situation encountered.
2. Intellectual maturity aids a child to formulate effective preplanning decisions as a skill sequence is begun.

3. During and at the completion of a skill, the intellectual maturation of the child brings better decisions concerning the evaluation of what has just happened. With successive performances of a given skill, the older and more intellectually adroit child will leave out skill components that have not helped and add those that are likely to enhance an action or actions. Following the completion of a task, the effects of effort are more likely to be evaluated well by older, more intellectually aware youngsters.

4. Furthermore, the intellectually more able child is more likely to seek out and copy effective models, and also to search for and take advantage of more obvious and formal opportunities to acquire skill. A boy who was on two Olympic gymnastic teams during his formative years, extending back into late childhood, was seen to travel from gymnasium to gymnasium in the Los Angeles area getting the best coaching available in the various events. During high school, he even promoted a fundraiser in order to buy a video tape player so that he might gain even more improvement in his chosen sport.

PLANNING FOR EFFECTIVE SKILL ACQUISITION

The primary focus of this text is on describing various signposts of motor development, as well as the various influences on these changes in action patterns seen at various ages. At this point, however, it is important to discuss briefly principles that seem appropriate when devising programs, teaching strategies, and environments intended to stimulate the acquisition of skills in infants and children. Information concerning the developmental perspectives that accompany the growing capacities of children to manifest skill would not be complete without at least a brief section devoted to the implications of these perspectives.

It has been suggested that near birth the infant, seemingly because of inherent dispositions, strives to seek information and to create novelty by exhibiting a large number of responses and response variations in movement qualities. Next, the child may begin to model, or subtly copy, others with whom he or she comes in contact. Further stages include informal and formal attempts by others to instruct the child, and finally the child acting as a self-instructor, devising increasingly sophisticated strategies and skill outcomes as he or she learns to engage in more effective self-instruction. A final stage may be reached as the child learns to think about thinking. These metacognitive behaviors may lead not only to better and better physical skills, but also to the formulation of plans of attack. A final point should be emphasized. These so-called stages in skill acquisition overlap in time; their appearance and disappearance may not be validly attached to specific ages. Rather, the ways in which they may come and go are often dependent upon the newness and difficulty of the task(s) facing the child.

Some of the principles these perspectives suggest are the following:

1. Early in the life of the infant, an environment should be created in which the infant is free to explore variability and novelty. The infant should be free emotionally as well as physically to express broad variations in actions, including those apparently intended, those that are reflexes, and those that are rhythmic stereotypes (see Chapter 3). Paren-

tal approval should be apparent when the infant simply wishes to kick and to otherwise explore movement capacities. Clothing should be unrestricted, and objects should be available in the environment (within restrictions suggested by safety and good sense) that enable the infant freely to explore capabilities and variations which seem to flow out of the child during the early months of life.

2. This seeking of creative variability should not be suddenly turned off as the infant is faced with some of the more formal self-care skills needed by society. Rather, it should be continued into early childhood and even later, as suggested in the often highly creative programs formulated by movement educators.

3. Most important, accidental acquisition of a skill due to chance actions occurring within random patterns should be brought to the attention of a child, repeated, and sometimes repracticed with intentions and outcomes made clear. During these bouts of variability, variability should be encouraged for its own sake, but at the same time when culturally useful skills accidentally occur their occurrence should be pinpointed and further exploited (Carson and Weigand, 1979).

4. A number of kinds of both specific and general models should be readily available to the infant and child even during the first year of life. These models should transmit both general emotions and ideas which accompany movement, as well as model specific skills needed by the society. The child should be exposed to general peer and adult models which portray the fact that vigorous movement is acceptable and joyful. Moreover, such general modeling should include the indication that often ballistic, random, and too-rapid action patterns may be placed under more restrained control, in order to accomplish skills of increasing usefulness and complexity required by the culture. During this phase, numerous attempts at precise teaching via well-thought-out demonstrations may not be as useful as simply presenting attitudes, emotions, and general tendencies and strategies (Leithwood and Fowler, 1971). Also during this modeling period, extending from birth until well into early childhood, the infant may be exposed to more specific demonstrations. These may take place daily as self-care skills are informally demonstrated, as well as during family outings, during which the child may observe recreational and sports skills important to the culture.

5. Formal instruction should be phased in and overlap in time formal and informal modeling. However, particularly during the formative years of early childhood, it should be remembered that the subject involved is hardly formal. The first tries at teaching a youngster a skill should be brief and relatively unstructured. "See me do it . . . now try also . . ." or simply "watch" might be phrases which accompany the first tries at teaching a young child anything. As maturity is gained, the child may be exposed to increasingly formal verbal instructions and demonstrations. He or she also should be gradually taught general strategies that may be applied to a number of skills and to other operations in classrooms, homes, and neighborhood, including social and academic skills. It should be remembered, however, that even during early and middle childhood, from 3 to 7 or 8 years of age, it may be more important to arrange conditions within the environment that permit the child to manipulate the environment in ways which are important to him or her. Educators were first puzzled when child development experts in England exploited the use of junk-filled playgrounds for children. Then it was realized that the child's efforts to manipulate the environment were more motivating in this kind of modifiable situation than were more formal climbing and play activities constrained by immovable playground equipment set in iron and cement.

6. During the engagement with these broad categories of response variability, modeling, and formal instruction, the sensitive educator should keep in mind that the content and opportunities afforded the maturing infant and child should be compatible with some

of the perceptual and motivational tendencies also outlined in this chapter. That is, the infant should not be exposed to tasks that contain too much complexity, and particularly to the presentation of too much simultaneous input. Let the children create their own skill complexity as they wish and are able; do not force too much input complexity at too early an age.

7. Those interested in motivating the child to move should realize that much of the motivation for early and later movement striving arises from the intrinsic need to move for movement's sake. The movements themselves and then the novelty and interest of the outcomes they create in the environment are motivation enough for most youngsters. These motives, coupled with mere parent interest, surprise, and approval, form a powerful complex of reasons to act with increasing effort, intensity, and complexity. The introduction of extrinsic bribes in the form of trophies, jackets, and medals may in early and late childhood quickly blunt the child's desires to partake in vigorous action for its own sake. Rewards of this latter kind should be afforded judiciously and sparingly at all ages, and then given only when true effort and achievement is realized, and not merely for participating.

SUMMARY

Numerous trends and variables contribute to the acquisition of skills in infants and in older youngsters. The child's cognitive and linguistic capacities, as well as the presence of social stimulation, are all likely to enhance or blunt the acquisition of skill.

Early in life infants evidence wide variations in the kinds of movement they express, as well as in the quantity they exhibit. With maturation, variability continues, but at the same time efficiency is achieved as skills are matched more and more with specific situations calling for action. A skilled child is one who exhibits the correct skill for the appropriate situation, not one who simply moves expansively and with apparently meaningless variation.

Children acquire skills and are motivated to do so because of several factors. Initially skills are acquired for their own sake; movement stimulates movement. Later the child begins to attend to models for actions within the environment, to copy others, and to do what others suggest.

Internal self-talk expands to serve as self-stimulation of appropriate learning strategies in later childhood. This internal speech tends to interact with more formal instruction extended by others.

Motor planning capacities improve. This improvement is due to better attention and neuromotor maturation, resulting in coordination improvement in middle and later childhood. With experience, children become able to (a) attend to more than one subskill at a time, and (b) put together ever-larger wholes as they engage in motor learning practice.

Those implementing motor skills teaching programs should provide not only for the exploration of a variety of actions, but also for help in the molding of precise, situation-specific skills needed at home, at play, and in school.

QUESTIONS FOR DISCUSSION

1. What implications does metacognition have for skill acquisition in middle and late childhood?
2. What differences are seen in the qualities of infants' movements versus those in children's actions that have implications for the stimulation of motor skills learning?
3. How does expressive and internal speech interact with the early expression of physical skills in the preschool child?
4. What changes in whole versus part perception influence skill performance and acquisition in younger and older children?
5. What implications do the presence of the infant stereotypes discussed in Chapter 3 have for the planning of a movement education program for children of 5 years of age?
6. How might you teach a child with a poor score on a motor planning test?
7. What rules might you follow for the teaching of a youngster with superior movement attributes?
8. What inherent characteristics were proposed? How do these interact with the acquisition of skill in infancy and in childhood?
9. What paradoxes or contradictions does the child confront when learning motor skills?
10. How might the awarding of jackets and trophies indiscriminately to children participating in competitive sport blunt motivation?

STUDENT PROJECTS

1. Help a child learn to throw a ball for accuracy. Plot variability of responses as well as accurate scores recorded on a target placed either horizontally or vertically.
2. Place one toy in front of an infant of from 6 to 10 months. Record how long he or she plays with it. Next add a second object, new to the infant. Record shifts to the new object, and duration of time spent with the familiar and the novel object.
3. Permit one child to explore a new skill without any formal instruction, such as kicking a ball toward a target. Contrast the progress of this first child to that of one given formal instructions in the same task. Draw implications as to what is best in this situation and for this type of child—formal instruction or exploratory behavior.
4. Discuss with an adolescent athlete how he or she mentally practices the skills of the sport when not actually engaged in physical practice. Contrast the responses you get to those received when you ask the same question of a more experienced university-level athlete.
5. Position yourself near a nursery school play yard, so that you can hear conver-

sations taking place. Are you able to pick up the kind of expressive self-talk accompanying skills discussed in this chapter? Under what conditions?

6. Begin teaching a child a new physical skill. First, give only one instruction; next, give two pieces of advice at nearly the same time; later, give three instructions; and so on. Find out how much information your child wishes to, or can, process at one time.

CHAPTER ELEVEN
VISUAL–PERCEPTUAL
DEVELOPMENT

The fathers of experimental psychology were intrigued by how infants and children begin to see and to interpret visual worlds (James, 1890). These early scholars believed visual abilities to be limited to primitive reflexes. When they speculated about how infants and children perceive visual information, it was usually thought that a mass of confusion surrounded the infant's first attempts to draw meaning from visual experiences.

During the first decades of this century, those trying to understand vision and its development in the child continued to confine their efforts to measuring simple visual reactions in the presence of color and form. Then, as today, most energies of experimentalists were confined to trying to determine how the infant within the first year of life functioned, rather than taking a more enlightened and comprehensive look at the continuing unfolding of vision and visual perception in early and later childhood.

In the early 1960s a marked shift occurred in how researchers viewed the early visual activity of the child. Studies emerged that used measures of duration of visual attention displayed by the newborn to various kinds of conditions and displays. The infant began to be looked upon not only as a simple reactor to stimulation, but as an individual who seemed to possess the ability to choose what to attend to (Fantz, 1961). Recently developed measures of visual scanning of infants have demonstrated that not only does the newborn engage in a vast amount of visual activity, but that early in life the young are active seekers of things to see in ways that appear to be innate (Haith, 1980).

Obtaining a clear and simple picture of how visual-perceptual abilities change from birth through childhood is an undertaking made difficult for several reasons. Precise demarkation between unfolding visual capacities and qualities that reflect how the maturing child forms judgments of visual space is not always possible. Finding out how well a child brings in a clear picture of an event to the retina does not always afford information on how well that same youngster is able to *interpret* visual-spatial events.

The numerous and diverse ways in which both visual and visual-perceptual abilities are measured makes summaries of how they change as a function of age even more difficult. Sometimes, for example, the scores obtained reflect judgments gathered while the child is a relatively passive observer. At other times the youngster is required to make various kinds of movement responses when confronted with visual stimuli and events.

Finally, a discussion of visual-perceptual development is complicated by the fact that a far larger percentage of the literature has traditionally focused upon infants and younger children, rather than upon individuals in middle and late childhood. Literally hundreds of studies have been published since the 1960s describing various parameters of visual behaviors in infants, while investigations of how children from 6 to 12 deal with moving missiles are more scarce.

What is clear, however, is that infants and children engage is a vast amount of visual activity, and that many of the processes underlying that activity seem innate. Untangling the meanings of changes in visual activity and visual-perceptual behaviors is a more difficult undertaking. However, gaining a hold upon the whys of perceptual development is beginning to be made easier because of the formation of several useful theories by modern researchers and scholars.

A number of conundrums abound when attempting to delve into the visual-perceptual qualities that interact with voluntary movement. At times certain perceptual qualities interact with specific movement qualities, and at other times vision and visual perception are quite independent of the accuracy of motor acts. Often it is apparent that visual-perceptual qualities mature in advance of actions that will later accompany them. For example, quite early in life the infant apparently is able to discriminate among triangles, circles, and squares. However, it is not until the fifth and sixth year that most youngsters are able to draw these same figures using the movements of their hands. To cite another example, children of about 3 seem able to identify various geometric figures that are presented within either an up or a down orientation. However, these same children will be unable to arrange letters in precise up-down and left-right relationships through their printing efforts on a page (Cratty and Martin, 1969).

Infants and children are seen gradually to build up qualities that will finally contribute to complex visual-motor-perceptual tasks in later childhood. For example, infants are able to engage in rudimentary visual tracking near birth, and by the sixth month can engage in this activity for prolonged periods of time. It is several years later, however, before children can catch balls with their hands, and even longer before a youngster can first watch and then position hands and body in ways that will result in a ball being caught within a playground game (Sadulis, 1985).

Visual-perceptual development does not proceed independent of cognitive and linguistic changes. Indeed, some have described three stages in visual-perceptual metamorphosis, including (1) an initial stage that is characterized by apparently "wired in" visual tendencies and perceptual searchings, (b) a second stage marked by more and more choice behaviors on the part of the child, and (c) a final stage in which visual-perceptual development is accompanied by symbolic linguistic qualities.

VISUAL CHARACTERISTICS OF THE NEWBORN

Recently, methodological advances have resulted in more precise evaluation of early visual behaviors. Simple measures of fixation times, popular in the 1960s, have been replaced by even more sophisticated electronic devices permitting us to peer into and out of the eyes of babies. The electroretinogram (ERG), for example, is a measure of the changes in electric potentials of the retina when it is exposed to light. Another direct measure of the eye's activity, the electrooculorgram (EOG), measures with precision movements the eyes make by plotting the pathways of the electric potentials that emerge from between the retina and cornea (Maurer, 1975).

Indirect measures of visual and visual-perceptual activity in the newborn are also coming into prominence. For example, changes in the infant's heart rate when exposed to various visual displays have been employed to assess both perceptual and cognitive judgment-making in infants within the first weeks of life. Finally, measures of brain-wave activity have been employed in direct responses to visual stimuli. This assessment of visually evoked potential (VEP) seems to afford insight into the brain's processing of visual stimuli (Karmel and Maisel, 1975; White et al., 1977).

Despite present knowledge of early visual behaviors, information about the exact ways in which the visual system matures physiologically is more limited. These limitations are caused by the difficulty of correctly interpreting physiological changes in the eye and the neurological tissues that support vision in newborns shortly after their expiration (Haith, 1978). Thus apparent knowledge of how the visual system develops physiologically and anatomically has been derived from studying such measures as nerve conduction velocities obtained in the visual systems of infant animals, notably kittens and rhesus monkeys (Parmelee and Sigman, 1976).

Partly because of the need to extrapolate from animal studies, there is disagreement about the maturity of the retina at birth. Initially it was believed that the center of the retina, the fovea, did not mature until around the fourth month. However, researchers in the late 1970s became convinced that the cells adapted for clear central vision are relatively mature even at birth (Haith, 1978).

The optic nerve of the infant is both thinner and shorter than that of the adult. Estimations of the completion of myelinizations range from three weeks to four months (Last, 1968; Duke-Elder and Cook, 1963). Generally it is believed that various peripheral (the retina) and supporting neural structures of vision mature in the order in which information is processed. That is, the retina matures first, and then deeper structures within the nervous system that receive and process visual information (Bronson, 1974). Thus the visual cortex is quite underdeveloped at birth (Conel, 1959). Indeed, fibers within the visual cortex are believed to continue to myelinate through the first ten years of life (Yakovlev and Le Cours, 1967). In addition to the gradual gaining of nerve sheaths during the first ten years of life, other evidence that the visual cortex is maturing comes in the form of changes in the size of cell bodies, length of axons, and dendritic branches, as well as in modifications of electric activity emerging from the visual cortex (visually evoked potentials) (Karmel and Maisel, 1975).

Despite the relatively sketchy picture available about neurological and physiological processes accompanying visual-perceptual maturation, there is no shortage of information about early visual behaviors. Indeed, the most striking kind of finding is the vast amount of visualization recordable in infants at and shortly after birth. Careful inspection of the number of visual fixations in the newborn places them at over two a second during 90 percent of the child's waking hours (Haith, 1980). Furthermore, the infant seems almost obsessed with obtaining as much information as possible, as evidenced by the fact that frequent visual fixations and searching occur even when the child is placed in the dark (Haith, 1980).

Within the first days of life, the visual system undergoes rapid changes, primarily in the form of increased flexibility of function. Accommodation that was apparently locked in at birth at a distance of about 7 feet from the face rapidly ex-

FIGURE 11.1
Infant eye movement recording apparatus. From R. N. Aslin and R. Salapatek, "Saccadic Localization of Peripheral Targets by the Very Young Human Infant," *Perception and Psychophysics, 17* (1975), p. 294. Reproduced with permission.

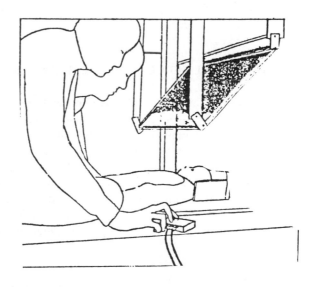

pands to permit the child to survey objects at various distances within the first weeks of age. Tracking responses in a similar manner change from those involving a relatively limited arc to pathways taken by the eyes that are more expansive and in various directions. Visual acuity measures, although depending upon the kinds of stimuli employed, generally undergo marked changes during the first days and weeks of life in normal infants. For example, in some studies visual acuity of infants has been found to approximate that of adult vision between the sixth month and first year of age (Teller, 1973).

Most important, however, are studies which indicate that the young infant's visual searchings seem governed by rather basic rules, built-in tendencies that seem part of the human make-up at birth (Haith, 1978). These rules, as one researcher names them, include the following:

1. If the infant is alert and awake, and the light is not too bright, the eyes are open and actively fixating.
2. In the dark the infant will similarly open the eyes even wider and actively scan for signs of information that may be dimly available.
3. The eyes will scan in searches for the edges of figures and will scan these edges once found. Contours and shapes are similarly sought for and found.
4. Infants attend in general ways; and when encountering worthwhile stimuli, they focus their attention and concern in more specific ways.
5. Most important, the infant is attracted to, and will tend to marshal, physiological-neurological forces when encountering movement within the space field. It has been found that different cell groupings are employed in the retina when various contours and angles are encountered. However, when movement is looked at, most cells within the retina are activated (Haith, 1980).
6. Functionally, both when tracking movement and when looking at lines at various angles, the human infant seems innately to prefer to move the eyes in a horizontal rather than in a vertical direction.

EARLY VISUAL-PERCEPTUAL PREFERENCES

The discovery by Fantz and others in the 1960s that infants displayed choices in what they spent their time looking at initiated a vast amount of interest in these preferences. Stemming from these investigations are rather straightforward findings, and also models and theories that purport to explain the genesis of visual-perceptual behaviors, and of how intellectual and linguistic abilities first appear.

Furthermore, as the technology used to collect visual preferences and fixations became more sophisticated, so did the data emerging from these investigations. More recent ones, for example, have demonstrated that not only do infants simply look at various shapes and configurations, but they move their eyes over parts of the stimuli confronting them in ways that depict not only interest but bore-dom and familiarity (Bronson, 1982).[1]

Numerous kinds of stimuli have been presented to infants, and fixation and scanning measures obtained. These have included the human face, as well as lines and contours of various types. Targets, grids, and geometric figures have also been favored by researchers.

Age and sex differences have been explored, as well as differences caused by habituation to previous stimuli and prior visual experiences (Fantz, 1966; Vurpillot, 1976). In addition to simply clocking fixation times and observing scanning behav-iors, researchers have also recorded concurrent physiological responses.

These have included changes or irregularities in respiration and heart rate, as well as pupil dilation and muscular tension changes. It has been found, for example, that attentive behaviors are sometimes accompanied by peripheral dilation of facial blood vessels, as well as by modifications in respiration and heart rate (Kagan, 1967).

In general, the evidence from studies of visual attention and preference in in-fants suggests the following:

1. More prolonged visual attention is often given to stimuli that are, for the infant, rea-sonably complex and novel (Fantz, 1963). Berlyne (1960), among others, has sug-gested that novelty is a key principle in directing attention. Sokolov (1960) has also suggested that a novel stimulus produces a kind of "What is it?" response.

2. Most of the time stimuli that resemble the human face elicit more attention than those that do not (Kagan, 1967).

3. Infants show marked changes in visual responses at various ages, particularly when different patterns are shown to them. An example of how scanning movements may change in infants at two ages, when exposed to both familiar and unfamiliar stimuli, is in Figure 11.2 (Zinchenko, Van Chizi-Tsin, and Tarakanov, 1962). As can be seen, younger children evidenced less activity when confronted with the stimuli shown. Their visual fixations clustered toward the center of the figure. The older children evi-denced two types of scanning movements, those linking up the edges and center, as well as those focusing upon specific features and the contours, as well as the center.

4. Early experience is likely to influence visual preferences. Some experimenters have suggested that the quality and selection reflected in measures of early visual preference and attention are likely to prove valuable in the early assessment of later intellectual functioning (Fantz et al., 1966; Haith, 1980).

Most encouraging are recent attempts to formulate theories and meanings from measures of attention and preferences obtained from infants (Haith, 1980). For

---

[1]The brevity of the treatment of this enormous amount of data here is caused by space limitations and by the emphasis in this text upon motor, and thus visual-motor, relationships. The interested reader may consult recent reviews by Haith (1980) and Bronson (1982) for contemporary information and theo-ries in this highly diverse and complex area of study. Reviews by Cohen and Salapatek (1975) and Vurpillot (1976) might also be useful.

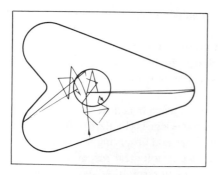
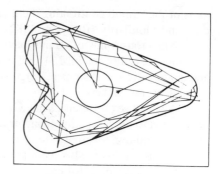
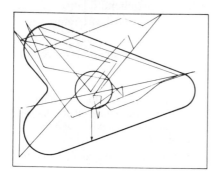
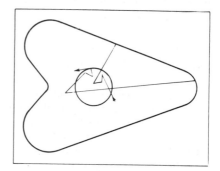

FIGURE 11.2   From V. P. Zinchenko, V. Van Chizitsin, and V. V. Tarakanov, "The Formation and Development of Visual Perception," *Soviet Psychology and Psychiatry, 1,* (1963), p. 4. Used with permission of the publisher, M. E. Sharp, Inc.

example, Kagan (1967) has suggested that infants look at things for two reasons (a) to somehow savor a pleasurable and novel experience, and (b) to place familiar objects into more and more precise and useful categories.

A shift in emphasis has been suggested by Haith in recent work (1980). He has proposed that infants are not simply "captured" by stimuli of various kinds, shapes, and configurations. Rather, he postulates it is the infant who does the capturing. He views the neonate and infant as an active seeker after visual experience and the meanings that may be derived from these experiences.

EARLY VISUAL-MOTOR INTERACTIONS

By the end of the first month, the infant begins to include other components of the muscular system when deploying the directioning musculature of the eyes. It is probable that as other muscular subsystems are added to searching behaviors, more and more information is being obtained about the visual world. Head movements, for example, are likely to accompany ocular tracking and fixations by the thirtieth day of life. In contrast, infants at birth often use eyes and head independently as they attempt to obtain first impressions of their world.

By the second and third months, the eye blink response to approaching objects is seen (Pieper, 1963). Generally the eyes first blink when objects approach from the front; only later will they blink when objects approach from the side. During the third month, and sometimes earlier, the infant will discover body parts and begin to spend a considerable amount of time inspecting them. At first these inspections will not be accompanied by movements of the hands and feet. Later the hands will be seen to open and close as they are watched.

Evidence obtained by Cruickshank in 1941 seemed to indicate that infants by about six months were able to organize depth cues when reaching for rattles. However, it remained for creative research efforts decades later to illustrate how well infants of an even younger age were able to make judgments about visual space, about missiles coming toward them, and even how the young child could be expected to make various motor reactions to often complicated spatial events.

In the 1960s, for example, White (1963) found that infants as young as 8 weeks blinked their eyes when stimuli approached. The apparatus in which this kind of study was carried out is shown in Figure 11.3. Studies in the 1970s continued to explore variables that seemed to contribute to the ability of extremely young infants to react to movement in visual space. Bower and his colleagues (Bower et al., 1970), for example, found that if infants are tested in an alert, upright position when objects are made to come toward them, they are likely to evidence both eye blink responses and defensive arm reactions. Even during the second and third weeks of life, the infants tested appeared to react to approaching objects that were real and were not simply responding to the apparent increase in size exhibited by approaching objects (Bower et al., 1970).

Studies in the late 1970s and into the 1980s indicate that within the first months of life, infants not only are able to predict where a moving object is likely to be at a future time, but may indeed make remarkably accurate interceptions of objects with their hands (DiFranco et al., 1978; Von Hofsten, 1980; Von Hofsten and Lindhagen, 1979). Moreover, it has been found that the infant is able to reach for stationary objects with reasonable success at about the same time that moving objects are intercepted (Von Hofsten and Lindhagen, 1979), at about the sixteenth to eighteenth weeks of age. These reaching abilities, coupled with the apparent visual-perceptual capacities required, have led several contemporary researchers to speculate that such visual-motor behaviors are apparently innate (Von Hofsten, 1980; Haith, 1980; Bower et al., 1970). Even during these early weeks, however, infants evidence individual differences in what has been termed *reaching styles* (Di Franco et al., 1978). Thus what is needed are longitudinal studies of the same infants following their visual-perceptual abilities from the earliest months of life through childhood. As will be seen later in the chapter, tasks requiring perceptual-motor abilities in interception have been studied more in infants than in older youngsters.

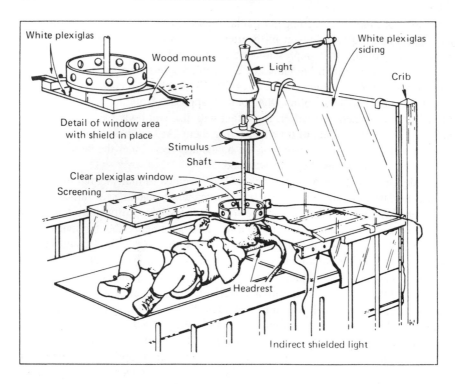

FIGURE 11.3   The blink-eliciting apparatus used by White (1963). From B. L. White, *Human Infants: Experience and Psychological Development.* Copyright 1971. Reproduced by permission of Prentice-Hall, Englewood Cliffs, N. J.

From the 1950s to the 1980s researchers have explored an important group of perceptual tasks that might be termed visual-perceptual-locomotor relationships. These studies were spurred by the classic work of Richard Walk, who exposed infants who could crawl to the visual cliff arrangement pictured in Figure 11.4. It was found that infants, and many lower animals, were reluctant to crawl over a transparent surface exposing them to a "visual cliff." This was taken as evidence that children, when mobile, had already become able to organize important cues relative to depth in their visual field.

More recent visual cliff arrangements have required infants to crawl along a gradually narrowing runway, thus reducing the number of infants who refuse to move in the experimental arrangement pictured. Walk and his colleagues (Walters and Walk, 1974) continued their work using motor responses other than locomotion (creeping). For example, in more recent work they have used the support response, moving seated infants toward visual cliffs and studying whether or not they reach out to support themselves. It has been found, for example, that infants between 8 and 11 months usually evidence the tendency to support themselves on apparently close solid surfaces, whereas most at this age do not reach out to touch a transparent surface over a visual cliff (Walters and Walk, 1974).

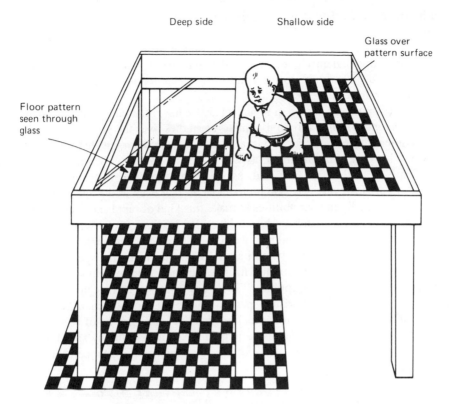

Deep side   Shallow side

FIGURE 11.4 The visual cliff. The infant crawled across a heavy sheet of glass toward his mother. Under the glass was a textured piece of checkered linoleum. For half the distance, the linoleum was just beneath the glass; for the second half of the distance, it was 3 ½ feet below the surface of the glass. At the midpoint, the infant was faced with a visual cliff. Adapted from *Monographs of the Society for Research in Child Development, 28* (1963), Figure 4, p. 11.

Perceptual abilities of children continue to mature and to improve throughout the early months and years of life. By 5 years of age, it has been found that children evidence a number of relatively independent (uncorrelated) perceptual abilities, most of which contribute in specific ways to their ability to deal with visual objects moving through space (Smith and Smith, 1966). These separate abilities or factors include (a) the ability to make judgments about depth relative to the position of the child; (b) the ability to make judgments about movements in space; (c) the ability to make judgments requiring the division of space, as for example when asked to determine what is halfway between the child and an object; and finally (d) the ability to make determinations of position with regard to the position of something (or someone) other than the child making a judgment. Overall, the evidence suggests that any coherent theory about visual perception in children should take into account at least three classes of variables, including (a) ocular characteristics, including measurable functions of the eye; (b) the manner in which various stimuli are interpreted by the child as they strike the retina; (c) qualities that are dependent upon learning.

Moreover, just as is true among infants, children by fifth year continue to evidence marked individual differences in so-called pure perceptual abilities, as well as those that probably contribute to the child's capacities for accurate movement in visual space (Cratty et al., 1973).

Using the apparatus shown in Figure 11.5, we have studied a perceptual quality called *dynamic visual acuity* in a number of studies over the years. Essentially the task is quickly to select accurate visual information from targets that vary in the speed with which they are presented, as well as in size. When children of various ages are exposed to this task, we find, as would be expected, that improvement occurs with age. However, it is also quite apparent that even at the age of 5 years children vary markedly in their abilities to make this kind of rapid and accurate discrimination. As a result of our work, we identified two perceptual types. One of these types consists of young children we named "velocity resistant." This first group is able to react well when stimuli are moved with increasing speed and can select information from these stimuli with the accuracy seen in adults. A second group we called "velocity susceptible." These are youngsters who can see clearly and are able to deal well with visual space when objects are stationary, but who have great difficulty making accurate judgments about the location of stimuli and their constitution when the targets to be judged are moved with any speed at all. Thus, any accurate survey of the nature of the development of visual perception in

FIGURE 11.5 From B. J. Cratty, E. Apitzsch, and R. Bergel, *Dynamic Visual Acuity: A Development Study*, Perceptual-Motor Learning Laboratory UCLA (1973).

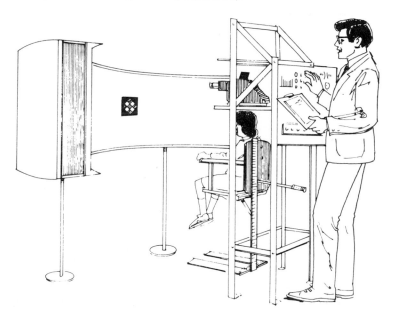

children should also come to terms with so-called norms reflecting visual-spatial judgments at various ages, and attempt to deal with individual differences of the type we and others have found in carefully conducted experiments (Cratty et al., 1973; Di Franco et al., 1978; Hellwig, 1972).

It is possible that individual differences in how well children can physically intercept moving balls etc, in subsequent studies (Stadulis, 1985), also reflect how well children can extract detail from moving targets as was evaluated in the investigation described.

QUALITATIVE CHANGES IN VISUAL-PERCEPTUAL DEVELOPMENT

In addition to the obvious improvement in visual and visual-perceptual performance measures, there are a number of qualitative changes in the ways in which children observe and make judgments about visual space. For example, at birth infants seem first to deal with various parts of their perceptual field. When given two objects to watch, for example, they will select one for inspection and to some degree ignore the other. Later they will be seen to look back and forth from one to the other, apparently engaged in comparative processes.

This same part and whole change occurs when the child's tendencies to both look at and deal motorically with visual space are compared. Initially, visual inspection of objects seems to take place independent of various movements seen in the same infant. Although various measures of physiological activation are often seen when the child is confronted with an object, voluntary movements seem to occur at first somewhat independent of whatever may be occurring within the child's space field. Later, however, the child spends a good deal of time joining information obtained from visual space and actions needed to deal with these new and intriguing spatial events.

The findings from an experiment by Elkind and his colleagues serve to illustrate this whole versus part shift in the perceptions of children (Elkind et al., 1964). When presented with the drawings in Figure 11.6, quite different reports were received from children of various ages, when asked "What are these?" For example, it was found that 4- and 5-year-olds would make statements indicating that they were dealing only with parts. They might report "I see vegetables," for example. At the age of 7 a shift in perceptual behavior was found to occur. Children at this age usually reported seeing the wholes, and might thus report that they saw a "scooter," or that "Here is a heart." At another time children of 7 might alternate in their statements and seem to see only the parts, without perceiving the wholes. Their statements might resemble those of younger children, as they would report seeing candy, or perhaps vegetables. By later childhood, from 60 to 78 percent of the children became apparently able to organize both parts and wholes at the same time. Their statements reflected this simultaneous ability to deal with parts and

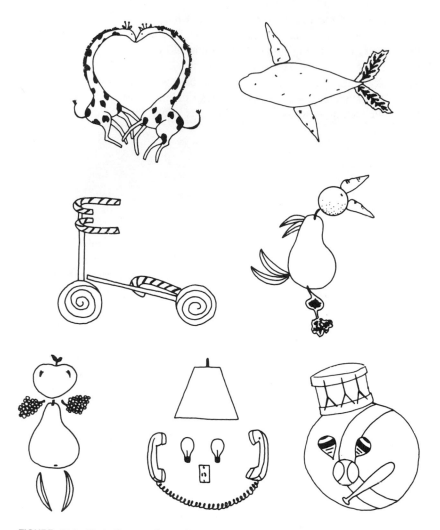

FIGURE 11.6 Illustrations used to evaluate whole versus part perception by Elkind. From D. Elkind, R. R. Koegler, and E. G. Koegler, "Studies in Perceptual Development: II, Part-Whole Perception," *Child Development, 35* (1964), pp. 81–90.

wholes; they might report "I see a man made of vegetables," or perhaps "There is a scooter made of candy."

In our laboratory over the years we have employed several tests with children of various ages, illustrating the concept of how, with maturation, children build up wholes from formerly apparently independent parts. In one of these, the children are asked to contact a ball with the finger as it swings in front of them on a string 15 inches long. Initially, children of 4 are able only to track the ball visually or to swing inaccurately at the string. They may also formulate the strategy of simply holding their arm extended so that the ball contacts their finger. However, when the task is presented to children of 6 and 7 years, a marked change is seen. By these ages, they are seen to coordinate the visual-perceptual qualities needed to determine where the swinging ball will be as it crosses their space field, move their arm and finger quickly to the correct spot, and successfully complete the task required.

A second task also illustrates this part versus whole principle of perceptual maturation. In this task the requirement is accurately to compile a multipart drawing as successive parts are demonstrated by the tester. First the child copies a larger square, then, first, the demonstrator, and then the child adds a figure to each of the corners. Younger children are able to execute geometric figures with some facility. Their squares and circles do not look the same, while at the same time they will attempt a triangle. However, it is seldom that a preschool child, or one of 5 or 6 years, will successfully integrate all the information needed to complete the figure correctly. It is not until a year or two later that the figure will be copied, segment by segment, as demonstrated by the tester.

Another important qualitative change in visual-perceptual development involves the ways in which children identify forms and the spatial orientations of various configurations. This dimension of perceptual maturation becomes particularly important as a youngster enters school and is faced with the job of identifying letter and word shapes, and also trying to determine the meanings and sounds attached to various asymmetrical letters and numbers. Before entering school, a pencil is a pencil no matter whether it rests on the floor or appears in a vertical position. When the 5- and 6-year-old is confronted with *E*s, *R*s, and the like, it becomes important that both the left-right and the up-down dimensions of figures and forms are correctly identified.

Infants at rather young ages are apparently able to discriminate visually between various geometric figures. Ling (1941), for example, found that by 6 months youngsters could differentiate between various figures, discriminations that were apparently not influenced by changes in the size of the stimuli. Several experimenters have found that three-dimensional shapes are easier to identify than two-dimensional forms (Hershenson, 1964; Johnson and Beck, 1966).

Infants a few weeks of age have been found not only to prefer to inspect the human face (or configurations resembling the face), but also to be able to differentiate between various orientations of the face. Watson (1966) found this ability appeared as early as the fifteenth week of age. However, it is probably true that early

FIGURE 11.7

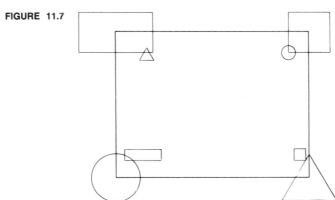

discriminations of the orientations of forms may depend upon how interesting and meaningful the figure is to the youngster. In this same study by Watson, his subjects did not respond with accuracy to the orientations of geometric figures that apparently had little attraction for them.

The available evidence indicates that as children mature, they seem to evidence a reasonably orderly sequence as they organize various dimensions of their space field. First to mature are judgments of the vertical dimensions, followed by the recognition and organization of the horizontal. The more complex oblique or diagonal dimensions of the space field are the last to become organized by the child (Jeffrey, 1966; Rudel and Teuber, 1963). Children of 2 years are as likely to look at many figures and pictures upside down as in an upright position. However, by the third and fourth year of age, preferences for upright pictures are usually seen. By the age of 6, the child is able not only to visually discriminate well between vertical, horizontal, and oblique lines, but also is able to draw these lines with some ease. Children are thus able to discriminate between upright and inverted forms at relatively early ages. However, their ability to discriminate between the asymmetries in such letter combinations as *b-d* and *p-q* often prove difficult even after the child has entered the first or second grade (Davidson, 1935; Ghent and Bernstein, 1961).

Confusions about the names, sounds, and meanings of various asymmetrical letters and numbers are common in children of 5 and 6. Davidson and others (Asso and Wyke, 1971), however, have found that the method used when asking a child to discriminate between various letter forms seems to be important. For example, it appears significantly easier for a child to copy a letter correctly than to either read a letter aloud in the right way or match letters visually (Table 11.1).

Numerous writers have asserted that the ability to make correct left-right judgments in space, sometimes called *directionality* is dependent upon how well the child is able to make various left-right discriminations about the body and its parts (Kephart 1964). However, when these two kinds of abilities are contrasted, no significant correlations are found (Ayres, 1964; Cratty and Martin, 1975). Both the ability to identify body parts correctly and the ability to make various discriminations about asymmetrical letters mature at about the same time of life, from six to seven years of age. However, with a single child, the prediction of how well one perceptual-cognitive discrimination is able to be made by surveying how well the other discrimination is carried out is a somewhat difficult undertaking.

TABLE 11.1 Percent of Children Evidencing Confusions in the Comparisons Shown in Kindergarten and First Grade

	n	d-b	d-p	d-q	b-p	b-q	q-p	q-b	q-d	b-d
Kindergarten	48	93	50	35	40	42	96	43	27	87
Grade 1	111	65	19	13	19	15	62	11	13	60

From Helen P. Davidson, "A Study of the Confusing Letters B, D, P, Q," *Journal of Genetic Psychology*, 47 (1935): 458–68. Reprinted with permission of the Helen Dwight Reid Educational Foundation. Published by Heldref Publications, 4000 Albemarle St., N. W., Washington, D.C. 20016, © 1985.

THE PREDICTION OF LOCATIONS OF MOVING STIMULI:
BALL INTERCEPTION

Visually tracking moving objects in horizontal and vertical planes is a basic and quite primitive quality in visual-perceptual functioning. This important ocular skill was needed early in our evolutionary past, and thus is a more primitive quality than is the focusing upon the printed page by bringing the eyes in toward each other.

Despite the importance of this kind of ability for numerous facets of a child's life, there is relatively little solid information about how it develops, particularly during the elementary school years. Literally thousands of investigations may be found describing the preferences infants evidence when simply inspecting immobile stimuli. However, how children acquire the ability to predict the location of balls on the playground as well as of dangerous cars on city streets is still not fully understood.

Part of the problem lies with the lack of funding available to explore dynamic visual and perceptual characteristics as they evolve in normal youngsters. Most of the emphasis has been placed on pathological ocular conditions by those who fund research, as well as by investigators themselves. The studies that are available often contain data and findings difficult to compare and interpret. These difficulties arise from the numerous and diverse kinds of experimental arrangements, ranging from tasks requiring the child to make various physical responses to balls to those in which relatively passive judgments are called for. An example of this latter type of investigation, for example, might require children simply to observe balls moving down ramps and then to make various judgments about their relative and/or future locations (Stadulis, 1971, 1985).

The identification of what qualities may contribute to success or detract from ball interception performance is also a difficult undertaking. At least four sets of factors are likely to be operative. These include various perceptual qualities, including the ability to predict the pathways of balls and to select the ball (the figure) from its background (the ground). Additionally, the child must possess or acquire various motor traits, including the ability to move to the predicted location, and the shaping and readying of the arms and hands. Still another important set of variables include those pertaining to learning and experience.

Virtually without exception, the results of studies of ball interception by children reflect improvement with age. It is suspected that the additional experience and learning that is expected in older children may override any kinds of motor and/or perceptual qualities that may be necessary in this kind of complicated task (Williams, 1968; Hoadley, 1941; Torres, 1966 . . .; Stadulis, 1985). To intercept a ball, a child must somehow turn on a rather complicated "ball interception" program involving the motor and perceptual qualities alluded to previously. Thus it is often found that a simple analysis of either perceptual or motor qualities in order to understand how this quality matures in children often elicits nonpredictive results (Hellwig, 1972).

Basically, the job of the maturing youngster is to process not only enough information about what is happening, but the correct information. Thus the younger child must learn how to learn or, more specifically, must learn how to attend and to what this attention must be given. It is not surprising, therefore, that when younger children are evaluated in ball catching situations, they may tend to look away at important times and to miss important cues (Deach 1950). Hellwig (1972) observed in a filmed analysis that the more successful children in her sample (6 and 7 years) tended to look longer at the ball in flight and essentially to "look it into their hands."

Overall, the research paints this picture of children at various levels of experience, as they try to intercept balls:

1. At from 4 to 6 years of age, when the child is first exposed to the problem, several characteristics are seen. Attention may be varied, not always watching either the person (or thing) projecting the ball or the flight of the ball itself. Their insecurities are heightened if balls begin to injure hands, or even the face, and as a result stress levels rise to make the task of accurate programming of interception movements even more difficult. At this age, as is true of others, sex differences are not likely to be present (Cratty et al., 1973; Williams, 1968; Stadulis, 1971). However, marked individual differences shortly begin to appear, even at this beginning level. These include actions that may be related to the previously discussed qualities of dynamic visual acuity, as well as to the degree to which a child at this level is able to obtain a meaningful, stressless experience. For example, when good versus poor ball interceptors of this age range are contrasted, marked differences are seen (Hellwig, 1972). The most successful will not only watch the path of the ball longer than will the inept, but will also focus more intently upon the person or machine releasing the ball.

Thus the more mature catchers will attempt to gain information for as long as possible from as many sources as are available. Good hitters in professional baseball gain a great deal of information about velocities and trajectories of the balls thrown at them by watching the pitcher carefully. It seems that younger children who are more successful in a similar way soon learn to watch the actions of those throwing balls their way, in a manner similar to major league hitters (Hellwig, 1972).

Several other characteristics mark the child at this first level. As a group, marked variations will be seen, but a single child may vary markedly from trial to trial in how he or she executes catching movements and how well he or she perceives the flight of balls (Hellwig, 1972; Cratty et al., 1973). Children at this age are still seeking what some researchers term appropriate *work methods*. Thus *what* they choose to look at, as well as *how* they move bodies and hands, will differ from attempt to attempt. This modification of technique as a result of experience is likely to override any kinds of perceptual qualities a child may possess at this age (Hellwig, 1972). However, even at this young age, the more successful interceptors of balls will be those whose techniques are more stable and consistent from trial to trial than is the case for those who are less able. Often the less successful at this first level will tend to act impulsively, moving too quickly to a hypothesized location of a moving ball that is in truth incorrect. Often at this age a child will simply look at a ball's early location and then look away while making a motor response, without any real attempt or effort being made to plot the trajectory of the missile (Randt, 1985).

Finally, at these early ages small balls of high velocities will simply not be dealt with effectively (Randt, 1985). This is the case particularly if the ball is traveling from left to right or right to left across the visual field with a velocity that requires careful computation. Likewise, balls coming directly at the child will also be difficult to intercept, because in this case the main cues the child will be able to utilize are those involving the increase in apparent size of the object (Cratty, 1973; Williams, 1968).

2. The second phase of ball interception in childhood arrives at about the age of from 7 to 9 years (Carriere and Bellec, 1981). By this time youngsters have gained experience. Those who continue to stand in the way of incoming missiles at least have an appreciation for the difficulty of the interception task. They no longer move to some hypothesized and incorrect location in the mindless manner often exhibited by younger children. Rather, they may pause and reflect before advancing to catch the ball, thus at times becoming late arrivals to the ball's final pathway (Williams, 1968). At this age it is typical to see marked improvements in interception abilities (Cratty et al., 1973; Williams, 1968; Hoadley, 1941). They will usually first inspect all cues, including those given off by the thrower in a given situation, and then with increased practice learn to compute ball trajectories with a decreasing number of cues.

They may, for example, tend to upset a coach, as they appear not to always look a ball through an entire trajectory. By this age some have, as is true with more mature ball players, learned to use a minimal number of cues to decide what future ball locations will consist of. In this way they are becoming increasingly able to deal with smaller balls at higher velocities and of smaller sizes than were their younger contemporaries (Davis, 1971; Bruce, 1966; Stadulis, 1971; Cratty et al., 1973; Randt, 1985). At this age also, as was true among younger children, sex differences are not found in the interception skills under discussion (Cratty et al., 1973; Williams, 1968; Stadulis, 1971). Randt (1985) suggests that more effective training in ball interception will occur at this stage if children are exposed to tennis-ball-size missiles.

3. At a third level, late childhood, continued improvement as the result of experience is likely to occur. Torres, for example, found significant differences in the abilities of 10-year-olds and 13-year-olds in ball interception tasks. This same researcher also found significant differences at these ages in selected measures of perception, including figure-ground perception (Torres, 1966). In late childhood the neuromotor system is relatively mature. It may be expected that many youngsters will evidence adultlike abilities to intercept balls. At the same time, as was true among younger populations, it is often difficult to predict the overall quality of ball interception by correlating scores of specific perceptual or motor abilities (Torres, 1966; Victors, 1961; Hellwig, 1972). At this final level youngsters, like adults, can often compensate and substitute stronger motor abilities for weaker perceptual

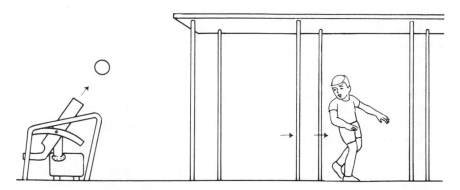

FIGURE 11.8 Children of various ages were evaluated by Williams in their ability to judge accurately the landing position of balls, when they were not permitted to see the final part of the trajectory (76).

traits. As might be expected, at these ages the visual apparatus, although not fully mature, enables the individual to deal even more effectively with missiles at increased velocities, and with balls of smaller sizes, than was true among younger children (Torres, 1966).

Finally, by late childhood and early adolescence, many youngsters need no longer pause when first seeing a ball that must be intercepted. They can, with experience, react quickly and accurately to the trajectories of balls, and can rapidly place their bodies and hands in positions that enable efficient interceptions (Williams, 1968). Randt has found more improvement in children after the age of 8 years when evaluating catching than was true when children of 4 and 6 years were compared, (Randt, 1985).

Figure 11.8 depicts a type of experimental arrangement that has been used to determine ball interception accuracy in children from 5 to 12 years of age. The task was for the child to run quickly to the suspected location of the termination of the ball, whose initial trajectory was seen by the child. Reaction time was computed by subtracting the time the ball was first projected from the time the child left a platform to move to the hypothesized termination of the trajectory (Williams, 1968).

TRENDS AND ISSUES

Although there is an increasing amount of experimental findings, numerous theoretical and practical questions remain about how infants and children mature relative to visual-perceptual functioning; what changes experience and learning play in age changes that are seen; how educators may, by offering useful experiences, modify visual-perceptual abilities; and finally the manner in which active movement may or may not modify visual-perceptual abilities and maturation changes. Theoretical models (Haith, 1980) seem to suggest that important cognitive qualities accompany the early visual searchings and scannings of infants. These same writers contend that instead of the infant being a passive receiver, or even a simple discriminator of stimuli, he or she is an active seeker of information, even within the early days, weeks, and months of life.

One encouraging contemporary trend evidences a useful and important shift in how visual-perceptual development may be assessed. Previous measures of so-called perceptual development traditionally employed movement responses, with drawing the most popular motor response employed (Frostig, 1963). Recent and more sophisticated efforts to evaluate perceptual changes in youngsters of various ages have used "pure" measures of visual-perceptual ability (Colarusso and Hammill, 1972; McDaniel, 1972). These measures, for example, simply ask a child to say or to point to answers to perceptual problems. Thus the "contamination" of possible motor ineptitude will not influence the results. In contrast, for generations, children have been condemned as having perceptual problems, when in truth they could not use a pencil accurately in so-called perceptual tests that were in truth assessments of hand-eye coordination.

Another important issue that has been present for decades within various educational programs of special education involves whether or not movement experiences contribute in positive ways to various visual-perceptual qualities. A review of these programs will not be undertaken here, as it has been accomplished elsewhere (Cratty, 1980; Meyers and Hammill, 1982; Kavale, 1983). Essentially, however, there are some encouraging signs that when either ideas or simpler perceptual tasks are combined with movement experiences, a different kind of encoding to memory may occur in children. It has been found, for example, that the learning of simple geometric forms may be enhanced through the use of activities of the larger muscle groups (Thornberg and Fisher, 1971). More recently, Saltz and his colleagues have found that memory of sentences was facilitated if the sentences were acted out motorically rather than simply recorded auditorily (Saltz, 1982; Saltz and Donnenwerth-Nolan, 1981). Even more useful are the strategies recommended by Meichenbaum and others for the enhancement of self-control through various movement tasks accompanied by useful cognitively oriented self-talk (Kendall and Finch, 1979; Cameron and Robinson, 1980; Cohen et al., 1981; Meichenbaum and Goodman, 1971; Cratty, 1985). The interested reader should consult these and other contemporary literature on the subject.

SUMMARY

Although psychologists in the last century became interested in the perception and visual abilities of infants, it was not until the 1960s that research was concentrated on early visual and visual-perceptual abilities. Studies that explored selective looking in infants have accompanied those looking more closely at more mechanical aspects of visual maturation.

Initially, "looking" studies seemed to indicate that the infant was somehow "captured" by various stimuli. More recently, it has been hypothesized that the infant is the one who "captures" information in ways that have been found to be relatively sophisticated and intense shortly after birth. The infant actively searches for information, even in the dark. Additionally, this intense seeking seems governed by several innate tendencies, or rules.

Shortly after birth, various components of the muscular system begin to accompany visual behaviors. Incoming objects are sometimes avoided by protective actions of the arms, for example. During infancy the head and eyes become coordinated, as more and more mature looking and searching is engaged in during the end of the first half-year of life.

Several stages have been identified in visual-motor integration. (a) First the visual and motor systems function somewhat independent of one another. (b) Second, visual-perceptual behavior and motor behaviors become closely paired—as, for example, when a young child both looks and manually contacts objects. (c) Finally, vision and movement again operate either together or independently, depending upon the type of task and the specific demands made upon the child.

In early childhood, more and more component parts of various tasks are brought together. Although visual following of stimuli is possible at birth, it is not until the third to fifth years that children both watch and attempt to intercept missiles through actions of their larger and smaller muscle groups. At first these efforts at contact are possible only with objects and balls that move relatively slowly. Later, however, the maturing children may not only move their bodies to the future locations of moving objects, but also begin to engage in other behaviors simultaneously.

QUESTIONS FOR DISCUSSION

1. What various measures are cited in the chapter for the evaluation of both visual and visual-perceptual maturation?
2. Separate, if you can, operations that include visual abilities from those that involve visual-perceptual qualities.
3. Justify the statement that "The infant at birth is an active information seeker."
4. What evidence is there that visual searching behaviors are innate rather than learned?
5. What is meant by whole versus part perception? How are these qualities seen in the maturing child?
6. What stages do children pass through as they begin to try to intercept balls moving within their space fields?
7. What kind of theoretical issues revolve around visual and visual-perceptual maturation?
8. What kinds of important questions underlie the establishment of programs intended to train perceptual abilities using movement experiences?
9. Why might tests of visual perceptual development employing drawing responses produce questionable data?

STUDENT PROJECTS

1. Play catch with two youngsters, one from 2 to 4 years old, and the second from 7 to 9 years old. What subtle differences can you ascertain relative to their visual attention, visual searching, and other visual or visual-perceptual behaviors as you contrast their behaviors?

2. Pass brightly colored objects, at various speeds, across the space field of an infant from 3 weeks of age to 6 months of age. What responses do you obtain? Are responses accompanied by or exclusive of attempts to act upon the objects motorically?

3. Discuss a standard visual examination with your local optometrist. What components of the examination might bear upon how well a child intercepts a moving ball?
   What components may be relatively independent of visual and visual-perceptual qualities needed when children engage in ball games?

4. Discuss what visual-perceptual qualities a local reading tutor or teacher feels are important when a child is first confronted with words on a printed page. Are any of these related to how well children can deal with moving objects and balls in playground games? What qualities seem comparable in both contexts? What qualities seem independent?

CHAPTER TWELVE
EXERCISE EFFECTS
AND PERFORMANCE
OUTCOMES

Children evidence an increasing amount of vigor at play after acquiring locomotor abilities during the second year of life. Expanding capacities to endure and to display strength and power are the outcomes of this increased effort on their part. The ability to sustain effort and to exert force are caused by interactions of the muscular-neurological and heart-lung systems. The functions of these systems are in turn undergirded by complex metabolic and biochemical reactions. Just as is true of adults, children who obtain more exercise evidence positive changes in cardiovascular processes, in the utilization of food fuels, and in the elimination of waste products within the muscles. These modifications in turn influence the child's ability to display strength, to engage in quick, powerful acts, and to exhibit prowess when exposed to prolonged endurance work.

However, there are some physiological and psychological processes connected with endurance and strength training and adaptations that are different in the child than in adolescents and adults. The child is a smaller and maturing "energy machine" in contrast to the more powerful and mature adult model. Although some of these differences are just beginning to be explored, they have important implications when exposing children to potentially stressful exercise regimes intended to improve endurance and/or strength. For example, there are differences in just how an adult and a child are likely to go about improving their fitness. Adults, for example, may engage in carefully monitored and planned programs containing bouts of exercise engaged in at exact intervals throughout a week. The child, on the other hand, is less likely to plan. Much of the time endurance activity is unconsciously embedded into daily play.

Even if an exercise session is carefully constructed for a child, he or she is less likely to tolerate the immediate discomfort caused by the effort, as well as to understand the long-range goals of the program, in contrast to the adult's ability to endure some immediate discomfort in order to gain long-range goals. Despite the apparent intolerance of young children for formal exercise programs, high levels of fitness may be acquired by them as they play vigorously, in both longer and shorter bursts of effort that may place useful stress on their heart-lung systems.

Understanding the nature of the way both organs and cells change due to exercise in the maturing child can be a perplexing undertaking. Sorting out the variables that contribute to a single child's failure or success in endurance and strength activities is made difficult by the number of possible influencers that may be involved. For example, in an endurance run there can be a number of contributors to performance, including changes in heart rate, amount of oxygen the child can process in a unit of time, biochemical efficiency of the child's arms, legs, and body moving in unison, motivation, the child's experience at pacing, previous training at the distance, as well as the type of muscle fiber that may predominate in the runner's neuromuscular system. Further difficulty is sometimes encountered when comparing children's performances to those of adults in a well-controlled laboratory environment. A child with endurance capacity equal to that of an adult may be outperformed on a treadmill test, because the child is likely to run with less biomechanical efficiency on this type of apparatus. On the other hand, scores may be more equal when both are tested on a stationary bicycle. The scores of a child may even exceed those of an equally fit adult if the younger subject has had specific training in bicycling.

Children, as is true of adults, evidence individual differences in exercise capacities and tolerance for stress, as well as in bodily make-up and biochemical and cellular level adaptations to exercise. Variations in the percent of body fat measured on three children may easily exert more influence on their exercise capacities than might be seen among three other children having similar body compositions but of different ages. Moreover, children obviously become larger as they mature. Thus the interpretation of the meaning of such qualities as heart rate, stroke volume, respiration rate and depth, as well as oxygen processing capacities (VO_2max), may be understood only if they are contrasted to the overall size of the children in whom these qualities are evaluated.

It is believed to be important to survey both age and sex differences in exercise effects and capacities. Although the data on some of the subjects within this chapter are sparse, it is important to discuss what evidence there is because of the increased number of children and younger adolescents in programs of vigorous exercise, as well as in competitive sports requiring sustained training and performing efforts. Assisting the interpretation of children's exercise capacities are data from recent studies comparing adult-child measures when both are exposed to comparable endurance loads.

Throughout the chapter, we will emphasize individual differences. Among these are variations in muscle fiber types, percent of body fat, oxygen-processing capacities, as well as differences in bodily and physiological changes that may occur when several children are exposed to a similar program of exercise. The chapter concludes with a list of principles appropriate to consider when formulating programs of vigorous training or sports competition. Adherence to important principles governing how the immature body may accommodate to exercise loads will result in quicker and more beneficial outcomes in youngsters exposed to them.

CAPACITY CHANGES

Sheer capacity changes in the functions of the major organs needed to support endurance and strength activities during childhood parallel similar changes seen in body size and muscular mass. The heart grows bigger during childhood. It becomes stronger with its increased size, as is true of most muscles, and thus can push out more blood at each beat as maturation occurs. This increase in volume per beat, or stroke volume, however, is needed to support the actions of an increasingly larger body (Figure 12-1). Although there are some data that after the age of 10 years heart rates in females are somewhat faster than in males, the differences are not great. Generally the heart rates during a typical day are more variable among a population of children than is true among a group of adults. The child's heart rate may descend

FIGURE 12.1   Age differences in heart rate. From A. Lliff and V. A. Less, "Pulse Rate, Respiratory Rate, and Body Tempature of Children between Two Months and 18 Years," *Child Development,* 23 (1952), pp. 237–45. Used with the permission of the Society for Research in Child Development.

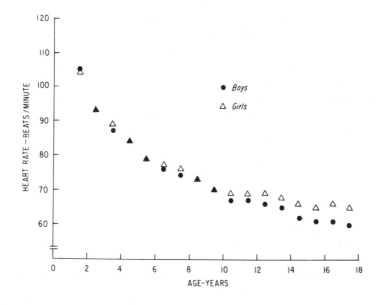

to 50 beats a minute or even less during sleep. During vigorous play, children's heart rates may rise to over 200 beats a minute for brief periods. It is probable that changes in resting heart rates at various ages are more influenced simply by the increase in the size and weight of the heart than by any subtle maturational factors. For example, in one study (Mautner, Luisada, and Weiz, 1941) it was found that heart rates in both animals and children were correlated closely with the size of the hearts in both the animals and children used in the investigation.

Blood pressure readings are not always easy to obtain in younger children. Encouraging the child to come to a truly quiet state may be difficult, while at times a too-large cuff may distort the reading obtained. In numerous studies of children of various ages, it has been found that there is a gradual rise in systolic blood pressure from the fifth year of age. Few sex differences are evidenced in blood pressure until the age of 14, at which time the systolic pressure continues to rise in boys but remains stable in girls (Rickey, 1931). In contrast, the diastolic blood pressure rises only slightly from the fifth year to the teens, and there are no significant sex differences. Differences in measures of systolic blood pressure during childhood have been linked to inherent maturational qualities reflecting early or late maturation, rather than simply chronological age (Rickey, 1931). Additionally, the time taken for the blood to circulate changes from infancy to adulthood. Although there are individual variations that range from 5 to 20 seconds, the mean times obtained for infancy are about 7 to 10 seconds; for children from 2 to 12, circulation time is over 11 seconds; and in adults the time can range from 1 minute to under 20 seconds, depending on the exercise effort being exhibited. It is possible the faster circulation times in younger children are due to the habitually higher levels of activity typically seen in infants and less mature children (Shock, 1966). See Figure 12.2.

Respiratory Functions

Respiratory measures correlate from $+.7$ to $+.95$ with such measures as height, weight, and surface area, just as is true when contrasting body size and various functional measures of the heart (Ferris, Whittenberger, and Gallagher, 1952; Tanner and Picco, 1960). Thus real changes in measures of respiration should be corrected and stated as ratios of respiratory function to body size, rather than being presented in absolute terms. Simply stated, as the child grows larger, the capacities of the lungs also expand (Figure 12.3).

In general there are regular changes in vital capacity between the ages of from 4 to 6 and adolescence (Ferris and Smith, 1953). This measure of the volume of a maximum expiration following a maximum inspiration evidences sex differences, with boys exceeding girls slightly during early childhood and more after the age of 12 years.

Maximum breathing capacity, measured by the total volume breathed during a 15-second period in which the child breathes as rapidly as possible, also increases in both males and females from the ages of 4 to 17 years, and then tends to drop off in adulthood. In contrast, measures of respiratory volumes and rates tend to drop in childhood when the children are evaluated in a resting state (basal state) (Shock and

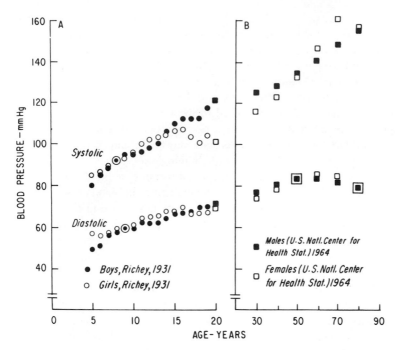

FIGURE 12.2 Age differences in blood pressure. From H. G. Richey, "The Blood Pressure in Boys and Girls before and after Puberty, Its Relation to Growth and to Maturity," *American Journal of Diseases of Children,* *42* (1931), pp. 1281–1330. Used with the permission of the American Medical Association.

FIGURE 12.3 Growth in vital capacity of boys and girls. From B. G. Ferris, Jr., and C. W. Smith, "Maximum Breathing Capacity and Vital Capacity in Female Children and Adolescents," *Pediatrics, 12* (1953), pp. 341–53. Used with the permission of the American Academy of Pediatrics.

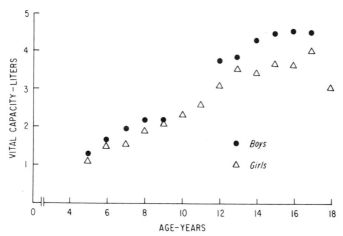

Soley, 1939). The sex differences found are probably due to differences in body mass.

These rather crude measures of respiration are of only marginal significance. For the most part, the most significant measure is how much, or what percent, of the oxygen is removed during a breath, and this can vary dramatically under various circumstances. For example, if a child holds his or her breath, the percentage of oxygen removed is far greater than if the same child is hyperventilating. Basal VO_2 uptake is about 4.3 milliter/per kilogram of body weight per minute. Thus as children grow larger, their uptake increases, and larger boys acquire more total O_2 than is true of smaller girls at various ages.

Power and Work Changes

More important than the consideration of relationships between heart-lung functions and age and size are measures reflecting if and how the child becomes a more efficient endurance-power machine as maturation occurs. Some of the basic questions that are beginning to be explored by contemporary researchers include those dealing with the questions of (a) whether age or training programs exert more influence upon the ability to do work, (b) how children's cardiovascular and muscular systems compare with those of adults when both are placed under similar exercise stresses and loads, and (c) the influences of such variables as fiber types, sex, and percent of body fat on children's capacities to engage in moderate and intense exercise.

As would be expected, regular exercise by children produces better endurance and generally reduces body fat (Parizkova, 1977). But it is not clear from the available evidence that laboratory exercise programs are more productive of cardiovascular improvement in children than would occur through normally vigorous play.

It is probable, however, that exercise capacities of children improve at least slightly as a function of age, and that exercise effects become greater as late childhood and early adolescence are reached. In a study published in the scientific literature from the German Democratic Republic (Harre, 1982), for example, marked changes in max O_2 uptake are seen after the age of 12, when exercised and untrained groups of boys and girls are contrasted (see Figure 12.4). Gilliam (1977) indicates somewhat less dramatic changes as a function of age earlier in childhood, in the study depicted in Figure 12.5. However, when contrasting these two investigations, it is difficult to compare the exercise loads imposed, and Gilliam's study involved few subjects.

It appears likely that experimentally introduced exercise stress must be rather intense to overcome the normally vigorous activity often seen in unsupervised children at play (Powers, 1984). For example, in two studies conducted in the 1970s in which intense exercise loads were employed, significant increases in work capacity and the ability to utilize oxygen quickly were obtained (Vaccaro and Clark, 1978;

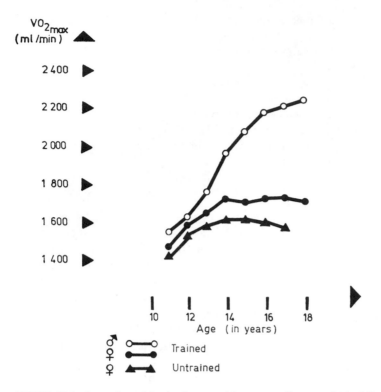

FIGURE 12.4 Comparison of the development of the age-specific oxygen intake (VO_2 max) of trained and untrained persons (based on published sources). From D. Harre (ed.), *Principles of Sports Training.* Berlin: Sportverlag Berlin (1982), p. 38. Used with permission of the editor.

Catch and Byrd, 1979).[1] In contrast, earlier studies in which less of a load was imposed resulted in no changes in work capacities beyond those expected through normal growth and maturation (Spryanova, 1966; Bar-Or and Zwiren, 1973).

Traditionally, the rate of displacement and rate of recovery of heart rate, blood pressure, and oxygen consumption following various types and intensities of exercise have been regarded as valid indexes of physical fitness. These measures are also considered by some as indexes of physiological maturation. Exercise has several physiological characteristics, including the increased delivery of oxygen and nutrients to contracting muscles and the removal of the waste products of exercise, including CO_2 and lactate. However, the responses both boys and girls make to achieve these physiological goals are exceedingly complex. The mechanisms by which oxygen uptake and CO_2 removal are increased include an increase in heart

[1]The most used measure of work capacity is maximum oxygen (O_2) uptake or (O_2 max). This reflects the milliliters of oxygen per kilogram of body weight per minute the body is able to utilize during some measured work. Training enables a child (and adult) to use more oxygen per unit of time, enabling the individual to *assume heavier maximal workloads* than their untrained counterparts.

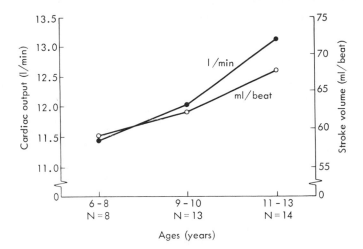

FIGURE 12.5 Comparison of peak cardiac output (1/min) and stroke volume (ml/beat) for three groups of children ages 6 to 8, 9 to 10, and 11 to 13 years. From T. B. Gilliam, et al., "Comparison of Peak Performance Measures in Children Ages 6 to 8, 9 to 10, and 11 to 13 Years," *Research Quarterly, 48* (1977), pp.695–701. Used with the permission of the editors.

rate and stroke volume and an increase in the arterial-venous difference for oxygen. For example, stroke volume peaks in moderate intensity exercise, increasing no higher as higher loads are placed on the individual. Heart rate continually increases until a maximum rate is reached. Arterio-venous differences increase continually until VO_2 max is reached. Regional shunting of the blood flow may also play a role, so that a greater proportion of the cardiac output goes to exercising muscles instead of to other less involved parts of the body.[2]

Most of these variables may be experimentally evaluated. However, the methods used with adults are not always adaptable to large numbers of children. Traditionally, earlier studies were limited to estimates of heart-rate recovery, blood pressure changes, and oxygen consumption, and only occasionally to changes in blood chemistry (blood lactate, pyruvate, Ph, and bicarbonate content). More recent studies have explored modifications of muscle fiber types, and even of how the nervous system changes as it sends messages to groups of muscle fibers being exercised.

The apparatus used when measuring children's exercise capacities can also make a difference in the results obtained, particularly when adult-child comparisons are sought. Using a bicycle ergometer with children is relatively easy. However, a treadmill run is influenced by other variables, including the child's running mechanics. So important are running mechanics when assessing endurance in children that often laboratory measures purporting to evaluate endurance correlate only slightly

---

[2]For example, it has been found that blood flow through the muscles may increase tenfold during exercise, from 1200 ml/min to over 12,000 ml/min. Threefold increases are found in the heart during exercise, while blood flow through the abdomen may be cut in half.

with so-called endurance runs conducted in the field (ranging from a 6-minute run to one of 600 yards).

However, even when using relatively scientific laboratory instruments such as the stationary bicycle, one must be careful when assessing children. A maximum workload on such a device for a 10-year-old boy weighing 95 pounds will not be comparable to the same workload applied to a 20-year-old of 165 pounds. Thus the fact that many physiological measures are influenced by workload, apparatus used when testing, as well as maturation in children makes one cautious when attempting to interpret the results of available studies. It is not surprising that different investigators have produced divergent findings when comparing the exercise capacities of children of various ages to those of adults. Astrand, for example (1952), could find no age or sex differences in maximum pulse rates after exercise. Maximum heart rate declines with age in both sexes. Therefore, it is to be expected that children will attain higher maximum heart rates during exercise than adults. In adults, heart rates are lower than those of children at any submaximal workload (Robinson, 1938), partly due to an adult's greater heart size and stroke volume, as well as because of age-dependent biochemical changes. At exhaustive work loads, an adult's heart rate may almost reach that of a child's. Under extreme exercise conditions, children's heart rates may change from between 170 to over 200 per minute, whereas adults' ranges are from above 140 per minute and may top off at about 180–190 per minute.

Shock (1944) has examined responses to exercise in children and early adolescents. Measures were taken before and for periods of from 40 to 45 minutes after exercise. Figure 12.6 indicates that youths of 17 years were doing more work at a greater rate than children of 13 years, presumably because of the greater body weight of the adolescents.

FIGURE 12.6   Age changes in pulse rate response to severe exercise, as shown by pulse rate one minute after excercise. The vertical line through each point indicates ± 1 standard error of the mean value. From N. B. Henry (ed), *43rd Yearbook,* National Society for the Study of Education (1944). Used with the permission of the editor.

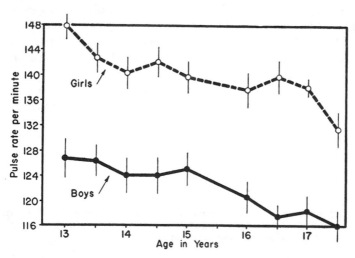

Shock and others have found that the maximum systolic blood pressure attained after exercise increases in boys after the age of 13 to 14, but not in girls. The same researcher found that after exercise, adult arterioles undergo less relaxation than those of children. This is based on the assumption that low diastolic pressures, increased pulse rate, and pulse pressures observed after exercise could be produced by vasodilation decreasing the peripheral resistance faster than the drop in the cardiac rate after exercise. There is thus evidence for more rapid response of the vascular systems of children to exercise than is true among adults (Ogden and Shock, 1935).

The maximum oxygen consumption during exercise is similar in boys and girls until about the age of 13. After the early teens, the increments are usually greater in boys than in girls. When the excess oxygen consumption is expressed as the percentage of increment over the basal level the sex differences disappear, but the increment as a function of age still persists.

In general, the rate at which recovery of physiological functions occurs after exercise diminishes with age. After moderate exercise, the heart has been found to return more quickly to resting level in young children than in adults, according to early studies on the subject (Jenss and Shock, 1936). In more recent investigations, the data suggest that marked differences in exercise adjustments between adults and children, as both reach a steady state[3] during the beginnings of exercise, may be absent or minimal (Figure 12.7).

Children under work conditions that require levels permitting their heart-lung systems to keep pace with demands of the task are said to be engaging in aerobic work, or work sustained by currently available oxygen intake and utilization capacities. Brief, intense tasks, including, for example, a 100-meter or perhaps a 400-meter run, often require that a child (or adult) engage in anaerobic work. Carbohydrate utilization becomes very rapid during this type of exercise, resulting in an inevitable buildup of lactic acid in muscle and blood. In this type of work, elevated blood lactate levels result in decreases in Ph (increased acidity) in blood and muscle, leading to rather rapid fatigue. Generally, preadolescent children demonstrate lower ability to engage in this kind of intense anaerobic work, in contrast to anaerobic efficiencies seen in adolescents and adults. However, with training even this kind of often painful work may be improved in preadolescent children (Eriksson, 1972).

The usual recommendation is to keep children away from this kind of intense anerobic output situation, rather than permitting them to train under more sustained workloads for relatively brief periods. The reasons for the diminished ability of children to engage in anaerobic work are still being debated. It has been suggested, however, that children may possess less of the important regulatory enzyme (phosphofructokinase, PKF) in carbohydrate catabolisms necessary to recruit quickly needed sugar energy from muscles than is true of older people. In general,

---

[3]*Steady state* refers to a plateauing of O_2 consumption reached at about 4 minutes into moderate rhythmic exercise, reflecting a balance between energy required by working muscles and production of fatigue products of work.

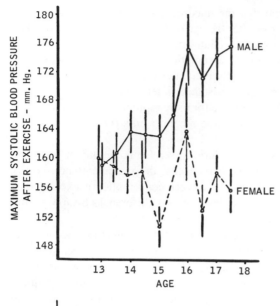

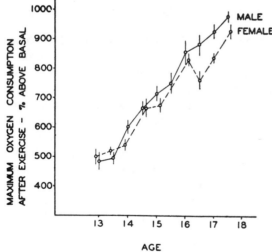

FIGURE 12.7

(a) Age changes in blood pressure response to severe exercise. The vertical line through each point indicates ± 1 standard deviation of the mean. (b) Age changes in metabolic response to severe exercise, as shown by the maximum oxygen uptake after exercise compared with the basal rate. The vertical line through each point represents ± 1 standard deviation from the mean. Both from N. W. Schock, "Physiological Responses of Adolescents to exercise," *Texas Rep. Biol. Med.*, 4 (1946), pp. 368–386. Used with permission of the editors.

however, available evidence suggests that maximal performance capacities shift as a function of age (Gilliam et al., 1977). As we will see in the following section, shifts upward in work carried out by the heart differ from the sixth to the thirteenth year of life.

EARLY ENDURANCE TRAINING AND LATER ADULT CAPACITIES

It is becoming increasingly clear, from a survey of contemporary evidence, that children react differently to exercise than do adults. For example, there are data which demonstrate that relatively more of the cardiac output during the exercise of children is distributed to the muscles than is true of adults (Bailey, 1978). Ericksson (1972) has also shown that training of children produced larger increases in stroke volume in boys than would be expected in adults.

Consideration of these data has led some researchers to speculate about whether or not endurance training in childhood would lead to larger stroke volumes in adulthood for the same subjects than would be true if there had been no prepubertal training. Although the data bearing on this intriguing question are rather sparse, the available evidence seems to indicate that preadolescent endurance will be effective in later life. For example, in a longitudinal study of 30 top Swedish female swimmers (Astrand et al., 1963; Eriksson, 1971), evidence seems to confirm the supposition that early endurance training will be effective later in life. When the girls were first evaluated, they were engaged in heavy training sometimes lasting 28 hours a week. Their mean oxygen uptake was approximately 46 percent greater than nontraining females the same age acting as controls. It was concluded initially that hard training had increased the size and capacities of the organs involved in oxygen transport.

After a 10-year period, these same females were evaluated, even though most had not continued their rigorous training. Most were housewives engaged in childrearing and work around the house. It was found that their aerobic power had decreased by about 30 percent over the years, perhaps due to detraining. In contrast, however, the size of their lungs and hearts were relatively unchanged. They thus appeared to have retained their organic capacities for high levels of endurance functioning, even though their actual O_2 uptake reflected reduced levels of activity. The investigators suggested that failure to continue activity by the subjects had resulted in a waste of available potential. It was further hypothesized that if endurance training engaged in in childhood is neglected later in life, it may not be possible to repair the resultant loss in capabilities in endurance tasks. That is, static values (volumes) may not change; whereas dynamic values (VO_2 max, cardiac output max, stroke/volume/max) may change (decrease) due to detraining. These young women apparently still possessed the basic machinery to do heavy work, but this machinery could no longer function at high levels of efficiency.

Continued effort in training in endurance activities is not only a matter of the physiological maintenance of various systems and subsystems; the person also needs to continue to be highly motivated to engage in grueling programs of swimming and running. In the study surveyed, for example, the female swimmers in later life had apparently been turned off to heavy exercise of all types by earlier exposure to heavy endurance training. Even though their apparent capacities, based upon static measures of heart-lung volumes, were more than 20 percent higher than untrained women their age, their measured aerobic capacities were about 15 percent *below* peers of the same age.

Sweeney (1973) describes another documented case of possible burnout due to lowered motivation in endurance activities. A New Jersey junior high school boys' running team had seven members who averaged miles of 4:47. Three years later, when this group was again surveyed, it was found that only one boy had continued to participate in distance running, and his time had improved only 22 seconds/mile over his junior high school time. These and other examples suggest the importance of early, well-motivated training by youngsters to produce sustained participation and thus adolescent and adult performances that represent continued improvement over earlier efforts.

Furthermore, the adult-child differences in anaerobic work characteristics have led some authorities to recommend that younger children should avoid longer sprints and the middle distances. Arthur Lydiard (Lydiard and Gilmore, 1967), for example, suggests that training focusing on distances of from 200 to 800 meters is unsuitable for children. Their advice is to limit young children to shorter sprints or to longer runs of from 1 to 3 miles. They contend that in the shorter sprints, although children will use all their reserves, they won't be forced beyond their limits by the urging of spectators and parents to try harder. At the longer distances, they believe, if children are activated by others, or by their own ambitions, they will slow their pace when becoming tired rather than hurting themselves by overextending their capacities.

Those urging caution in anaerobic middle-distance running generally point to a period of caution from childhood to the middle teens. Eriksson and Saltin (1974), for example, have found that the low blood and muscle lactate concentrations found in younger children generally change and reach almost adult levels by the middle of the fifteenth year. Astrand and Rodhal (1970) also point out that children's muscular strength is low, and the qualities needed for oxygen transport and uptake are not like those of adults.

It is important for those formulating and conducting endurance programs for children to be aware of these cautions. At the same time, a considerable amount of contemporary opinion suggests that young children, if carefully trained, can accommodate to anaerobic workloads reasonably well over time. Simply because they are not as able in this kind of effort should not, others contend, prompt trainers to withdraw them from expanding what capacities they do have at these younger ages. These contemporary experts suggest that we should not saddle children with programs that are too protective, and thus blunt their capacities and potentials.

Training in endurance activities does lead to improvement in both children and adolescents. These changes come about because of adjustments in the anatomical and physiological mechanisms discussed, as well as because of increased biomechanical efficiency that may be gained over time by children who are well taught. Furthermore, those conducting such programs should be aware that many of the field tests of endurance may actually be dependent at least as much upon basic cardiorespiratory capacities as they are upon how efficiently the child is able to run, walk, or bicycle (Cureton, 1977).

Contemporary evidence makes it clear that various factors reflecting high risk of cardiovascular problems in adulthood are seen rather early in life, even during childhood (Thorland and Gilliam, 1981). Furthermore, it is apparent that regular well-planned exercise in childhood is likely to reduce these unwanted qualities at the time the exercise is undertaken, and thus to produce fewer of these qualities later in life. Exercise has been found, for example, to reduce hypertension, high lipids, and obesity in children, all factors that may later contribute to high-risk conditions among adults (Thorland and Gilliam, 1981). From a preventive standpoint, all children should be exposed to vigorous programs of physical activity in ways that encourage them to persist in useful activity throughout the childhood, adolescent, and adult years.

BODILY CHANGES DUE TO EXERCISE

In addition to changes in exercise capacities in children due to exercise, changes in body shape and composition are likely to occur. These changes are linked to possible psychological feelings the child may possess about his or her body and its capacities for movement.[4] *Body composition* refers to the degree to which a child evidences body fat, usually expressed in some percentage. The total body mass, from which the percentage of body fat is subtracted, is referred to as the *lean body mass*. In children the nature of body composition fluctuates according to age, sex, and exposure to exercise programs.

More and more within recent years, the roles of exercise and diet have been explored in the reduction of childhood obesity. Obesity is usually expressed as an excess of body fat on a child, with standards of normality usually set at 20 percent or under of body fat in boys, and at or under 30 percent in girls (McArdle, Katch, and Katch, 1981).[5]

The amount and distribution of fatty deposits seem to be genetically determined in both children and in adults. The number of fat cells may evidence increases at various times in life. Earlier studies suggested that the periods of most rapid fat cell growth were in infancy and during adolescence. More recent and more accurate measurement techniques applied to fat-cell numbers present in children in-

---

[4]The modification of the body image as a function of its shape and capacities for movement are covered more thoroughly in Chapter 3.

[5]At times, exact estimates of the number of fat cells on a child are obtained by computing the average weight of a fat cell, by weighing many, computing an average weight, and then dividing it into the percent of the total body weight made up of fat.

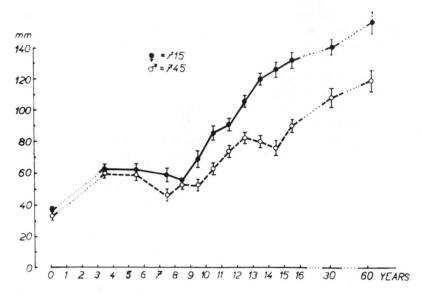

FIGURE 12.8 Development of subcutaneous fat, expressed as the sum of skinfolds measured at ten sites. From J. Parizkova, "Impact of Age, Diet, and Excercise on Man's Body Composition," *Ann. N. Y. Acad. Sci.,* 110 (1963), pp. 661–74. Used with the permission of the editors.

dicate that fat cells may increase in numbers throughout the life span, rather than at critical periods, as was once believed.

Fat is not useful weight to the exercising child and prevents quality endurance activity, just as would be true if an obese child was carrying a heavy pack of dead weight on his or her back while moving. Fat cells surgically drawn from a portion of a child's body quickly return to their original location, attesting to the inherent nature of the location of fatty deposits. However, it seems that the number of cells and their tendency to be added at various critical periods in the life of the child are subject to diet and sustained exercise habits. Body fat generally increases as children grow older and is greater in girls, particularly after the age of 10, than in boys. Using skinfold thicknesses collected at various locations, Brozek (1965) and Parizkova (1963) have documented these differences, as shown in Figure 12.8.[6]

The presence of more fat on girls has been hypothesized by some to be an aid to endurance activities by females, although most experts believe this assertion to be false. Excess fat on the female (in contrast to the male) is a liability in endurance activities, with the possible exception of endurance swimming in cold water, in which case fat provides insulation that prevents hypothermia. In general, girls who do not maintain a reasonable level of body fat (usually placed at between 10 to 20 percent) as they approach adolescence are likely to experience a delay in the onset of menstruation (Frisch and McArthur, 1974). Indeed this kind of delay is not infre-

---

[6]The usual standards for these kinds of skinfold evaluations are those formulated by Tanner and Whithouse (1962).

quently experienced by young prepubescent girls exposed to rigorous programs of ballet, gymnastics, and endurance running. A rise in percent of body fat is accompanied in adolescent girls by a parallel decrease in basal metabolism, a condition triggered by the production of estrogen. Thus in girls the general level of body heat (metabolism) is lowered, and at the same time more bodily fat accrues. As males reach adolescence, basal metabolism either remains constant or rises, while body fat may decrease as the result of testosterone production.

As has been pointed out, body composition, as reflected in percent of body fat, is modified by exercise in children just as is true among adults. However, the young seem to be able to release more fatty acids from adipose tissue than is true among older individuals. Figure 12.9 indicates changes by age, as well as by sex, in lean body mass and fat deposits during the growth years.

Generally both adults and children have higher lean body mass when they exercise than under sedentary conditions. In children during the growing years there seems to be a chicken-and-egg effect between skill, body build, and exercise seeking. That is, children with higher skill and exercise potentials exercise more than their less skilled and inherently less enduring counterparts. During the childhood years individual differences in measures of percent of body fat may become more marked in groups of children when physiologically active and sedentary children are contrasted. In one of the more impressive longitudinal studies of growing boys, Parizkova (1973) confirmed the relationships between exercise and body composition. She took a variety of measures in 96 growing boys between their eleventh and fifteenth years. They were divided into four groups, each exposed to a different level of exercise intensity. Overall, during this period no differences were found in heights and bony girths between the groups. However, there was a slight tendency for the height of the boys in the group exercising most to be slightly greater.

FIGURE 12.9 The development of body composition (percent of lean body mass and depot fat, body density) during growth. From J. Parizkova, "Body Composition and Excercise," *Physical, Activity Growth, and Development*, L. Rarick, ed. New York: Academic Press, 1973. Used with the permission of the editors.

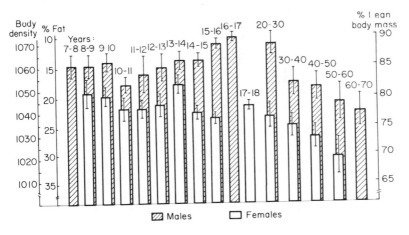

During the first year of this five-year study, no significant differences were seen between groups when body composition measures were contrasted. During the second through the fifth years of the investigation, lean body mass was significantly higher in the group exercising most. The group exercising the least evidenced higher levels of body fat at the close of the program. These differences persisted in 41 of the boys who continued to be followed for an additional three years. However, the greatest differences between the groups exposed to varying amounts of exercise appeared between the fifteenth and eighteenth years, when apparently the boys' interest in exercise was the greatest (Figures 12.10 and 12.11).

Other measures taken of the boys in this comparative study by Parizkova indicated that measures of aerobic work capacities tended to parallel changes in body composition. Just as was true in the case of body fat, no significant differences were seen between the groups during the first years in max O_2 uptake. By the third year, differences in this measure of exercise capacity did appear in the data and persisted until the final year of the study. This researcher found moderate relationships between aerobic power and total body weight at the ages of 11 and 12 years. Between 13 and 15, however, correlations were higher between measures of lean body weight and work capacity (Figure 12.12).

FIGURE 12.10 Changes in relative (%) and absolute (kg) amounts of lean body mass in groups of boys with different physical activity (I–IV) from 11 to 15 years (1961–1965). From J. Parizkova, "Body Compositions and Excercise," *Physical, Activity Growth, and Development*, L. Rarick, ed. New York: Academic Press, 1973. Used with the permission of the editors.

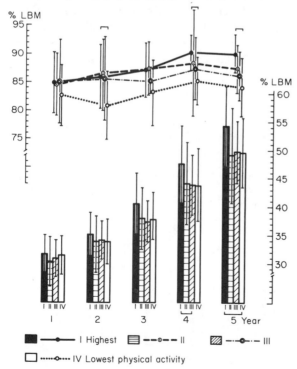

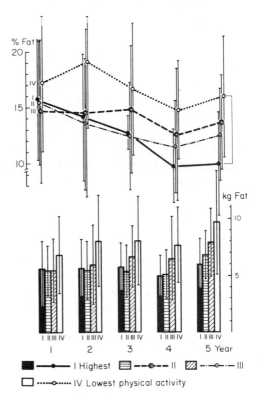

FIGURE 12.11
Changes in the relative (%) and absolute (kg) amounts of depot fat in groups of boys with different physical activity (I–IV) from 11 to 15 years (1961—1965). From J. Parizkova, "Body Composition and Excercise," *Physical, Activity Growth, and Development,* L. Rarick, ed. New York: Academic Press, 1973. Used with the permission of the editors.

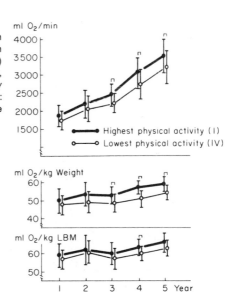

FIGURE 12.12
Changes in absolute and relative (per kg total and lean body weight) values of maximal oxygen uptake in groups of boys with different physical activity (I and IV) from 11 to 15 years (1961–1965). From J. Parizkova, "Body Composition and Excercise," *Physical, Activity Growth, and Development,* L. Rarick, ed. New York: Academic Press, 1973. Used with permission of the editors.

In more recent work Parizkova has found similar relationships between percent of body fat and activity levels encouraged by parents and through programs applied to preschool children. Generally this industrious Czechoslovakian researcher found that children whose parents reported exposing them to higher levels of physical activity and recreational opportunities evidenced less body fat than did the children of parents who apparently were providing a more sedentary environment. Likewise the preschool children who were apparently engaged in more prolonged programs of physical education were also the lighter in body build, and as expected more proficient in physical activities. These more active and leaner children even during the third to fifth years also exhibited postures that reflected more than adequate muscle tone (Parizkova, 1984).

Essentially, just as true in adults, exercise intensity correlates with reduction of body fat. Also, as is similar in adult populations, if a child terminates exercise, more body fat will likely appear. Parizkova, for example, studied a girl gymnast who terminated training. Her lean body mass fell and her percent of fat rose as a result. As more evidence is gathered, it is apparent that at least part of the cure for childhood obesity is the imposition of an intelligently applied exercise program. Programs of exercise lasting as little time as 7 to 8 weeks, for example, have been shown to reduce percent of body fat in children by 10 percent (Mayer, 1965). With sustained exercise, obese children will be found to reduce their body fat a significant amount, as indicated in Figure 12.13, which shows changes in obese children after exposure to a special summer camp designed to promote weight reduction. Coupled

FIGURE 12.13 Changes over a 4-year period in fat proportion (%) and lean body weight (kg) of obese boys before and after treatments in special summer camps(↔). From J. Parizkova, "Body Composition and Excercise," *Physical, Activity Growth, and Development,* L. Rarick, ed. New York: Academic Press, 1973. Used with the permission of the editors.

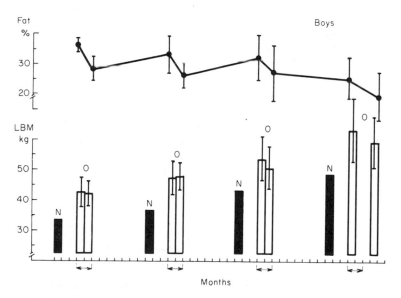

with these weight losses are increased capacities for sustained aerobic work in these same obese children.

FIBER TYPE

Another important quality emerging in research in the mid-1970s involves qualities within the muscles that seem to enhance either endurance or strength efforts of both children and adults. It has been found that individuals differ according to whether their muscular system contains fibers that enhance prolonged endurance efforts or short, powerful bursts of strength. Fiber types supporting endurance activities are termed type I; those supporting strength are termed type II.[7]

Not only do various muscle groups contain a predominance of one fiber type or the other, but individuals differ according to the percent of either slow (endurance) or fast (strength) twitch fibers they possess. For example, the soleus (larger) muscle of the calf contains about 90 percent slow twitch (type I) fibers, while the quadricep muscle of the upper thigh contains a larger percentage of fast twitch fibers. Furthermore, as might be expected, the percentage of either fast or slow twitch fibers possessed by a child may facilitate performance in tasks corresponding to either fiber type that may be present. Training will enhance performance regardless of fiber-type dominance, at any level of competition.

Training enhances the quality of all fibers that are recruited during regular exercise in the child, due in large part to the enhanced production of muscle components called mitochondria. Fibers subjected to endurance training, for example, will increase the quantity of mitochondria, which in turn aids aerobic metabolic reactions. These changes due to training also include enhanced anaerobic capacities by increasing anaerobic enzymes, especially phosphofructokinase. The enhancement of anaerobic enzymes with training is particularly evident in the child in contrast to the adult, because the child has a lower anaerobic capacity to begin with.

Children vary according to the percent of either fast or slow twitch fibers available, and variations generally range from 20 percent of one type to 80 percent of the other. In general, it has been found that there is less variability of fiber type in females than in males. It is possible that the possession of more extreme fiber types by some males permits them to excel in activities requiring high levels of endurance, as well as sports needing short strength bursts. It is possible that younger children who vary the kind of play they engage in from sustained slow activities to bursts of effort will promote a wider range of fiber types in their make-up than children who evidence little variation in the strength and endurance activities engaged in. The same may be true when formal exercise programs are engaged in by children. Regimes that promote a variety of activities including both strength and endurance efforts are likely positively to affect the broad range of fiber types present in

[7]Investigators have recently concluded that there are three types of fibers: slow oxidative (type I), mostly involved in aerobic work; fast oxidative (type IIa), involved in both aerobic as well as anaerobic work; and fast glyclytic (type IIb), involved mostly in anaerobic work.

a youth's muscular make-up. Thus while it is true that athletes at higher levels usually possess a predominance of the fiber types needed in their sport (Astrand and Rodell, 1977), children may benefit from training both in strength and endurance activities in ways that improve the quality of the muscle fibers they possess.[8] At the same time, a child with a predominance of fast twitch fibers (80 percent) will easily outsprint a child possessing only 20 percent fast twitch fibers. Because most efforts in early childhood involve short, fast bursts, the fast-twitch fiber type may excel early in life. However, as children are increasingly exposed to programs containing specialized activities designed to promote endurance, those possessing more slow twitch fibers are likely to come to the forefront, besting their stronger peers.

SUMMARY

Overall the following principles and findings seem to be valid relative to relationships between exercise and the maturation of children.

1. General increases in the size of the organs involved in cardiovascular functioning, and the work they do, is seen from early to later childhood. The heart grows larger and stronger and expels more blood at each stroke as a result.

2. Respiratory capacities change, as does blood pressure. However, overall efficiency in work capacities is dependent upon the relationships of these work measures to the overall size of the child and to the nature of the child's body composition.

3. Children acquire increased capacities to do physical work from early to late childhood. However, other factors, including opportunities to engage in vigorous play, body build, training, fiber type, as well as body composition, are likely to exert more marked influences upon work capacities than is age.

4. So-called endurance measures, including timed runs, are not always closely related to basic measures of physiological capacities, but are influenced markedly by motivation, as well as by the mechanical efficiency of the child.

5. Few sex differences are apparent in the ability to engage in endurance activities during early and middle childhood. As adolescence approaches, however, more marked sex differences emerge.

6. Differences in fiber types possessed by children are likely to cause obvious performance differences to the extent to which the children are exposed to either strength or endurance tasks. Training, applied intelligently and containing varied strength-endurance activities, will influence the quality of both the fast and slow twitch fibers a child may possess.

7. Differences in percent of body fat present are seen at adolescence when females and males are compared. Females exposed to exercise programs reducing their body fat much below 20 percent are likely to experience a postponement of menstruation.

---

[8]Generally both types of fast twitch fibers are innervated with nerves of larger diameters than is true of slow twitch fibers. Nerves connected to fast twitch fibers thus evidence more rapid conduction velocities, firing impulses at rapid rates and enabling rapid forceful contractions of the muscles. At the same time, this fast-firing nerve tends to fatigue rather quickly. In contrast, the slow twitch fibers are innervated by axons with smaller diameters whose slower delivery of the message to the muscles results in slower fatigue of the nerve and of the muscles it (they) innervates.

8. Marked differences are not seen, except in levels of performance, when adults and children are compared relative to the manner in which their bodies adjust to aerobic work. However, child-adult differences are apparent in how their bodies react to anaerobic work. In general, children are unable to dispel quickly the fatigue products of short bursts of effort requiring anaerobic work. Thus there is some question whether training in middle-distance running is advisable for children before the age of about 15 years.

9. In general, well-designed endurance training for preadolescents is likely to have more positive than harmful physiological effects, including the reduction of body fat and the increase of work capacities. However, transfer of the positive effects of this early training to efforts in adolescence and adulthood will occur only if the early training has been well motivated, and if attention is paid to maintaining the child's continuing interest from childhood to adolescence and beyond.

10. When running, physiological adaptations in adults and children are remarkably similar if sustained effort is expended. However, small children utilize available energy expensively due to the lower efficiency of the work they produce because of less effective running mechanics, higher stride frequency, and shorter leg length. Thus pure laboratory measures of cardiovascular efficiency in both adults and children are not always highly predictive of various so-called endurance activities carried on outside the laboratory, including cycling and running.

11. The number of red blood cells (erythrocytes) and amount of hemoglobin increases throughout childhood and continues to increase in boys as adolescence is reached. Lower hemoglobin in children as compared to adults, however, indicates that the blood's binding capacities are lower in the younger endurance athlete.

12. While cardiac stroke volume is of course lower in children, when expressed in units based on ratios between stroke volume and height (cubed), the stroke volume in children and adults is remarkably similar.

13. The amount and quality of early endurance activity to which children are exposed is a likely predictor of the presence of factors posing a risk to efficient and healthy cardiovascular function in later life. Early signs of high-risk qualities, including high lipids, obesity, and hypertension, are seen in children and may be reduced through regular exercise. Reduction of these in childhood is likely to produce a physiologically more efficient adult.

QUESTIONS FOR DISCUSSION

1. What gross anatomical changes influence cardiorespiratory modifications from early to late childhood?

2. What are static and dynamic measures of cardiorespiratory functioning? In what ways are the latter more valid measures of work efficiency?

3. What general statements may be made about relationships between fiber type and strength-endurance performances in children?

4. In what ways are children and adult cardiovascular adaptations to exercise similar? In what ways do the child's adaptations differ from those of the adult?

5. What findings are available that support the continued exposure of a child to endurance exercise throughout life?

6. In what measures of running (distances) might children and adults tend to differ most, relative to their adaptation to training?

7. What differences and similarities are there between how the two sexes adapt to prolonged exercise programs?

8. What evidence suggests that short-term exposure to an endurance program is not as beneficial as long-term exposure to such a program, relative to the reduction and control of body fat?

9. What is aerobic versus anaerobic work? What implications do these terms have when designing exercise programs for children of various ages?

10. What do you see as needed studies within the subject areas covered in this chapter?

STUDENT PROJECTS

1. With the help of an exercise physiologist and/or physician, design a six-month exercise program for yourself, carefully monitoring exercise increments, loads, and caloric intake. Carefully plot indexes of improvement of cardiorespiratory function during this period.

2. With the help of a physiologist or physician, design a program of endurance training for children from 6 to 8 years of age. Obtain sound advice on initial evaluative criteria, initial loads to be imposed, and how you might determine how and when you will increase loads. Plot their progress for a time period, using measures similar to those suggested in the chapter.

3. Obtain measures of percent of body fat among the members of a group of children. Interview them relative to the amount of time and the intensity with which they engage in vigorous physical activity each day, week, and month. Are you able to draw any relationships between the interview data and the measures you obtained relative to body fat?

4. Attempt to obtain interview data as to why a group of children may have dropped out of a competitive swimming or track program. What conditions and accommodations might have encouraged them to continue participation? What caused them to drop out?

CHAPTER THIRTEEN
SOCIAL DEVELOPMENT

Important social milestones achieved by the maturing infant and child are often inseparable from parallel signposts that signal the acquisition of physical skills. When the infants achieve the ability to pick up and release objects, they acquire the means by which they may begin to learn the give-and-take of social life, as toys are able to be given to and received from a friend nearby. Physical play affords children the opportunities to experiment with rudimentary social abilities and to observe and assess their own social impact on others. Still later, the adolescent may earn varying degrees of social status by competence exhibited on high school and college teams.

Motor activity and physical skills thus provide the means through which several important social qualities may be exercised and developed. (a) Physical actions make many social contacts imperative; they force social interactions. (b) Physical activity and play provide a testing ground for experimenting with interpersonal interactions that will be carried out later in less vigorous environments. (c) Various physical tasks engaged in early in life begin to introduce infants and children to the alternating give-and-take with others that mark conversations and more mature encounters with others.

Social pressures and demands also exert their influence on physical activities. Each culture places unique demands on the maturing infant and child. Early demands involve various self-care skills and the mere physical "answering" of the actions of another. The mother's smile should be answered, just as the ball should be rolled back when it is moved toward the child. Later, each culture rewards or punishes a child and adolescent in rather precise ways for acquiring or not gaining skills in various crafts, in sports, in driving a car, or in hunting. It is for these reasons that the studies of movement accompaniments to social interactions often produce different results when conducted within different cultures and ethnic contexts.

The first part of the chapter contains ideas gleaned primarily from recent research that pairs early physical actions and reactions with rudimentary social competence. This literature is characterized by an incredible devotion to detail and to subtle behaviors emitted by infants and their parents. Also interesting has been a rich body of research depicting early actions and reactions between two infants. The latter portions of the chapter view social skills in play groups and in sports exhibited by children in early and later childhood. The outcomes of these kinds of data have been efforts to make the early environment of the infant more conducive to both physical and emotional-social growth. Parents exposed to this information should also become more sensitive to the early and profound influences even their most minute behaviors are likely to have upon their newborn child's liking for and confidence in moving and in exploring his or her social world.

INFANCY

Several contemporary scholars have postulated that the infant's early social influences begin to make their impact before birth. Scales developed in the 1970s have as their primary focus the evaluation of the infant's social and emotional behaviors, behaviors that many feel are being molded while the fetus is still within the mother's womb (Brazelton, 1973). Contemporary research and researchers also make the important point that the infant is not merely a reactor to things that happen to him or her during the first days of life, but in fact exerts powerful and profound influences on the behaviors of those who first hover over the crib. However, even during these first days, weeks, and months of life, it is often difficult to determine just what behaviors *cause* what kinds of emotional-social and physical responses; or conversely, to determine what kinds of social events are likely to trigger various physical actions on the part of the infant. Several behaviors or actions may have a common, single purpose. Or a single, observable response on the part of an infant or mother may serve more than one need.

With these limitations in mind, the following discussion contains a brief survey of only a small portion of the contemporary literature on the early socialization of the infant. Particular attention is focused on variables that mold physical actions, or physical actions, abilities, and qualities that in turn are likely to modify various components of the social climate, including the behaviors of peers and family members.

The infant enters a world possessing only a visual channel with which to interact socially with the mother or father. Then looking blends into actions that are gradually acquired; interactions with close family members become expanded to include other babies and infants who may be available. The degree to which the infant is likely vigorously to explore his or her environment is greatly dependent upon the initial secure base provided by the mother and father. Likewise, the infant's first exposures to actions, and the approval and encouragement of these actions by others, will exert a rather profound influence upon further explorations, both social and motoric.

Basically the infant, upon entering the world, must deal with two kinds of objects, people objects and inanimate objects. The former are highly interesting to the newborn. He or she apparently has more difficulty controlling them but attempts to do so with variations in expressions and cries that are quickly acquired. The interactions with inanimate objects come later, and often in conjunction with the "people objects" experienced earlier. Objects the child can handle and otherwise influence provide numerous early opportunities for social interactions, as we shall see. In the following sections we discuss the infant's early exposures to mother, father, and peers. The later portions of this section on infancy, the first two years of life, focus on object availability and other emotional components that are integral to the social unfolding of the infant through and with movement experiences.

The close integration between motor behaviors and social development during the early months prompted Stechler and Carpenter (1967) to coin the term *sensory-affective* to replace the sensory-motor concept. That is, early motor behaviors they suggest are so closely intertwined with social development that at times they become inseparable.

PEOPLE INFLUENCERS OF EARLY MOVEMENT BEHAVIORS

The Mother: A Primary Caretaker

Traditional studies of infant-mother interactions adopted a one-directional approach. It was assumed that invariably the mother influenced her offspring in various ways. Contemporary research, however, is based on more complex models. It is assumed that (a) not only is the infant highly likely to affect maternal behaviors, but also that (b) to fully understand the nature of mother-child interactions, the entire family, including the father, must be studied (Lewis and Lee-Painter, 1974).

A most important concept when studying the ways in which mother-child interactions influence and are influenced by the movement characteristics and abilities of the latter involves the notion of *synchrony*. Increasingly, mother-child behaviors are seen to work in increased harmony, and in relationships that interact more closely in time as maturation occurs. First, these kinds of mutually influential and closely intermeshed behaviors include the ways in which an infant may choose or not choose to cuddle by molding his or her body against the mother. The mother may in turn reciprocate, depending upon the movements and postural adjustment of the infant, and either relax or become tense when handling her own infant

(Brazelton, 1973). Another interacting chain of events that involves close interweaving between mother and child are their smiles. Rudimentary smiles, usually while drowsing, are detectable in the child as early as the second month of age. However, it is the infant's later efforts at smiling at the mother that are rewarded by the same facial response by the caretaker. Absent, late, or abnormal smiles, postures, or other signs of motoric incompetence emanating from the infant may initiate similar negativism from the mother. These anomalies in behaviors may thus begin to trigger further chains of undesirable mother-infant interactions, that if persisted in may cause and magnify later emotional and social problems in the lives of both (Ainsworth et al., 1972).

Infants differ in many ways that influence mothers' behaviors. An infant who attends to the mother visually is likely to elicit visual attention in return. Korner (1970) and Fries and Wolff (1953) were the first of several to recognize what might be termed an infant's *congenital activity type*. In subsequent studies (Wolff, 1971), it was found that differences in muscle tone, motility, duration of alertness, and general vigor contributed a great deal to the mother's reactions to her infant. However, it was also suggested that the mother's unique expectations, and the acceptability of various of these movement qualities and tendencies, combined to formulate and influence the overall reaction of maternal caretakers to children of various types.

Essentially the mother provides, to varying degrees, an emotional base for the child during the first two years of life. It is a base whose degree of security then influences whether or not the child feels able to engage in vigorous motor activities with others who might be present, and with play materials in both familiar and unfamiliar situations. Early in life the mother's visual attention to physical acts and to objects themselves serves to direct the infant's attention to these same objects and actions and to give them status and importance. As maturation occurs, the mother moves from a social position that is close to the child to a more distant one, permitting and encouraging the child to make social and physical forays into his or her life space that become increasingly independent of maternal protection (Lusk and Lewis, 1972).

Among the factors that influence this shift from a proximal to a more distant role for the mother is the increased physical maturity of the infant, including changes in the child's physique. Heightened agility on the part of the child, as well as an increase in interest in the social aspects of the environment, further accelerate this striking out by the infant and child (Moss, 1967). Conversely, the infant and child who evidences physical immaturities remains more closely bonded socially with the mother for a more prolonged period of time (Kempe, 1976).

The more secure the social base the mother provides, the more the infant will move outward socially. However, the mother still serves as an emotional support, even when it may not appear so. In numerous studies, for example, it is found that a child will tend to play more in unfamiliar situations and with peers when the mother is present than when she is absent. At the same time, with maturation the child tends to become more vocally active with the mother, while becoming physically more active with other children (Vandell, 1976).

The mother thus provides the child with (a) the first object, which may be tugged on, pulled, and otherwise manipulated; (b) a secure emotional base from which the child moves both socially and emotionally; and (c) a model of interest in and attitudes about objects to be manipulated, as well as about the desirability of action itself. Infants confront their mothers with differences in activity needs, muscle tone, alertness, and physical stature and maturity. These differences in turn contribute to an ever-expanding chain of mother-child behaviors that persist into childhood and adolescence, and that in turn are potentially powerful molders of later movement capacities and inclinations on the part of the child, youth, and adult.

When attempting to predict later physical behaviors from earlier tendencies to move, care must be taken to specify just what kind of movement qualities and attributes are being compared and contrasted. Such variables as general activity level and variability of activity, as well as motor maturation and physical skills, have been used. The research on this subject has often provided findings that are extremely thought provoking to those interested in motor activity and physical development. For example, Kagan and Moss (1962) in their classic longitudinal study found that restless, impulsive motorically "too active" youngsters below the age of 3 tended to be less involved in intellectual pursuits, as did Halverson and Waldrop (1975). Bell (1975) has proposed an inversion of intensity hypothesis which suggests that infants who were more tranquil during the newborn period are those who are more likely to be actively involved in games and more assertive during the years immediately preceding entry into school. Indeed, differences between cuddlers and noncuddlers in infancy, it has been suggested, are predictive of later physical qualities. Schaffer and Emerson (1964), exploring this dichotomy in infants, suggested that cuddlers enjoyed, accepted, and actively sought out physical contact of all kinds. Noncuddlers, on the other hand, were likely to be more restless and intolerant of physical restraints during their second year of life.

The Father

It has only been within the past several years that adequate attention by researchers has been paid to the social influence of a potentially powerful member of the family constellation, the father. Despite the fact that in most cultures fathers are not viewed as likely to be as interested in the newborn as the mother, some evidence suggests that the father may be an equal, or even a more powerful, interactor with the infant than the mother. Lamb (1977), for example, observing fathers in the home setting, found that infants seem more attached to them than to their mothers. Clarke-Stewart (1977) also found that there are no apparent differences in the kinds and quality of attachment behaviors directed toward father, as compared to these same behaviors beamed toward mothers.

Additionally, the available information suggests that father's early role is critical when surveying parental behaviors that serve as antecedents to later motor activity, physical abilities, and attitudes about actions by children. For example, it is a uniform finding that fathers not only engage in more play with their offspring, but also evidence qualitative differences in the type of play activities expressed. Generally it is found that fathers spend from 10 to 20 percent more time in play with children, while mothers engage more in caretaking activities, including feeding (Kotelchuk, 1976). Fathers spend about three times more hours playing with their children than with so-called caretaking activities (Rendina and Dickerscheid, 1976). It is thus not surprising that the father's very presence may tend to blunt the interactions between infant and mother (Parke and O'Leary, 1972). The father is therefore both a direct and an indirect influencer of the interactions that take place around the home.

The quality and type of the play engaged in by the father is likely to differ from the play encouraged by the mother. The father's actions and those he encourages are generally more rough and tumble than those occurring between child and mother (Lamb, 1977). Mothers, on the other hand, instigate playful actions more likely to consist of verbal and tactile experiences.

Both the mother and the father differ in several other important ways relative to early social influences on motor development. The father generally prefers a boy baby, and when viewing the male child will attach more attributes involving physical coordination to him, than will the mother (Rubin et al., 1974). This early tendency toward sex-typing continues, and is evidenced in how both mothers and fathers play with female versus male offspring. Fathers tend to play more vigorously with their male children than their female children. They tend more to cuddle their girls. The reverse is often true of the female caretaker, who is seen more to cuddle and hold her male infant, while relating more in play situations to the girl of the family. These differences in how mothers and fathers deal with their youngsters are not great when engaging in basic caretaking activities. However, when at play the differences are striking and persist during the first year of life (Park and Sawin, 1977). This tendency of different treatment for male offspring by the father has been seen in many cultures and occurs even in primate families (Gewirtz and Gewirtz, 1968; Redican, 1976). The differences stem from very early sex typing by fathers of both their male and female newborn, self-imposed stereotypes that persist and may influence differences in how girls and boys later function in both play and sport situations.

Other Infants

The heightened interest in peer relations is part of the general resurgence of concern about social interaction seen in journal articles published in the 1970s and early 1980s.

The role of physical activity is a vital one to study in relation to social development and peer interactions, because play and other forms of mutual interaction often force social interactions. Physical interactions also provide ways in which the infant and child may assess the social impacts they have on others as well as the degree to which they may control others. For example, a child might use a pull toy in the presence of another. The second child, noticing the toy moving across the floor, might begin to follow it. The first child, noticing the second child being influenced, may change direction and thus exert control over the follower. The chain of events may thus continue, with the two children stopping the action and continuing to vocalize, to their limits, the excitement generated by the situation.

For the most part, peers begin exerting their influence over the physical actions of each other shortly after the mother's behaviors do so. As early as 2 months of age, two infants may begin to notice each other, while by 6 months one infant may smile at another. Visual regard of another child occurs before touching, which may happen at about the middle of the first year. By the sixth month, a child may offer an object to or take one offered by another. At the beginning of the first year, social imitation is seen to occur, and at the same time objects are used in ways that interweave the behaviors of two toddlers in meaningful ways (Eckerman et al., 1975; Mueller and Brenner, 1977).

A number of influences may heighten the quantity and quality of peer interaction at play. Two toddlers present, during the first two years, are more likely to encourage interaction than is a group. The familiarity of the peers, their previous association, is likely to exert a positive influence upon social interactions at play. The presence of a mother-caretaker with whom a child feels secure will likely expand the social horizons seen in actions toward another child who may be in the room.

Often objects will heighten peer contact, as will the nature of the ratio between objects and children in a room. For example, less than one object for each child may engender hostilities, while a single object for each child will not do so. Objects that hold great novelty and interest for a child will sometimes block the child's tendencies to play with others in a situation.

Most interesting are individual differences seen during the first two years of life when the play of toddlers is studied. For example, it has been found that there were marked differences between what were termed *frequent initiators* and *infrequent initiators* of peer interactions at play (Bronson and Pankey, 1977). Additionally, the popularity of youngsters during these formative years seems related to how

FIGURE 13.1 One twin shares a special secret with his brother at six months of age.

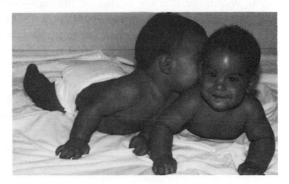

adroitly they initiate social contacts at play, and how well accepted these overtures are seen to be by their playmates.

Other differences revolve around the early friendliness and aggression seen at play. It has been found, for example, that generally both sharing and fighting are seen to be moderately correlated in the same children when youngsters are competing for materials. However, with maturity children are seen to increase friendly interactions at play over the aggressive ones (Muste and Sharpe, 1947).

With maturation and experience, the young child will begin to move toward others physically and emotionally and away from the caretaker mother. However, obvious differences will remain as to how children play with each type of play companion. Children tend to be more motoric or physically active when playing with peers than with their parents in early childhood. When playing with a parent, children tend to express themselves more vocally than physically during the second, third, and fourth years of life (Vandell, 1976).

The success or failure experienced by the youngster during these early excursions into parts of the world separate from parents is likely to mold further bravery and risk taking at play, and later in sport. Individual differences in social risk taking, together with the children's capacities for movement, combine to produce (a) a child who is confident and physically able; (b) a youngster who evidences an average amount of confidence in play situations; or perhaps (c) a child who rejects and withdraws from physical activity as new play companions and situations are encountered.

OBJECT AVAILABILITY AND USE

The increasingly complex ways infants become able to manipulate objects is covered in Chapter 8. Of interest here are the ways in which object availability and use triggers important social milestones. In a similar way, social maturity influences the increasingly complex ways in which objects are exchanged with others in a play context.

The developing infant and child is faced with two types of objects. On one hand, highly interesting and animate objects—people—initially confront the newborn. Within the first six months of life, however, the infant also learns not only how to handle inanimate things, but how to influence various social situations and people through the use of objects that the child must exert his or her own efforts to change. The first object the infant is likely to tug at, pull, and otherwise manipulate is the mother. This type of behavior peaks at about the seventh month of age (Mahler et al., 1975).

Object exploration during the early months of life is likely to result in the initiation of a number of kinds of chains of behavioral events. For example, object handling during the first months of life is often accompanied by babbling and other primitive vocalizations. These vocalizations in turn are likely to trigger vocal feedback from the mother, words that in turn will encourage the child to gain even more complex sounds, thus contributing to later speech (Yarrow, 1972).

Research points to the critical roles objects play in various qualitative and quanitative measures of social behavior. It has been estimated that objects are present within from 60 to 80 percent of the social contacts and behaviors seen in infants and children during the first two years of life (Mueller and DeStefano, 1973; Mueller and Bremer, 1977). For the most part, social interactions during the formative months and years of life do not exist in a vacuum. Objects and people must be present in order for socialization to run its normal developmental course.

Based upon studies of twins, Lichtenberger (1965) has suggested that during the first two years of life, social behaviors involving objects pass through seven overlapping phases. A given child may engage in several of these stages during the same day, depending upon the conditions and people present. The stages include the following:

1. In the first period, lasting from birth to the sixth month, the infant, while attracted to objects, is not likely to initiate social contact with them, even if another infant is present. It is during this period that the mother is a primary object to manipulate (Mahler et al., 1975).

2. The second period, called the first conflict period, lasts from about 5 to 9 months and is marked by one twin taking a toy from the other, but with no obvious distress seen in the deprived member of the duo. The infant acquiring the object is not focused upon the peer, but upon the object.

3. The third period is marked by more gamelike exchanges and lasts until about 11 months. During this period, exchanges were marked by the children's awareness of the other and were also likely to be accompanied by primitive vocalization. Vincze (1971) has found that at the end of the first year of life, the use of objects seems to peak within social interactions and exchanges; objects are present in over 90 percent of the social interactions he recorded in children of this age.

4. Lichtenberger (1965) also identified a second conflict period, lasting into the beginning of the first year and beginning at about 9 months. This period contains exchanges of objects that are unlikely to be accompanied by positive emotions, but instead by conflict and anger. The twins evidenced the acquisition of the notion of possession at this point, and often hid objects from their acquisitive peer.

5. Between 8 and 17 months, Lichtenberger suggests, is a period that contains object exchanges of a less volatile nature. Voluntary offers of objects are increasingly apparent in children of these ages. Eckerman (1975) has also documented the tendency of children from 12 to 24 months to evidence the taking and receiving of toys without undue conflict or stress.

6. The final periods identified by Lichtenberger are marked by the use of objects in tandem in meaningful ways. *Yours* and *mine* become attached to objects by infants during the second year of life. Furthermore, exchanges become increasingly likely to be accompanied by verbal labels. As a child of 18 months hands another an object, for example, the exchange is likely to be accompanied by "da" ("there").

Historically, block play has been used to study the social interactions of young children, particularly competitive behaviors (Greenberg, 1934). Thus objects provide important ways in which insights about evolving social behaviors emerge in playgrounds, where two or more children are present.

It also seems that during the second and third years of life, social behaviors become less likely to be accompanied by objects. That is, the child may acquire the ability to instigate and even maintain rudimentary social contact with words rather than actions. Vincze (1971), for example, noted that after the eighteenth month, objects were present in only about 70 percent of the social contacts of the children he studied, rather than in 90 percent of the interactions, as recorded during the first year of life.

TWO YEARS AND AFTER

Familial Influences

By the end of the second year, the child has begun to acquire serviceable speech and language. Parental influences continue to exert strong influences on movement and sport preferences. Furthermore, the parents' attitudes about recreation and sport are likely to contribute to the recreational and sport opportunities they afford their maturing offspring. It has been found, for example, that the early drawings of toddlers and their fantasies about animals reflect both fear and admiration of their parents (Bender and Rappaport, 1944). Parents also continue to exert an important influence upon the child's self-concept. Several researchers have found that children scoring high on measures of self-esteem possess parents who were classified as loving (Schaefer, 1961). As was true during the first two years, parents continue to mold and to be concerned about the aggression expressed by their charges. Confusion about child rearing patterns and practices in the family is likely to produce overly aggressive youngsters. Although most parents demand moderate retaliation against other children when their own child is insulted, they are far less tolerant about aggression toward them (Schaefer and Bell, 1957).

Parents continue to influence the kind of physical activity engaged in by their children in ways that are quite operational. The amount of physical control exerted by the parents appears to influence the acquisition of movement attributes by children between the ages of 2 and 6 years. The amount of physical mobility permitted by mothers, as well as how often the child is "checked" while at play, varies markedly among parents. Sears, in a study of this component of child rearing, found that about 50 percent of the mothers studied restricted children of 5 and 6 years to their immediate neighborhood, and 11 percent restricted their children to the yard. Only 1 percent of the parents surveyed admitted imposing no restrictions on their child's geographical play areas.

This same investigation polled mothers concerning the frequency with which they located their children while at play. It was found that about 36 percent of the parents monitored them occasionally, if they had not heard their voice for an hour; 25 percent checked fairly often, at half-hour intervals; 8 percent constantly oversaw their children; and only 10 percent practically never became concerned about their children's whereabouts (Sears et al., 1957).

It seems apparent that parents exert early and direct influences that mold children's inclinations for action and the amount of vigorous activity they consistently express, as well as their emotional expressions as they engage in various structured and unstructured play situations. As Sears points out, the child's personality is "the cluster of potentialities for action," and among the primary determiners of a child's personality are the dimensions of his or her parents' personalities (Sears et al., 1957).

Parental Attitudes and Children's Performance Attributes

Parental attitudes about physical activity continue to influence attitudes about activity on the part of their children into middle and late childhood, as well as into adulthood.

Data I have collected revealed that by the age of 18, performance differences may be obtained between students whose parents place a high value on physical education versus students whose parents are not as favorably inclined toward motor activities. There is relatively little information, however, on this same relationship for younger children (Cratty, 1967).

Heathers published an interesting study in 1955 in which dependency behavior was evaluated in a stressful performance situation. Children aged 6 to 12 years were blindfolded and asked to walk an unstable, narrow plank 8 inches above the ground. The experimenter offered help to all the children. It was noted who accepted and who rejected help. Children who accepted help tended to have parents who had encouraged them to depend on others rather than themselves (Heathers, 1955).

Rarick and McKee published a study in 1950 that explored differences in children exhibiting extremes in motor performance. Among the data collected were indices of parental participation in physical activity. In general it was found, as would be expected, that the parents of superior children were active in sports, whereas very few parents of children in the inferior group participated in any type of vigorous physical activity. Additionally, the parents of the inferior group did not participate with their children, whereas 80 percent of the children in the superior group had their parents sometimes accompany them in play (Rarick and McKee, 1950).

Data of this nature, of course, do not indicate that parental attitudes *cause* performance fluctuations in their children, but they are highly suggestive. Further investigations in which data are collected longitudinally should illuminate the factors that influence these high correlations. For example, successful performance by a child may engender more positive attitudes toward physical activity. Conversely, positive attitudes by parents may lead them to encourage children to become physically active. This, in turn, is likely to elicit good performance. Whether parental physiques and attitudes toward activity, or success, which is probably influenced by physique and performance capacities, is more important in the molding of the off-spring's physical performance skill needs to be determined.

PHYSICAL MATURITY AND PERFORMANCE AS PREDICTIVE OF SOCIAL SUCCESS

It is a common assumption that children, particularly males, who perform well physically enjoy more status among their peers than do underdeveloped, poorly functioning youngsters. Studies among schoolchildren affirm the findings derived from older populations that social success is related to the ability of some people to distinguish themselves in desirable ways from the group. And as physical perform-ance is valued to varying degrees by maturing children of both sexes, distinguishing oneself in this area may lead to increased social acceptance. According to innumera-ble studies, friendships are usually formed by people who are in close physical proximity for prolonged periods of time and who perceive themselves to be similar in various attributes. The same finding is echoed in the literature dealing with child development. Similarities of physical maturity, along with IQ, are found to be more important indices of affiliation among youngsters than more subtle personality traits (Pintley et al., 1937; Challman, 1932).

Status is usually conferred on children who perform above accepted group norms in various physical tasks. In a number of studies by Mary Jones and her col-leagues at Berkeley, it was found that physically accelerated boys are more accepted and treated more favorably by both peers and adults. This status leads to positions of leadership in the school community and persists in measurements of personality traits made during adulthood. Hardy also found that the best-liked pupils were supe-rior to other pupils in tests of physical achievement, with 70 percent of them scoring above the group mean (Jones, 1948; Hardy, 1937).

The effects of motor ability, as might be expected, are more marked on the social acceptability of boys than girls. Similarly, as boys progress from elementary through secondary school, social status increases as a function of athletic ability. At the same time, with increased association, the effects of athletic ability on social status may be diminished, as boys perhaps begin to look for less obvious personality qualities on which to base their friendships (Hardy, 1937; Anastasiow, 1965; Davitz, 1955).

It is difficult to separate the effects, particularly among boys, of early maturity versus athletic proficiency on social acceptance and positive personality traits. Ma-turity begets superior physical performance, and thus early-maturing boys appear to form a base of success at play upon which to rest a positive self-concept. At the same time, early physical maturity on the part of males results in a physique that is more attractive to adults and peers with whom the child comes in contact. Thus, drawing direct causal relationships between social and physical proficiency during infancy, childhood, and adolescence becomes an even more difficult undertaking.

SOCIAL CHARACTERISTICS OF CHILDREN AT PLAY

After the age of 2, the child begins to move outwardly even more and becomes able both to initiate and to respond to the overtures of others with increasing sophistication. The play groups become larger, and leadership and followership roles and patterns emerge. More and more, the child becomes judged socially upon what he or she can do; the movement competencies possessed become of more importance in social acceptance, approval, and self-acceptance.

Several variables have been assessed by observing children of various ages at play. The complexity of the group in which the children choose to play, its size, leadership patterns, and the nature and vigor of the efforts they expend have all been subjects of various amounts of experimental attention. Usually such measures are collected via a technique whereby an individual child is observed for a period of time at regular intervals, and notations are made on his or her methods of gaining group recognition, leadership attempts, vigor of activity, the influence of various play materials on play characteristics, and similar assessments (Goodenough, 1930; Goodenough, 1928).

Using such a technique, it is usually noted that as children grow older, they tend to form more complex and larger social systems when at play (Crum and Eckert, 1985). At the same time, the nature of the leadership patterns seen in these groups becomes more complex and more directly related to group goals. Sex differences in the vigor of activity, as well as in the nature of the social attributes evidenced, also seem related to age when children are observed in systematic ways while at play (Cockrel, 1935; Parten, 1933; Hurlock, 1934).

During the preschool years, children stimulate each other in indirect ways by their very presence. More vigor as well as more expressions of joy while at play is usually seen when more than one child is present in a play situation. The nature of this mutual stimulation during the nursery school years, however, is relatively nonspecific in nature. And the typical play patterns include either solitary participation or what has been called *parallel play*.

In this latter pattern, children engage in similar tasks but are not directly interacting with one another (Figure 13.2). They seem to be affecting one another by indirect imitation, rather than by direct physical and/or verbal interactions. Sex differences in play characteristics have been noted by several observers of preschool children. Girls are seen to engage in less vigorous activities during these years and to engage more in verbal social interactions than in contacts involving some overt physical output (Bridges, 1931).

The usual size of the group children 2 to 3 years of age will form when playing consists of two individuals, playmates of the same sex. The presence or absence of play materials at this age will apparently exert a significant influence on the amount of social contact the child will evidence. Deprivation of play materials will result in a child's paying more attention to himself than to others, according to research by Cockrell (1935). The presence of play materials, as might be expected, will generally encourage a wider variety of play behaviors in preschool children.

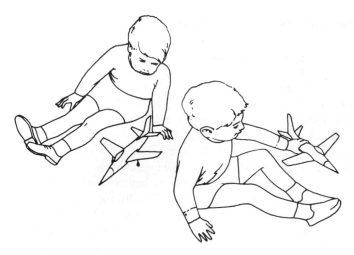

FIGURE 13.2 Parallel play in which each child is working independently but at similar tasks. Each is apparently receiving social stimulation from the other.

At about the age of 4 years, however, children seem to begin to seek the direct companionship of at least one other child while at play. If such a friend is lacking, they will tend to make up imaginary friends to fulfill their apparent need for social interaction. As children grow older, they tend to watch less and participate more, to engage in imitative activity less and in group play more. Rudimentary attempts at leadership may emerge at the age of 4, as some children through direct and indirect means are seen attempting to manipulate the actions of others. These attempts at gaining leadership at play have proved to be highly correlated with a child's general social competence.

As children enter grade school at about the age of 5, they begin to seek more and more companions to play with at one time and will more often seek members of the opposite sex with whom to associate, although still preferring members of their own sex when engaging in various play activities (Crum and Eckert, 1985). The range of activities decreases, particularly in the case of boys, perhaps as various cultural sanctions as to what kinds of activities are given value become more exactly known by the participants.

During middle childhood, various aspects of the subculture in which the child resides begin to exert a more marked influence on the modes of play as well as the type of activities selected. For example, rural boys of from 8 to 10 years were found by Lehman to engage in more activities than town boys of the same age. Boys in a city environment, Lehman hypothesized, are more restricted by their environment in their selection of play interests than are boys who grow up on farms (Lehman, 1927).

The influence of type and number of siblings begins to exert itself on play characteristics in middle childhood. Children tend to prefer either older or younger playmates, according to whether they have older or younger brothers and sisters at home. Moreover, the roles children assume at play are likely to be tied to their birth order in the family. Stoneman and her colleagues (1984), in studying this problem area, identified several types of roles children assume at play. These included teacher, learner, manager, and managee, as well as playmate. Overall, they concluded that younger children willingly accepted the manager roles of their older siblings while at play; the role of teacher was more often assumed by older siblings, as would be expected. Differences were found in the assumptions of the various roles they identified when different group sizes were contrasted. A group of three containing one friend and two siblings, for example, was more likely to elicit cooperative subordinate behavior on the part of the younger sibling (Stoneman et al., 1984).

SOCIAL REINFORCEMENT

As has been pointed out, subtle reinforcers influence the first primitive behaviors of the newborn. These reinforcers may even be as subtle as prolonged visual inspection by the mother. Various rewards for children's physical performance in childhood have also been explored.

Several developmental trends can be discerned in the literature on the influence of various kinds of social reinforcement on the motor performance of children (Keiley et al., 1964). For example, during the early years of life, prior to the age of 4, when confronted by verbal encouragement from another or by the presence of an audience, children seem to become generally excited and aroused. But this increase in activation does not usually translate itself into improved performance scores.

Missiuro, for example, studying the effects of social reinforcement on several motor tasks, concluded that before the age of 6 general tension was increased in children because of social stimulation, but rarely were performance scores improved (Missiuro, 1964). Philip, in a similar study in which the effects of strangers and friends utilized as competitors on kindergarteners' performance was studied, also concluded that the type of pairing did not influence the mean efficiency at a marble-dropping task, but it did affect the quality of the response. "Strange" pairs resulted in relatively unexcited, quiet performance on the part of the 5-year-olds studied, and "preference" pairs elicited noisy and excited performance. Even though children become aware at an early age of the presence of onlookers, their performance is not affected positively by this kind of social stimulation until about the age of 6, judging from the available research evidence (Philip, 1940).

Patterson also found that with increased age children became more responsive to various social reinforcers. Using a marble placement task, this researcher found more marked changes in older subjects when they were reinforced for their efforts by friends than was true when younger children were exposed to the same experimental situation, despite the fact that children at early ages become aware of and perform more vigorously for friends than for a neutral peer (Patterson and Anderson, 1964).

The period of childhood during which verbal encouragement and various other kinds of social stimulation appear to affect performance most is between 6 and about 10 or 11 years. After this time, children seem to become relatively sophisticated and tend at times to block off various kinds of social reinforcers, becoming more sensitive to the difficulty and intrinsic interest of the task itself. For example, in a study by Lewis and others it was found that, in a lever-pressing task, social reinforcement—the experimenter's directly indicating a correct response—was more motivating to first-graders than to sixth-graders and more motivating than indirect correction of the response. Allen also found that younger children (5 years of age) remained longer under conditions of social approval in sorting, drawing, and puzzle tasks than was true when children of 10 were asked to perform under the same circumstances. It was found by Allen that when adults' comments differed from the children's evaluation of their performance, they would remain longer on the task, tending to "cast off" this kind of verbal reinforcement. Similarly, the children in this investigation tended to evidence fewer effects of social reinforcement as the tasks became more difficult (Allen, 1965; Lewis et al., 1963).

The effects of social stimulation in children, similar to the findings of studies with adult subjects, tend to vary as functions of the complexity of the task and the personality of the child. Arousal-producing conditions, as might be expected, will tend to elicit faster responses but may block the production of accurate responses in children (Latané and Arrowwood, 1963).

Similarly, the state of habitual arousal in the child, the anxiety level, may interact with various social reinforcers in the modification of performance in various motor tasks. Again, using a marble-dropping task, Cox (1965) found that boys evaluated as evidencing low levels of anxiety improved more in the presence of their mothers, a peer, teachers, and a strange female, whereas boys with high levels of anxiety already present in their personality trait complex performed best when only the experimenter was present in the testing situation. In a similar context, Latané and Arrowwood found that emotionally arousing a teenage girl by berating her verbally did not influence her ability to execute a simple task, but did tend to disrupt her responses on a complex task, such as pushing buttons to light cues (Latané and Arrowwood, 1963).

Another important variable is the sex of the onlookers as compared to the sex of the performer. For example, Stevenson found in children the same "cross-sex effect" sometimes seen in studies of adults. Testing by a member of the opposite sex, Stevenson concludes, increases competiveness, anxiety, and desire to please, and this effect is more marked when male experimenters are dealing with female subjects (Stevenson, 1961).

Children perform motor tasks better, on the whole, when in groups with both obvious and subtle social stimulation present than when performing alone. Mukerji suggests that this effect is more marked in the case of boys than girls. The direction and influence of the presence of other people on performance scores are functions of the number and social proximity of the onlookers and whether they heap praise or blame on the performing child, as well as the complexity of the task (Mukerji, 1940; Zigler and Kanzer, 1962; Noer and Whittaker, 1963).

Important evidence about what motivates children in physical activity and sports are data that indicate children exposed to reinforcers which are too plentiful and which come from sources other than their satisfactions with the physical tasks, and sports themselves, are likely to blunt effort in physical activities. A child who at first derives pleasure from actions in and of themselves begins to stop and to think that engaging in physical activity must indeed be work if the adult community needs to offer extensive rewards in the form of trophies, jackets, and the like for his or her participation. It is only if the child is selectively and carefully rewarded for real effort and marked improvement in late childhood and adolescence that he or she is likely to persist and to find pleasure in engaging in physical activity for its own sake. Too plentiful external rewards are likely to blunt the pleasures derived from sports participation and from engaging in vigorous recreational activities (Gerson, 1978).

Contemporary evidence has also made it clear that children often participate in physical activities and sports in order to satisfy important social needs. Richard Alderman, studying incentive systems of children 11 to 14 years engaged in sports, found that affiliation needs were most important followed by needs to be excellent in the task, followed by "striving for success." Affiliation was defined by Alderman as the assurance that one is worthwhile and accepted by peers, and the maintenance of existing friendships (Alderman, 1978).

SUMMARY

Some believe that before birth social factors influence rather basic qualities in the newborn, qualities that reflect physical vigor or passivity, alertness or apathy, as well as apparent motor maturation versus blunted physical abilities. At birth, the parents quickly exert both obvious and subtle influences on the child. The father quickly seeks out positive values in the child reflecting physical competencies, while the mother may look for other qualities in the newborn child. The child, in turn, depending upon the degree he or she radiates physical vigor, begins rather quickly to mold parental expectations.

At birth, the child seems concerned only with immediate visual stimulation, and with parts of his or her body. Shortly afterward, however, the child begins to relate socially first to the mother and father, and then to peers. Objects, when rudimentary manipulatory abilities emerge, become important vehicles through which the infant may instigate, receive, or force primitive social overtures with peers. As toys and objects are played with, the child learns to interweave social responses, first responding and then awaiting a further response from a young playmate. This reciprocal interweaving of social and physical behaviors is later reflected in the same give-and-take in both primitive and then more sophisticated verbal exchanges.

Early social actions at play permit the maturing child to try out his or her social impact upon others, and at the same time acquire follower skills. These early movements and play activities also help the child to place aggression into proper focus as maturation and experimentation take place.

Early childhood signals the emergence of the child from the secure shelter of the family, and play groups of increasing complexity and size are formed. These groups, at the ages of 5 and 6, begin to reflect role differentiation. Some children learn and practice leadership skills; others revert to more passive support roles in play groups. With the advent of games containing more codified rules, still more social complexity is seen, particularly as different roles are designated for various players in popular sports within various cultures.

Throughout infancy and childhood it is virtually impossible neatly to separate actions and behaviors that signal social growth in which physical activities are involved, and those that denote emotional and intellectual change and maturation. The infant and child experiment with play materials and gain emotional maturity. At the same time, experiments with interpersonal qualities such as aggression, competition, and cooperation in play groups and teams contributes to expanded intellectual vistas on the part of the participants.

QUESTIONS FOR DISCUSSION

1. How do the behaviors of the mother and the father differ toward both male and female offspring? How do differences in maternal and paternal behaviors influence the movement capacities of infants?

2. What genetic differences seem to exist in relation to the activity levels of infants? How might these differences influence the responses of both parents?

3. What roles do objects play in early infant socialization? What is the behavioral content of the stages infants pass through relative to the use of objects in a social context?

4. How do the size and constitution of children's play groups differ from 2 to 8 years of age? How do the play forms they engage in differ between these same ages?

5. What recent findings about infant-infant relationships have implications for the design of play environments and play objects?

6. What patterns of competition are seen in infants and children? What variables and social conditions are likely to heighten competitive behaviors?

7. What factors are likely to heighten aggressive behavior as children play?

8. What types of leadership patterns are seen in the play groups of younger and older children?

9. What early family influences are likely to produce a self-confident versus a withdrawn child at play in the middle childhood years?

10. How does play seem to contribute to verbal-linguistic skills? To intellectual development?

STUDENT PROJECTS

1. Observe children of 2 at play in a group of two or more. Attempt to determine the types of social behaviors that are displayed. Try to count and codify these behaviors, if possible.

2. Do a case study of a child evidencing a lack of self-confidence and/or coordination problems at the age of 7. Try to determine what in his or her early life might have contributed to the physical backwardness shown in middle childhood. Try to determine what kind of program would ultimately aid the child, including how you would arrange the social conditions for such a program.

3. Discuss a child who is playing organized sports with his or her father and/or mother. Try to determine from your conversation how the parents encouraged competitive sport behavior in their offspring. Formulate a list of useful questions before the interview, based partly upon materials in this chapter.

CHAPTER FOURTEEN
THE EVALUATION OF
MOVEMENT QUALITIES

A brief glance by an interested adult at a vigorously active youngster is likely to be accompanied by thoughts reflecting evaluation. "Isn't that cute!" or perhaps, "My isn't he/she doing well!" are among the exclamations that emanate from a caretaker and reflect the fact that some kind of informal assessment is taking place. The visibility of movement capacities in the newborn make them criteria most likely to be used by parents and friends as they evaluate the newest member of a family. Even by middle childhood, a child's abilities to engage in useful play are used by peers to formulate various social assessments and pronouncements.

For over a hundred years, members of the scientific community have been measuring the physical abilities and capacities of maturing members of the human race. These measurements began in the 1830s, when a longitudinal study of children's heights was published by Quetelet, a Belgian astronomer and statistician (Scammon, 1927). Efforts at the measurement of physical dimensions of children continued through the nineteenth century and were added to by more broadly based assessment instruments during the later part of that century and the first decades of the next. Formulators of more recent measurement devices based their efforts on philosophical assumptions about the nature of maturation and mental-motor relationships. Virtually all scales purporting to evaluate either general or specific development contain a large number of motor items. Thus the data emanating from these tools, and from the studies they have inspired, have contributed a great deal to our knowledge not only of developmental processes themselves, but of the ways in which various movement qualities and motor task performance evolve in infants and children.

Students of motor development should be aware of the contents of these instruments, and of the assumptions on which they are based in order: (a) to understand the ways in which various motor qualities are assessed and gain a thorough understanding of such abilities as static balance, agility, and the like; (b) to implement programs of motor development in ways that are professionally meaningful in the form of pre- and postevaluations and useful interpretations of these assessment procedures; and (c) to obtain a clearer awareness of just how various movement capacities are interwoven within the other qualities exhibited by the unfolding personality of the infant, child, and adolescent.

Trends in motor development assessment have included the evolution of measures of simple height and weight and the like into more broadly based tests evaluating the ways in which the child moves himself or herself and how interactions with objects begin to take place. Assessment instruments proliferated in the 1930s and 1940s and into the 1970s as successive observer-researchers became dissatisfied with their predecessors' basic assumptions, norming procedures, and/or test content. Direct and straightforward measures of motor development as seen at various ages, developed in the 1920s by such pioneers as Arnold Gesell, are supplemented by tools developed by those seeking to predict later intelligence of the child by early sensory-motor qualities (Cattell, 1940), as well as those who saw in infant behaviors a way to foretell the quality of a child's later social-emotional interactions with others (Brazelton, 1973).

Recently, the maturational-learning model proposed by Piaget has inspired more than one researcher to formulate scales of early intelligence containing many items that might be described as manipulative and thus motor in nature (Corman and Escalona 1969; Uzgiris and Hunt, 1975). Still another contemporary trend has resulted in two thrusts in the motor testing movement. Evaluative instruments are appearing that generally display a great deal of scientific backup in the form of adequate norms, validity studies, and attention to rigorous principles of good test construction. On the other hand, there has been an upsurge in instruments based on simple, strightforward observation of children's movement capacities in specific situations. The latter instruments may be used with a handicapped population, and may enable an observer simply to check off whether or not the child uses a designated playground apparatus in one of several possible ways. This kind of tool contains useful face validity and seemingly is unencumbered by the necessity for various kinds of reliability and validity checks. These instruments are sometimes called *criteria-referenced* tests.

Instruments that contain opportunities to evaluate the motor abilities of young humans often differ markedly both in content and in philosophical base, depending upon whether they are directed toward infancy or childhood. Scales used to evaluate children and infants below the age of 2 years are often directed at a rather broad developmental assessment of the child, and may contain sections devoted to the measurement of the emergence of language and social behaviors, as well as both larger and smaller muscle function. In childhood, however, the motor tests available are often separate from testing instruments focused upon other qualities.[1] Just as the child's ability profile becomes diffused in the later years (Chapter 1), so do the available evaluation tools. Tests in early and middle childhood used to evaluate movement capacities are easily separable from those directed toward the assessment of cognitive, linguistic, perceptual, and/or social-emotional qualities.

In the discussion that follows, scales and testing tools are briefly discussed within a time frame encompassing three periods: (1) *the neonatal period,* lasting during the first month of age; (2) *infancy,* from end of the first month until about the end of the second year of life, and (3) *childhood,* from about the age of 2 years until adolescence. Some of the instruments discussed pertain only to one of the periods, others extend over two or more periods. Overall we will focus on the movement qualities and abilities contained in the more common of the available scales.

THE NEONATAL PERIOD: BIRTH TO 30 DAYS

Some of the readers of this text are not likely to participate directly in the evaluation of the newborn. However, an awareness of what is testable during this period of early organization should provide a more penetrating picture of motor development processes and capacities in the weeks, months, and years that follow. Several approaches have been taken to assessment during the early days of life. A number of programs of reflex testing are found in the literature (Parmalee, 1974; Prechtl and Beintema, 1964). Their intent has been to evaluate the strength, quality, and balance of reflexes, including those described in Chapter 3. The intent of these schedules has been to identify the general neurological integrity of the infant, and thus to pinpoint high-risk infants. Specific neurological conditions are also sometimes the focus of this early evaluation.

Other instruments involve a more general look at the newborn. The Apgar Scale (Apgar, 1953) is now used throughout hospitals in the United States to evaluate the general condition of infants from 60 seconds to 10 minutes after birth. Among the five signs given a rating of from 1 to 3 is muscle tone. The other four are reflex irritability, color, respiratory effort, and heart rate. An infant who resists the straightening of flexed arms and legs is given a 2 in muscle tone, for example; a newborn who displays completely flaccid muscles receives a 0. The total Apgar score is predictive of infant mortality and related to the difficulty of the delivery by the mother (Apgar and James, 1962). At times, correlations of this simple screening test are not high when contrasted to the results of later neurological examinations. However, Drage et al. (1966) found that an Apgar at 5 minutes after birth was a predictor of neurological abnormality at 1 year of age. The size of the Apgar has

---

[1]Gaussen (1984) has recently written a useful, practical, and philosophical overview of early development scales illustrating their uses and limitations, particularly in the prediction of later verbal and academic achievement.

also been found to be roughly predictive of data from the motor part of the Bayley scale, obtained from infants at 8 months of age (Serunian and Broman, 1975). Both mental and motor components of the Bayley scale were lower at 8 months of age for neonates testing within the 0 to 3 range at birth than was true for infants scoring from 7 to 10 on the Apgar. Prediction of later intelligence from this brief survey of neonatal health does not seem possible, given the available evidence (Serunian and Broman, 1975; Edwards, 1968; Shipe et al., 1968).

Mothers throughout history have told whoever would listen that *their* infant was behaving in unique ways, evidencing a personality of his or her own within the first days of life. It was not until the 1940s that researchers in child development seemed to agree (Fries, 1944), and several years later before assessment instruments were formulated to capture these unique social, physical, and emotional traits of the newborn (Rosenblith, 1961; Brazelton, 1973). These contemporary instruments have as their thrust the assessment of individual differences in social-emotional interactions with conditions and with people in the world infants have just entered. One cannot help but be impressed with the precision and care that has been taken in the formulation of these latest attempts at capturing the essence of the newborn. Their content includes many items that reflect both momentary and possibly long-term motor functions. The most elaborate and the one that has seemingly inspired the most research is the Brazelton Scale.

The major premises underlying the Brazelton include conceiving of the newborn as a complexly organized whole whose adaptations include defending himself or herself from negative stimuli and interacting to varying degrees with social stimulation, including various mothering behaviors. It arose from a belief that traditional neurological evaluations lacked important social-emotional-behavioral dimensions. Furthermore, those who formulated the scale believe that the measures it contains are important criteria from which to predict later social-emotional adjustments, as well as signposts to evaluate developmental delays and to make useful intercultural comparisons.

Giving the scale requires special training. However, those who are proficient in its use evidence high levels of agreement (90 percent) and at the same time retain their abilities over time. Although containing traditional reflex testing procedures, the scale is differentiated from other neonatal scales by the presence of 11 items that are elicited by the examiner and scored on a 1 to 9 scale. Among these items are motor qualities involved in movement capacities required as the examiner pulls the infant to a sit and defensive movements taken as the infant's face is lightly covered with a cloth. An additional 16 items on the Brazelton are general behaviors scored as overall impressions by the examiner gained over the course of the evaluation. Among those pertinent to the theme of this book are general tonus, hand-to-mouth facility, and motor maturity. A number of subtest scores may be grouped together under the label motor capacities. The contributors to this general category of function include how well the infant is able to maintain adequate muscle tension and tone during the evaluation, how well he or she controls motor behavior, and how well he or she can perform integrated motor activity, including bringing the hand to the mouth and inserting the thumb or finger.

Other qualities that are scored include how well the infant is able to be quieted or can self-quiet after some kind of upset is experienced. An important predictor emanating from this scale is how well and how quickly the infant is able to recover overall organization after the trauma of birth (Tronick and Brazelton, 1975). It is suggested that the first evaluation using the Brazelton be done at about the second or third day after birth, after the stresses of delivery, including medication, have worn off. A second adminstration is desirable at about day 9 to 10, after the neonate has adjusted to a home environment. Throughout the testing, repeated administrations are recommended, as the intent is to obtain the best qualities the infant is capable of displaying, rather than an average. The Brazelton appears more accurate in the identification of later abnormalities than standard neurological evaluations (Tronick and Brazelton, 1975). Likewise, consistent interracial differences are seen in neonates from different cultures (Freedman and Freedman, 1969).

Several researchers have used the Brazelton to predict later motor competencies with some accuracy. Bakow et al. (1973), for example, found that motor qualities and the infant's temperament at 4 months were moderately correlated. Powell (1974) also found that at 6 months dimensions of the Brazelton correlated .67 with motor scores obtained from the Bayley Scale. The implications of the Brazleton are wide-ranging for those interested in early infant motor development and the stimulation of the neonate and infant. Moreover, the volume of research stimulated by this and similar scales is extensive. Recent reviews of this work should be consulted for those focusing upon this period of life and upon motor development as well as other aspects of neonatal and infant development (Als, 1979).

Several more traditional scales begin their surveys of behaviors, and specifically of motor behaviors, during the early days of life. The most prominent of these include the Gesell Developmental Schedules, the Bayley Scales of Infant Development, Griffiths' Mental Development Scale, as well as the Graham and the Graham/Rosenblith Test for Neonates. (Several of these will be reviewed in the next section on motor assessment during infancy.) Most important, however, is the indication that generalized emotional states and motor qualities are seen early in life. Further, with training these qualities may be evaluated reliably and are predictive of later movement abilites. Finally, these early neonatal measures indicate that movement qualities are often inseparable from social and emotional measures obtained during the same first days of life.

INFANCY

Infancy is roughly that period following the first month of life until the child begins to gain speech and language at about the age of 2 years. During this period, the most rapid explosion of movement capacities is seen, together with emerging social and emotional behaviors that contribute or detract from effective movement. It is a period of time from which many believe one may identify behaviors, motor and otherwise, predictive of later intelligence and academic success. Most developers of scales on which to assess infants have, however, conceived of early development in general terms rather than formulating testing instruments to predict later cognitive qualities.

The Gesell Scales

Historically, the first developmental scales used in America were those published in the 1920s by Gesell. They were designed to assess development of infants within several areas. The latest revisions of these scales by Knoblock and Pasamanick (1974) have included items such as adaptive behaviors, language, and personal-social abilities. Although Gesell had no models of test building to copy, he conceived that his tests resembled the steps identified by the embryologist and geneticist in the development of all growing organisms. His identification of physical growth and the emergence of behavior thus was similar to the slides studied by the human biologist (Gesell, 1925).

The first version of the scale published in 1925 consisted of 144 items divided into four general fields. The types of items grouped into *motor behaviors* included postural control, locomotion, prehension, drawing, and hand control. An additional division labeled *adaptive behavior* also contained a preponderance of tasks requiring motor abilities, including hand-eye coordination, object recovery, and the like. The original assessment contained testing points at ages 3, 6, 9, 12, 18, and 24 months. The recent revision of the scales by Knoblock and Pasamanick consists of selected items suited to testing infants at from 4 to 56 weeks and children at 15, 18, 21, 24, 30, and 36 months. In various of the original and revised versions, it is found that the presence of motor items changes in versions designed for children and infants of various ages. For example, motor items comprise about 45 percent of the items at the 4-month level, while language is only 3 percent at that level. However, by the twenty-fourth month, motor items constituted only 11 percent of the test, while language grows to 21 percent (Yang, 1979).

The Gesell schedules have been continually subjected to the criticism that they are inadequately normed, and that averages that do appear do not encompass children from an ethnically diverse population (Yang, 1979). The scales have also been criticized for the fact that they are not predictive of later IQ. However, Gesell conceived of the scales as reflecting *development* in general rather than being used as predictors of later scores on IQ tests.

Several factor analyses have been conducted using Gesell items that have been relatively unchanged since the inception of the test in 1925. They have concluded that the tests are heavily laden with motor factors. As Richards and Nelson pointed out (1938) after inspecting the Gesell items, it is an "obvious fact that all behavior at this early level is . . . motor." More recently, the placement of items at various ages has been improved, as have descriptions of successful performance on some subtests (Knoblock and Pasamanick, 1974). Today the tests are used primarily in doctors' offices rather than at the core of research because of the questionable nature of the averages available and the reasonably lengthy administration time. Cattell, among others who wished to use early developmental milestones as predictors of late intelligence, have formulated scales of this nature purportedly more free of the contamination of motor qualities (Cattell, 1940). The more recent of these latter types of scales have been influenced by the theories and ideas of Piaget (Uzgiris and Hunt, 1975). But even these, reflecting Piaget's notion of the early sensory-motor period, contain coordination tests in parts intended for infants under the age of 1 year (Corman and Escalona, 1969).

The Bayley Scales

In 1933 Bayley published scales originally intended to evaluate the mental development of the infant. Two years later, they were followed by a motor scale copied after the items in the Gesell. Both these initial scales have been revised (Bayley, 1969), producing scores that are now termed both a mental development index and a psychomotor development index. The present motor scale is made up of 81 items. Correlations between the mental and motor parts of the scale range from +.78 at the younger ages to +.24 at the older ages, as would be expected from a consideration of the diffusion model of abilities described in Chapter 1. Inter-rater agreement of infants using the Bayley usually exceeds 90 percent. The number of infants used to norm the scale has inspired more confidence from researchers than has the Gesell, and numerous studies have been conducted using the instrument. The most common of them have been longitudinal studies of the status of suspect infants, as well as those reflecting various intercultural differences in infants. Hofstaetter (1954), factor-analyzing the battery, found that two kinds of qualities seemed to be present at two ages. Initially he felt that sensorimotor alertness was an important contributor to success in the items at about 12 months of age. The second factor identified was persistence, or the tendency to perform without being distracted by interfering conditions, present at from 20 to 40 months.

One of the more ingenious uses of the Bayley Scale has been to compare identical versus nonidentical (dizygotic) twins (Wilson, 1974; Nichols and Broman, 1974). The higher correlations between identical (monozygotic) twins of +.84, compared to dizygotic twins (.55) and siblings (.22), suggest that there is a substantial genetic influence on the scores obtained. Relationships between the quality of maternal care infants receive and test performance have resulted in mixed results.

The age range for the current Bayley Scales is from 1 month through 2.5 years. The items are arranged in an order that reflects how 50 percent of the children on whom the test was normed accomplished each one. The more valid norms and the ease of administration of the Bayley Scales have tended to prompt their use more in research requiring precision and validity within recent years than has been true of the Gesell.

Other Scales

Numerous other scales purporting to evaluate either development or mental development during the early months and first two years of life include sections of motor items. Griffiths' Mental Development Scale (Griffiths, 1954), for example, is divided into five sections, two of which are labeled locomotor and eye-hand. Other groups of items on such scales invariably include movement competencies, despite their location in such categories as social-emotional, performance, and the like.

The Denver Developmental Survey. A recent and flexible survey instrument emerged from the state of Colorado during the 1970s. Normed on Anglo as well as children with Spanish surnames, the scale is less dogmatic when placing a given task at a specific age than is true of the earlier scales, including the Bayley and the Gesell. An item in this scale is represented by a bar, which suggests the *percent* of infants at a given age who might successfully accomplish it. Thus, the bar suggests at what age 25, 50, 75, and 90 percent of the children might successfully complete each task. Again, the content of the items is more heavily laden with movement qualities in the part of the scale assessing competencies during the first 10 months of life. The Denver, however, contains two sections labeled fine motor adaptive and gross motor.

The Denver is a survey instrument from which a more detailed evaluation might be carried out, using the Bayley, for example, if some problem area is detected. After testing, the child's performance is characterized as normal, abnormal, or questionable. Early versions of the test have been criticized as inadequately normed (Herkowitz, 1978), but more recent versions have included children from diverse ethnic backgrounds, so the test should hold up well as a screening instrument if all 105 items are employed.

The Brigance. The test developed by Albert Brigance consists of two main parts: an inventory of early development, taking the child from birth to 7 years, and a second part evaluating children into adolescence. The first part contains a predominance of motor items within four sections labeled pre-ambulatory motor skills and behaviors, gross motor skills and behaviors, fine motor skills and behaviors, and self-help skills.

The Brigance Inventory of Early Development is a criteria reference test based on the author's survey of the literature rather than on norms specifically obtained for the instrument. Its age-specific criteria, however, seem well founded, and if interpreted correctly by an evaluator, the tool is a useful one for screening early motor competencies of both the preschool child and the child during the first two years of elementary school (Brigance, 1977).

The Koontz Child Developmental Program. This useful evaluation instrument is based also on a compilation of the data of others (Koontz, 1974). Its value, however, lies in the precision with which an evaluation may be applied, as well as in the fact that adjacent to each developmental signpost are suggestions for the enrichment and/or remediation of the quality assessed. Like many of the infant scales, the breakdown of items is more frequent within the first year of life; then developmental milestones are located further apart up to the fourth year of life. Reported inter-rater reliability is high, over 90 percent. This instrument involves a survey that may be useful to the preschool teacher, but its precision may preclude its use by researchers. It contains both gross and fine motor sections. Like the Denver, a more precise evaluation may be indicated after the application of the Koontz.

Motor Problem Assessment in Infancy

Highly useful instruments are available to the medical or paramedical with which to evaluate infants within the first two years of life who are suspected of displaying motor problems. Special neurological schedules have been constructed for the identification of these special infants (Touwen and Prechtl, 1970). Most interesting and ingenious, however, are two scales reflecting the interweaving of infant reflexes and early voluntary motor behaviors. These scales depict the interdependence of these important motor qualities in ways that indicate (a) what kinds of reflexes must be phased out in order for what voluntary behaviors to take place, and conversely what basic response patterns must mature in order to support even more mature reactions. The first of these instruments was published in the 1960s as a result of the efforts of two Italian pediatricians (Milani-Comparetti and Gidoni, 1967). Special training, and the supervision of a qualified therapist physician, is necessary for its use. The graphic depictions of how important early movement behaviors are interdependent, and how the presence, delay, or absence of these interactions is likely to portray either normal or abnormal motor development during the first months of life, are essential to the early detection of movement problems. A more expanded scale of this nature has also been published more recently by two physical therapists in the United States, Hoskins and Squires (1973).

MOTOR EVALUATION IN CHILDHOOD

Early and later childhood present new challenges for those formulating testing measures, evaluation programs, and assessment tools with which to evaluate motor competencies. As they pass their third and fourth birthdays, children can be evaluated on more diverse kinds of abilities than was possible with the relatively straightforward observational scales used for infants and neonates. Moreover, some of the movement qualities children begin to evidence by the third and fourth year, notably printing abilities, are critical precursors and predictors of early school success.

It is probably that much of the relative success of preschool children in any test, motor, mental, perceptual, or social, is at least partly due to the maturation of the nervous system, particularly that component aiding attention and control capacities. It is not unusual to obtain higher correlations between measures of impulse control ("How slowly will you draw a line for me?") and a movement task than may be obtained when two or more motor tasks are contrasted when assessing children during the preschool and early school years (Cratty and Gibson, 1985).

If one is to believe the considerable evidence that the movement personalities of children become more diverse as one samples scores at successively higher ages, as is indicated in Chapter 1, then it follows that one should probably plan to use a somewhat larger number of subtests when attempting to evaluate the motor abilities of children of 5 and 6 than might be employed with younger children. Still another decision to be made when formulating a program of motor evaluation is the scope of the testing program relative to the selection of tests that may display other important qualities associated with movement capacities. It is sometimes useful, for example, to include assessment tools capturing such qualities as self-concept and self-control, as well as those evaluating fine motor abilities including printing and writing, with groups of instruments more traditionally expected in an examination of movement competencies. The addition of these associated testing instruments should be dictated by (a) the tester's competencies and background, including ability correctly to interpret test results that may reflect other perceptual, social, and/or emotional qualities; and (b) the availability of other evaluative personnel, including psychologists, social workers, and child development specialists, as well as physicians, nurses, physical and occupational therapists, and speech pathologists.

For the most part, the motor expert should consider himself or herself part of an evaluative team, and indeed he or she usually functions in that manner. Care should be taken to adhere to tests and subtests that match the background and expertise of the examiner, and that furthermore are in line with reasonable objectives and goals for the type of motor development program being formulated. The growing tendency of some movement specialists to engage in the assessment of visual functions has been encouraged by some test makers, as well as some theoreticians. However, this kind of overstepping of one's professional bounds is likely to produce from moderate to disastrous outcomes. The naive movement person giving and trying to interpret a test of visual functioning and/or visual perception, may produce what is termed a false-negative or a false-positive. That is, they may falsely pronounce that nothing is wrong with the child's visual functions, when indeed there may be a progressively worsening eye condition present (a false-negative). Conversely, the motor development specialist may unduly alarm parents and others by identifying a nonexistent perceptual problem, when in truth the test result obtained is an invalid indicator. This latter misinterpretation is labeled a false-positive, and often occurs when movement experts are too quick to identify a visual or perceptual problem on the basis of a drawing test, a strategy that often evaluates *movement,* rather than perceptual competencies.

Another basic principle to be observed involves matching program goals, stated objectives, and testing instruments and subtests. It is surprising how often those who formulate programs for change incorporating movement experiences fail to provide tests that match their claims; at other times, claims made for the program are not reflected in the nature of the activities engaged in. Finally, and this is less likely, more tests are included in the battery than are necessary, taking into consideration the number and type of stated objectives and the makeup of the program itself. Failure to adhere to this matching principle may lead to one or more of the following outcomes: (a) Objectives are being formulated for which no provision is made either in the testing program or in the program content. (b) Something is tested for, and thus it is implied that it will be improved, and yet no provision is made for its improvement in the program. (c) Provisions are made in the program to improve a quality that is not reflected in the test battery, and thus the program workers do not receive formal evaluative credit for the possible improvement of the quality. Adherence to this principle of matching will produce a professional testing program, coupled with a plan well undergirded by reasonable claims and accompanied by a meaningful program.

As children become capable of being tested more precisely, with methods of increasing formality, the insertion of and adherence to formalized testing procedures and criteria should take place. That is, the infant who passes a hand-to-mouth item on an infant checklist is accomplishing a task that has obvious face validity. On the other hand, the insertion of a subtest purporting to evaluate balance on a scale for older children should be able to pass a validity check of a stricter nature. One should be able to answer the question of whether the latter test really measures (is a valid measure) of balance.

The consistency with which a test or a test battery evaluates whatever it says it is assessing should be of concern, just as was the reliability of the infant scales covered in the first part of the chapter. As the children themselves become more consistent and thus reliable in response, it is reasonable to expect that testing procedures and testers confronting older children should in a similar manner contribute more and more to the overall consistency of the scores obtained. The tester is not able to blame the capricious responses of the immature child on variations in test scores when dealing with children in middle and late childhood, as can be true when trying to capture accuracies of movement and task performance in the younger infant.

Batteries of motor tests should, for efficiency's sake, consist of subtests that evaluate relatively independent qualities. The critical user should look for the quality of factor purity when selecting tests and test batteries. To obtain this type of battery, one often has to select useful subtests from more than one battery. The overtesting of children in tests that successively evaluate almost the same quality (pushups and pullups both evaluate dynamic arm-shoulder strength) is wasteful of time, money, and effort that might be better focused on the formation and application of program content.

Finally, and this is most important, the nature of the tests applied should be appropriate to the nature of the age, sex, ethnic make-up, and geographical location of the subjects involved. For the most part, available tests do not have sufficient norms even for middle-class Anglo children. Thus great care should be taken during the selection of tests and their pairing with children of diverse ethnic-racial make-up; even more care should be taken when the results of such testing efforts are interpreted for school authorities, parents, and other interested consumers. When more and more tests of increasing sophistication are available, individual differences seen even in the results obtained from infant scales will be accommodated to and explained via test results. Failure to follow this principle of matching the test make-up with the make-up of the population served can cause a number of problems between test giver, school authorities, and parents, as children are mislabeled, misclassified, and otherwise burdened with interpretations not valid for that part of the human group from which the child-client comes.

Oseretsky: The Test and Those That Followed

Historically the first professional effort to evaluate the motor abilities of children sprang from the Moscow Neurological Institute and was formulated by Oseretsky. Searching for what was called "motor idiocy," this evaluative instrument contains items intended to evaluate both large and small muscle control. Over the decades, a number of translations followed, including several in English (Sloan, 1955; Bailer, Doll, and Winsberg, 1973; Bruinick, 1978). Stott has used a highly modified Oseretsky to develop a scale pointed specifically toward the identification of the physically awkward child, as was Oseretsky's original intent. Overall, these recent versions (Bailer et al., 1973) contain items to assess the motor development status of children from 5 to 12 years. About two-thirds of the items involve hand and arm movements, evaluating speed, dexterity, coordination of two arms, and rhythm. The gross motor items involve balance, jumping abilities, and the like.

Controversy has continued, after repeated factor analyses, as to just what qualities the test measures (Thams, 1955). The more recent versions are reliable, but often normed on exceedingly few children at each age level (Bruinick, 1978). Some authorities (Herkowitz, 1978) consider recent modifications of the test valuable tools for studying the motor performances of school-age children. However, the absence of subtests involving ball skills, including throwing and kicking, often renders them less than useful in some school settings in which these skills are important (Bailer et al., 1973). The early form of the Bruinick's revision of the Oseretsky required a great deal of equipment, and thus a short-form (Beitel and Mead, 1980) is probably more useful. At present, the well-researched and factor pure tests by Fleishman published in 1965 offer a well-normed battery. However, the averages from 20,000 subjects contained in this instrument are for youth from 10 to 14 years of age.

Charlop-Atwell Scale of Motor Coordination

This scale was developed to assess some aspects of gross motor coordination in children from the fourth to sixth year. The test requires little equipment but has been standardized on a relatively few children (201). Although proponents suggest that it is useful for evaluating children from various subcultures, the lack of subjects in the norming attempts make one skeptical. Its validity and reliability have been obtained, and it appears a relatively sound instrument statistically (Charlop and Atwell, 1980).

The Hughes Test

One breath of fresh air in the otherwise stale environment of motor assessment instruments for children is offered by the test developed by Jeanne Hughes of the University of Colorado. It has been normed for children from 6 to 12 years, factor-analyzed, and is a potentially useful instrument. The test contains items intended to evaluate balance, locomotor items, throwing, and other ball-handling skills, including dribbling. Reliability of over .9 has been reported, and norms have been based upon 90 children at each age and of each sex. Although norms apparently fail to include a percentage of children from various ethnic groups, careful interpretation of the results by a tester could yield useful information and provide a basis for discussion when working with parents of children displaying movement problems (Hughes, 1979).

Ohio State University Test

Loovis and Ersing (1979) have also developed a criteria-referenced test for the evaluation of motor competencies of children in middle childhood. Eleven basic motor skills are covered, including locomotor activities, ball skills (kicking and striking), and the like.

Each basic skill is scored within one of four levels, ranging from least mature performance to level 4, "mature functional pattern" of that skill. A clinician is provided with a descriptive assessment of a child's current gross motor functioning for all the tests. This test may help those formulating programs of remedial motor activity for physically awkward youngsters of elementary school age.

Fine Motor Control, Printing, Writing

During the preschool and early elementary school years, there is often a need to include tests of fine motor control, as well as of printing potential, in batteries of motor development instruments. Among the more useful of these are the perceptual-motor component of the Vane Kindergarten Test, which yields a perceptual-motor quotient as the result of a figure-copying subtest. Norms from 4 to almost 7 years are available, and this test is a reasonable starting point when dealing with potential printing problems during early childhood (Vane, 1968).

Originally developed as a test of visual-perceptual development, the Frostig Developmental Test of Visual Perception contains subtests that are useful in evaluating drawing and printing potential and accuracy (Frostig, 1964). The norms are well developed, and the test is quickly administered.

Interpretations may be and have been made of children's inability to draw well and/or to copy figures (Bender, 1938; Harris, 1963; Koppitz, 1973), ranging from perceptual problems through intelligence, brain damage, and emotional problems, as well as problems with motor coordination. It should be noted that a drawing test probably evaluates perceptual and motor abilities, as well as the abilities needed to integrate perceptual input with motor output in some combination. Recent tests that evaluate visual perception in a straightforward manner, without the need for the child to display motor coordination, have produced scores that are not correlated with measures taken from drawing tests traditionally used to evaluate visual perception, such as the Frostig. Professionals wishing to evaluate visual perception should perhaps use instruments such as that developed by Colarusso et al. (1973).

On the other hand, the evaluation of the hand-eye coordination needed to print well is critical to early school success and should be dealt with using some of the instruments suggested.

Other Instruments

It is beyond the scope of this discussion to survey all the potential instruments that may be used as adjuncts to a motor testing program, including self-concept tests (Piers and Harris, 1964), tests of body image (Berges and Lezine, 1965), as well as measures of other subtle perceptual and movement qualities, including the sensory awareness of various body parts and motor planning, as well as activity level and impulsivity (Cratty and Samoy, 1984; Cratty and Sibson, 1985; Connolly and Stratton, 1968). Moreover, an increasing number of tests are available to tap the movement abilities, self-care skills, and movement-related competencies of various handicapped populations (Cratty, 1980). An extremely well-made contemporary test for the evaluation of awkward children should be consulted if one desires to conduct this kind of screening of school-age children (Stott, 1975). Containing different types of tests at various ages, the test by Stott evaluates five different movement qualities in children from 4 to 13 years.

A CONTEMPORARY APPROACH TO MOTOR EVALUATION

Several contemporary writers have advocated a rather broad approach to the evaluation of physical abilities and skills in the maturing youngster (Cratty, 1975; Herkowitz, 1978; Gallagher, 1984). It is advocated that a given motor act be looked at from several angles, rather than simply scoring performance success. This comprehensive approach involves the inspection of how a given act is executed, the relative success achieved in performance, as well as the presence or absence of other qualities imbedded within the overall intent of the child. Thus the act of throwing a ball would be assessed with a view to distance as well as to the efficiency of the mechanics the child exhibits as he or she releases the implement.

This same throwing task may be analyzed with regard to other movement qualities, including (a) the degree to which extraneous movements or tensions may be exhibited in other parts of the body, overflow that does not contribute directly to the success of the task; (b) the degree to which the act exhibits correct symmetry or correct asymmetry—that is, the throw would be viewed as to whether the other arm acts in a complementary manner, and whether the throwing arm seems unrestricted in its use; (c) the degree to which the body parts are correctly integrated in the act—in this case, the role of the legs in the throw. Still further evaluation and analysis of the task might include the resistance of the skill to social stresses, such as the presence and/or pressure of onlookers. Finally, the task may be analyzed relative to its usefulness and appropriateness to the culture and subculture in which the child is attempting to function. These latter two qualities may have to be described in para-

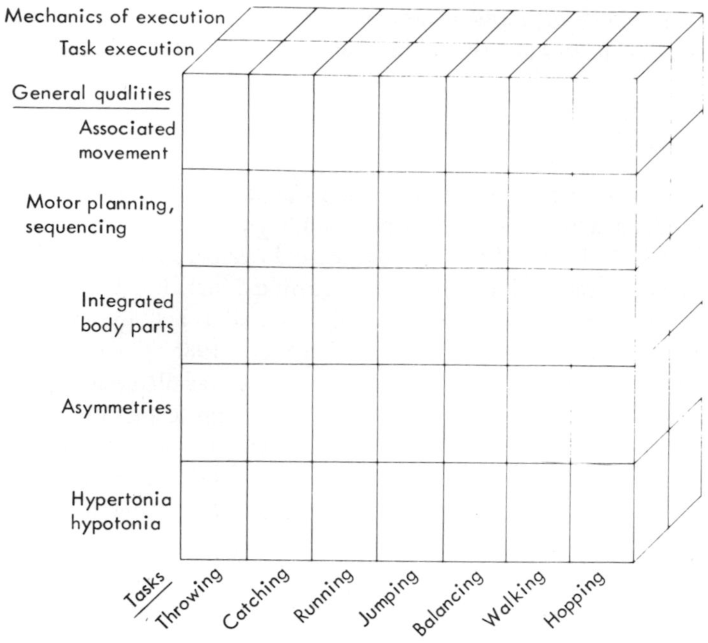

Mechanics of execution
Task execution
General qualities
Associated movement
Motor planning, sequencing
Integrated body parts
Asymmetries
Hypertonia hypotonia

Tasks / Throwing / Catching / Running / Jumping / Balancing / Walking / Hopping

FIGURE 14.1

graph form, rather than being reduced to some kind of index number. Task analyses carried out using some or all of the above criteria present problems involving scientific veracity. At the same time, the patterns of information, descriptions, and measures emerging from this type of thorough look at skills often provide more important information than numbers emerging from some poorly normed test.

Viewed diagrammatically, this type of approach may be depicted as in Figure 14.1. Using this approach, differences in the way in which various tasks are evaluated may take place. For example, some tasks may lack a symmetry dimension. At the same time this evaluation of process (mechanics of execution) as well as product (task execution), together with more subtle qualities of the task described in Chapter 9, might prove to be a helpful contemporary road to follow when evaluating children's motor competencies in the 1980s and afterward.

SUMMARY

Assessment instruments intended to evaluate the motor qualities of humans may be found in scales designed to test infants, children, adolescents, and adults. For the most part, early development scales contain a preponderance of items evaluating movement capacities, but these are often called developmental scales rather than tests of motor development.

Many of the contemporary instruments intended to evaluate infant development also contain items intended to evaluate the early social-emotional personality of the infant in ways that are likely to predict how that infant will behave physically, and in turn how that infant is likely to be reacted to socially and physically by adults.

A number of preschool assessment scales are available, most containing motor components intended to evaluate both fine and gross motor skills and abilities. Such scales also contain many motor items in such categories as adaptive behaviors and self-care skills. These scales are useful in the assessment not only of nonhandicapped preschool youngsters, but also of developmentally delayed populations.

There is a shortage of well-normed motor ability scales applicable to the measurement of physical skills during the elementary school years. Those that are available, if their results are interpreted well, can prove to be useful when counseling parents of children who are suspected of displaying motor problems.

Contemporary approaches to motor assessment can include the administration and interpretation of ancillary tests including those evaluating performance self-concept, impulsivity, and other qualities. A modern trend seen in the literature is to evaluate the product of the effort (how far did the youngster throw?), the biomechanical appearance of the throw (the process), as well as other more subtle qualities that may have been evidenced, including overflow of excess tensions, asymmetries, the integration of body parts, and how well the action was planned.

QUESTIONS FOR DISCUSSION

1. What are criteria-referenced tests? How might they be used? What advantages and drawbacks might they have?
2. What early personality qualities seen in infants, after assessment on such instruments as the Brazelton, might contribute to the child's later acquisition and display of motor skill?
3. What does a factor-pure test mean? What are the advantages of such a test?
4. What does the principle of matching mean?
5. What problem might occur if the principle of matching is not observed?
6. What tests might you use when formulating a battery to assess the child entering school at 5 years of age? What tasks might you require that are independent of any test?
7. What tests are available to assess the motor skills of a child entering junior high school (about 12 to 13 years of age)?
8. How might you formulate a data collection sheet to evaluate the process as well as the product of various motor skills deemed important in middle childhood?

STUDENT PROJECTS

1. Using Chapters 5 and 13, develop a checklist to assess the motor competencies of a child (female) of 7 years, a boy of 8 years.

2. Using a partner in your class, observe a child at play, and independently score his or her abilities. Find the percentage of inter-observer agreement on the various tasks you included on your assessment instrument.

3. Using some of the tests, or their parts, discussed in the chapter, formulate a battery of motor tests appropriate when assessing children entering kindergarten (5 years of age). What allowances, modifications, and so on might you make when assessing the abilities of various ethnic-racial groups of 5-year-old children (see Chapter 4)?

4. Using a child to whom you have access (a family member), evaluate his or her motor competencies using a checklist (pass-fail) approach. Be sure you obtain parental permission. Formulate an ideal program of motor activities, sports participation, and so on for the child as a result of your evaluation. If needed, what remedial activities might be useful?

5. Test two children of equal abilities under different motivational conditions (one alone, the other in the presence of an encouraging parent or peer). What differences might you obtain, or did you obtain, in the results?

6. Assess a large number of children of various ages in a large number of motor tasks—galloping, skipping, throwing, and the like. Develop a developmental sequence of activities as a result of your assessment, arranging tasks in order of difficulty—the most difficult were passed by the fewest children, the easier by a larger percentage, and so on. What implications might such a sequence of activities have for program planning?

REFERENCES

CHAPTER 1

BAYLEY, NANCY, "Behavioral Correlates of Mental Growth—Birth to Thirty-Six Years." *Amer. Psych., 23* (1968): 1–17.

BOWER, T. G. R. *Development in Infancy*. San Francisco: W. H. Freeman, 1974.

BOWER, T. G. R., AND WISHART, J. G. "The Effects of Motor Skill on Object Permanence." *Cognition, 1* (1972): 165–72.

BOWER, T. G. R. *Human Development*. San Francisco: W. H. Freeman, 1979.

BROADHEAD, G. D., MARUYAMA, G. M., AND BRUININKS, R. H. "Examining Differentiation in Motor Proficiency Through Exploratory and Confirmatory Factor Analysis," in Clark, J. E., and Humphery, J. H. *Motor Development*. Vol I, Princeton, N.J.: Princeton Book Co., 1985.

BROWN, G., AND DESFORGES, C. *Piaget's Theory—A Psychological Critique*. London: Routledge & Kegal Paul, 1979.

CARPENTER, AILEEN. "The Differential Measurement of Speed in Primary School Children." *Child Development, 12* (1941): 1–7.

CLARKE, A. D. B., AND CLARKE, A. M. "Constancy and Change in Growth of Human Characteristics," *Journal of Child Psychology and Psychiatry, 25* (1984): 191–210.

CLAUSEN, J., *Ability Structure and Subgroups in Mental Retardation*. Washington: Spartan Books; London: Macmillan, 1966.

COHEN, D. *Piaget—Critique and Reassessment*. New York: St. Martin's Press, 1983.

CRATTY, BRYANT J., *The Perceptual-Motor Attributes of Mentally Retarded Children and Youth*. Monograph, sponsored by Mental Retardation Services Board of Los Angeles County, Los Angeles, 1966.

_____ . *Movement Behavior and Motor Learning*, 3rd ed. Philadelphia: Lea and Febiger, 1973.

_____ . *Perception, Motion and Thought*. Palo Alto, Calif.: Peek Publications, 1969.

_____ . and Martin, M. M., *Perceptual-Motor Efficiency in Children*. Philadelphia: Lea and Febiger, 1969.

CUMBEE, F. Z. "A Factorial Analysis of Motor Coordination." *Res. Quart., 25* (1954): 412–28.

CZIMENTHALYI, M. "Self-Awareness and Aversive Experience in Everyday Life." *Journal of Personality, 50* (1982): 15–29.

DECARIE, T. B. "A Study of the Mental and Educational Development of Thalidomide Children." In *Determinants of Infant Behavior,* VI, B. Foss (ed.). London: Methune, 1969.

DENNIS, W. "Infant Development under Conditions of Restricted Practice and of Minimum Social Stimulation: A Preliminary Report," *J. Genet. Psycho., 53* (1938): 149–58.

DONALDSON, M. *Children's Minds.* New York: Fontana, 1978.

DYE, N. W., AND VERY, P. S. "Growth Changes in Factorial Structure by Age and Sex," *Genet. Psychol. Monogr., 78* (1968): 55–88.

FANTZ, R. I. "The Origin of Form Perception." *Scientific American, 206* (1961): 115–25.

FLAVELL, J. H. *The Developmental Psychology of Jean Piaget.* New York: Van Nostrand, 1962.

FLEISHMAN, EDWIN A. *The Structure and Measurement of Physical Fitness.* Englewood Cliffs, N.J.: Prentice-Hall, 1964.

————, AND HEMPEL, WALTER E., JR. "Factorial Analysis of Complex Psychomotor Performance and Related Skills," *J. Appl. Psych., 40* (1956): 2.

FRENCH, J. W. "The Relationship of Problem-Solving Styles to Factor Composition of Tests," *Educ. Psych., Measmt., 25* (1965): 9–28.

GARRETT, H. E. "A Developmental Theory of Intelligence." *Amer. Psych., 1* (1946): 372–78.

GELMAN, R. "Cognitive Development." *Harvard Review of Psychology, 28* (1978): 297–32.

GINSBURG, H., AND OPPER, SYLVIA. *Piaget's Theory of Intellectual Development.* Englewood Cliffs, N.J.: Prentice-Hall, 1969.

HEBB, D. O. *The Organization of Behavior.* New York: Wiley, 1949.

ILLINGWORTH, R. S. *The Development of the Infant and Young Child,* 3rd ed. Edinburgh and London: Livingstone, 1967.

INHELDER, B., SINCLAIR, H., AND BOVET, M. *Learning and the Development of Cognition.* Cambridge, Mass.: Harvard University Press, 1974.

JOHN, E. ROY. *Mechanisms of Memory.* New York and London: Academic Press, 1967.

JUDD, C. H. "The Relationship of Special Training to General Intelligence," *Educ. Rev., 26* (1908): 28–42.

JUURMAA, JYRKI. "On Interrelations of Auditory, Tactual and Visual Spatial Performances." Helsinki, Finland: Reports from the Institute of Occupational Health, No. *54,* September 1967.

KALM, S. B. "Development of Mental Abilities: An Investigation of the Differentiation Hypothesis'." *Canad. J. Psych., 24* (1970): 67–71.

KEPHART, NEWELL C. *The Slow Learner in the Classroom.* Columbus: Charles E. Merrill, 1960.

KILPATRICK, F. P. "Two Processes in Perceptual Learning." *J. Exp. Psych., 36* (1946): 187–211.

KONORSKI, JERZY. *Integrative Activity of the·Brain—An Interdisciplinary Approach.* Chicago and London: University of Chicago Press, 1967.

MONTESSORI, MARIA. *Dr. Montesorri's Own Handbook.* New York: Frederick A. Stokes, 1914.

MURRAY, F. B. (ed.) *The Impact of Piagetian Theory on Education, Philosophy, Psychiatry, and Psychology.* Baltimore: University Park Press, 1979.

PIAGET, JEAN. *The Child's Conception of the World.* New York: Harcourt Brace and World, 1929.

————. *The Consruction of Reality in the Child.* New York: Basic Books, 1954.

————. *The Early Growth of Logic in the Child.* New York: Harper and Row, 1964.

————. *The Origins of Intelligence in Children.* New York: International Universities Press, 1965.

————. Foreword in M. Schwebel & J. Raph (eds.), *Piaget in the Classroom.* New York: Basic Books, 1973.

RARICK, G. LAWRENCE, AND DOBBINS, D. ALAN. "Basic Components in the Motor Performance of Children Six to Nine Years of Age," *Med. and Science in Sports, 7* (1975): 105–10.

ROBINSON, M. E., AND TATNALL, L. L. J. *Intellectual Functioning of Children with Congenital Amputation.* Clinical Proceedings of the Childrens Hospital, North Carolina, 1981.

ROSENTHAL, R. "Early Human Experience." *Developmental Psychology, 18* (1982), 36–41.

SCHMIDT, RICHARD A. "A Schema Theory of Discrete Motor Skill Learning." *Psych. Rev., 82* (July 1975).

SMITH, OLIN W., AND SMITH, PATRICIA C. "Developmental Studies of Spatial Judgments by Children and Adults." *Percept. Mot. Skills,* Mono. Suppl. 1–V22, 1966.

TREVARTHEN, C. "Communication and Co-operation in Early Infancy." In M. Bullowa (ed.), *Before Speech.* Cambridge, Mass.: Cambridge University Press, 1979.

WHITE, BURTON L., AND HELD, RICHARD. "Plasticity of Sensorimotor Development in the Human Infant." In H. Harlow and C. Woolsey (eds.), *Biological and Biochemical Bases of Behavior.* Madison: University of Wisconsin Press, 1958.

WILLATTS, P. "The Stage IV Infant's Solutions of Problems Requiring the Use of Supports." *Infant Behavior and Development, 7* (1984): 125–34.

ZAJONC, R. "Hot Cognition." Paper read to the American Psychological Association, New York, August 1979.

CHAPTER 2

BERENBERG, S. R., CANAIRIS, M., AND MASSE, N. P. (eds.). *Pre and Postnatal Development of the Human Brain.* New York: Karger, 1974.

BLAKEMORE, C. "Development of Functional Connections in the Mammalian Visual System." In Brazier (ed.), *Growth and Development of the Brain.* New York: Ravens Press, 1975, pp. 157–69.

DOBBING, J., AND SMART, J. "Vulnerability of Developing Brain and Behavior." *British Medical Bulletin, 30* (1974): 164–68.

HERSCHKOWITZ, N. AND ROSSI, E. "Critical Periods in Brain Development." CIBA Foundation Symposium, *Lipids, Malnutrition, and the Developing Brain.* New York: Associated Scientific Publications, 1972.

LEMIRE, R., LOESER, J., LEECH, R. AND ALBORD, E. *Normal and Abnormal Development of the Human Nervous System.* New York: Harper and Row, 1975.

LOU, H. C. *Developmental Neurology.* New York: Ravens Press, 1982.

MOLLIVER, M., KOSTOVIC, I., AND VAN DER LOOS, H. "The Development of Synapses in the Cerebral Cortex of the Human Fetus." *Brain Research, 50* (1973): 403–7.

MOORE, K. *The Developing Human: Clinically Oriented Embryology.* Philadelphia: Saunders, 1982.

PURPURA, D. P. "Pathobiology of Cortical Neurons in Metabolic and Unclassified Amentias." In R. Katzman (ed.), *Congenital and Acquired Cognitive Disorders.* New York: Ravens Press, 1979.

RORKE, L., AND RIGGS, H. *Myelination of the Brain in the Newborn.* Philadelphia: Lippincott, 1969.

WILLIAMS, H. "Growth and Development of the Nervous System." In *Perceptual and Motor Development.* Englewood Cliffs, N.J.: Prentice-Hall, 1983.

YAKOLEV, P. I. AND LECOURS, A. The Mylogenetic Cycles of Regional Maturation of the Brain. In A. Minkowski (ed.), *Regional Development of the Brain in Early Life.* Philadelphia: F. A. Davis Co., 1967.

CHAPTER 3

ADAMS, N., AND CALDWELL, W., "The Children's Somatic Apperception Test". *J. Genet. Psych., 68* (1963): 43–57.

ANDERSON, H. H., AND H. F. BRANDT. "Study of Motivation Involving Self-Announced Goals of Fifth Grade Children of the Concept of Level of Aspiration." *J. Soc. Psych., 10* (1939): 209–32.

ATTNEAVE, FRED, AND MALCOLM D. ARNOULT. "The Quantitative Study of Shape and Pattern Perception." *Psych. Bull., 53* (1956): 452.

AYRES, JEAN. "Patterns of Perceptual-Motor Dysfunction in Children: Factor Analytic Study." Monograph Supp. *Percept. Mot. Skills, 1* (1965): 335–68.

BARRY, A. J., AND CURETON, T. K. *Research Quarterly 32* (1961): 283–88.

BENTON, ARTHUR L., *Right-Left Discrimination and Finger Localization.* New York: Paul Hoeber, 1959, p. 14.

BERGÉS, J., AND I. LÉZINE. *The Imitation of Gestures* (transl. Arthur H. Parmelee). London: The Spastics Society Medical Education and Information Unit in Association William Heinemann, 1965.

BOOKWALTER, K. W. "The Relationship of Body Size and Shape to Physical Performance." *Research Quarterly, 23* (1952): 271–76.

BRENGELMANN, J. C., "Expressive Movements and Abnormal Behavior." In H. J. Eysenck (ed.), *Handbook of Abnormal Psychology.* New York: Basic Books, 1961, chap. 3, 69–75.

CACOURSIERE-PAIGE, FRANCOISE. "Development of Left-Right Concept in Children." *Percept. Mot. Skills, 38* (1974): 111–17.

CLARKE, H. H. *Physical and Motor Tests in the Medford Boy's Growth Study.* Englewood Cliffs, N.J.: Prentice-Hall, 1973.

CLEVELAND, SIDNEY, AND SEYMOUR FISHER. "Prediction of Small Group Behavior from a Body Schema." *Human Relations, 10* (1957): 223–33.

COLLINS, J. K. AND PROPERT, D. S., "A Developmental Study of Body Recognition in Adolescent Girls." *Adolescence, 18* (1983): 768–73.

CRATTY, BRYANT J. *Perceptual-Motor Attributes of Mentally Retarded Children and Youth.* Los Angeles County Mental Retardation Services Board, 1965 (Monograph).

————— . *Social Dimensions of Physical Activity.* Englewood Cliffs, N.J.: Prentice-Hall, 1967, chap. 3.

————— . *Active Learning: Games to Enhance Academic Abilities,* Englewood Cliffs, N.J.: Prentice-Hall, 1985.

————— , AND WILNER, M. "The Effects of a Three-Month Training Program upon Children with Moderate Perceptual-Motor Dysfunction." Unpublished study, 1967.

CRISP, H. H. "Some Psychobiological Aspects of Adolescent Growth and Their Relevance for the Fat/Thin Syndrome (Anorexia Nervosa)." *Inter. Jour. of Obesity. 1* (1977): 231–38.

DIBIASE, W., AND HJELLE, L. A. Body-image Stereotypes and Body Type Preferences among Male College Students." *Percept. Mot. Skills, 27* (1968): 1143–46.

DILLON, DONALD J. "Measurement of Perceived Body Size," *Percept. Mot. Skills, 14* (1962): 191–96.

DWYER, J., AND MAYER J. "Variations in Physical Appearance during Adolescence (part 2 girls) *Postgrad. Medicine, 42* (1967): 91–97.

FALKNER, F. "The Development of Children: A Guide to Interpretation of Growth Charts and Developmental Assessments: A commentary and future problems." *Pediatrics, 29* (1962): 448–86.

GALLIFRET-GRANJON, N. "L'elaboration des rapports spatiaux et al dominance laterale chez les enfants dyslexiques-dysorthographiques." *Bull. Soc. Alfred-Binet, 6* (1959): 452.

GARN, S. M. "Fat Thickness and Growth Progress During Infancy." *Human Biol., 28* (1956): 232–38.

————— "Fat, Body Size, and Growth in the Newborn." *Human Biol. 30* (1965): 265–70.

————— "Body Size and its Implications," in L. W. Hoffman and M. L. Hoffman (eds.) *Review of child development research* (Vol 2), New York: Russell Sage Foundation, 1966.

GUGGENHEIM, K., POZNANSKI, R., AND KAUFMAN, N. A. "Attitudes of Adolescents to their Body Build and Problem of Juvenile Obesity." *Inter. Jour. of Obesity, 1* (1977): 135–49.

HACAEN, H. AND DE AJURIAGUERRA, J. *Left-Handedness, Manual Superiority and Cerebral Dominance,* New York: Grune & Stratton, 1964.

HAMACHEK, D. E., *The Self in Growth, Teaching and Learning,* Englewood Cliffs, N.J.: Prentice-Hall, 1965.

HAMMOND, W. H. "The Determination of Physical Type in Children." *Human Biology, 25* (1953): 65–70.

HARTER S., AND PIKE, R. *The Pictorial Scale of Perceived Competence and Acceptance for Young Children.* University of Denver, Colorado, 1981. Unpublished Monograph.

HEATH, B. H., AND CARTER J. E. L. "A Comparison of Somatotype Methods." *American Journal of Physical Anthropology 24* (1966): 87–99.

————— "A Modified Somatotype Method." *American Journal of Physical Anthropology, 27* (1967): 57–74.

HENDRY, L. B., AND GILLIES, P. "Body Type, Body Esteem, School, and Leisure: A study of Overweight, Average, and Underweight Adolescents." *J. of Youth and Adolescence, 7* (1978): 181–95.

HEWITT, D. AND ACHESON, R. M. "Some Aspects of Skeletal Development through Adolescence: Part I Variations in the Rate and Pattern of Skeletal Maturation at Puberty." *American Journal of Physical Anthropology, 19* (1961), 321–31.

HOWARD, I. P., AND TEMPLETON, W. B. *Human Spatial Orientation,* New York: Wiley, 1966.

ILG, FRANCES L., AND AMES, LOUISE B. *School Readiness,* New York: Harper & Row, 1966.

JERSILD, A. T. *In Search of Self,* New York: Teachers College, Columbia University, Bureau of Publications, 1952.

JOHNSON, W., FRETZ, B., AND JOHNSON, J. "Changes in Self-Concept During a Physical Development Program." *Res. Quart., 39* (1968): 560–65.

JONES, MARY C. "The Later Careers of Boys Who Were Early or Late Maturers." *Child Dev., 28* (1957): 113–18.

KRETSCHMER, E. *Physique and Character,* Trans. W. J. H. Sprott, New York: Harcourt, 1921.

KUCZAJ, S. A., AND MARATSOS, M. P. "On the Acquisition of Front, Back and Side," *Child Development, 46* (1975): 202–10.

LERNER, R. M. "The Development of Stereotyped Expectancies of Body-build Relations." *Child Develop. 40* (1969): 137–41.

LONG, A. B., AND LOOFT, W. R. "Development of Directionality in Children," *Developmental Psychology, 6* (1972): 375–80.

MALINA, R. M. "Biosocial Correlations of Motor Development During Infancy and Early Childhood," In L. S. Green and F. E. Johnson, *Social and Biological Predictors of Nutritional Status and Neurological Development,* New York: Academic Press, 1975.

MALINA, R. AND RARICK, G. L. "Growth Physique and Motor Performance," in Rarick G. L. (Ed.) *Physical Activity, Human Growth and Development,* New York: Academic Press, 1973.

MARESH, M. M. "Bone Muscle and Fat Measurements". *Pediatrics, 28* (1961): 971–75.

McCANDLESS, B. R. *Children and Adolescence,* New York: Holt Rinehart and Winston, 1961.

MIZUNO, T. AND HIRATA, H. "Ideal Body-builds of Present-day Youths. *Research Journal of Physical Education,* (Japan), *9* (1966): 398–405.

MIZUNO, T., HIRATA, H., AOYAMA, S., CHAN-SHI, J. AND ISHIKAWA, N. "An International Comparative Study on Body Concepts of Youths." *Research Journal of Physical Education* (Japan), *12* (1968): 141–46.

MUSSEN, P. H. AND JONES, MARY C. "Self-Conceptions, Motivations and Interpersonal Attitudes of Late and Early Maturing Boys." *Child Dev., 28* (1957): 243–56.

PARIZKOVA, J. *Growth, Fitness and Nutrition in Pre-School Children.* Prague, Czechoslovakia: University of Prague Press, 1984.

————— "Impact of Age, Diet, and Exercise on Man's Body Composition," *Ann. NY Acadm. Science, 110* (1963): 661–75.

PARNELL, R. W. *Behaviour and Physique, An Introduction to Practical and Applied Somatometry,* London: Arnold, 1958.

PETERSEN, G. *Atlas for Somatotyping Children.* The Netherlands: Royal Vagorcum Ltd. Pub. Assn., 1967.

PLATZER, W. S. The Effect of Perceptual-motor Training on Gross Motor Skill, and Self-concept of Young Children." *Am. J. of Occupational Therapy, 30* (1976): 423–28.

PRYOR, H. N. "Charts of Normal and Body Measurements and Revised Width-Weight Tables." *J. Pediatrics, 68* (1966): 615–25.

ROTCH, T. M. "A Study of the Bones in Childhood by the Roentgen Method." *Trans American Association of Physicians,* v. *24* (1909), 603–30.

ROWE, A. A., AND CAMPBELL, W. E. "The Somatic Apperception Test." *J. Genet. Psych., 68* (1963): 59–69.

SCHILDER, P. *The Image and Appearance of the Human Body,* London: Routledge and Kegan Paul, 1935.

SEAGRAVES, R. T. "Personality, Body-build, and Adrenocortical Activity," *British J. Psychiatry, 117* (1970): 405–11.

SHELDON, W. G., AND STEVENS, S. S. *Varieties of Temperament,* New York: Harper and Bros, 1942.

SHELDON, W. G., DEPERTUIS, C. W., AND McDERMOTT, E. *Atlas of Men: "A Guide for Somatotyping the Adult Male at all Ages."* New York: Harper and Bros., 1954.

SHELDON, W. B., STEVENS, S. S., AND TUCKER, W. B. *The Varieties of Human Physique,* New York: Harper and Bros, 1940.

SHIRLEY, M. M. *The First Two years; a Study of Twenty-five babies. 1,* Minneapolis: University of Minnesota Press, 1931.

SPIONNECK E. Unpublished Study in Hacaen, H. and De Ajuria-guerra, J. *Left-Handedness, Manual Superiority and Cerebral Dominance,* New York: Grune Stratton, 1964.

STAFFIERI, J. R. "A Study of Social Stereotype of Body Image in Children." *Journal of Personality and Soc. Psych., 7* (1967): 101–04.

STAGER, S. F. "A Reexamination of Body-Build Stereotypes." *Journal of Research in Personality, 16* (1982): 435–46.

STECHLER, G. AND CARPENTER, G. "A Viewpoint on Early Affective Development." In J. Hellmuth (ed.), *The Exceptional Infants,* Vol 1, Special Child Publications, 1967.

STILES, D. B. "Comparisons of self-estimated height and width of children of 10 months to 10 years 9 months under static and dynamic conditions." M. S. thesis, Purdue Univ., 1975.

TANNER, J. M., AND WHITEHOUSE, R. H. "Standards for Subcutaneous Fat in British Children," *Brit. Med. J., 1* (1962): 446–50.

————— *Fetus Into Man,* Cambridge, Mass.: Harvard University Press, 1978.

TODD, T. W. *Atlas of Skeletal Maturation: Part I The Hand.* St. Louis: C. V. Mosby, 1937.

TUCKER, L. A. "Self-concept: A Function of Self-perceived Somatotype." *J. of Psychology, 113* (1983): 123–33.

WALKER, R. N. "Body-build and Behavior in Young Children; Body-build and Nursery School Teacher's Ratings." *Monograph of the Society for Research in Child Development, 3* (1952), 27–84.

WALTERS, ETTA. "Prediction of Postnatal Development from Fetal Activity." *Child Dev., 33* (1965): 801–8.

WEAR, C. L., AND MILLER, K. "Relationship of Physique and Developmental Level to Physical Performance." *Research Quarterly, 33* (1962), 615–20.

WIGGINS, R. G., "Differences in Self-perceptions of Ninth Grade Boys and Girls." *Adolescence, 8* (1973): 492–95.

WORSLEY, A. "Teenagers' Perceptions of Fat and Slim People." *Int. J. Obesity, 5* (1981): 15–24.

WYLIE RUTH C., *The Self Concept,* Lincoln: University of Nebraska Press, 1961.

CHAPTER 4

ALBERTS, C. L., AND LANDERS, D. M. "Birth Order, Motor Performance, and Maternal Influence." *Research Quarterly, 48* (1978): 661–70.

ALS, H., TRONIC, K. E., ADAMSON, L., AND BRAZELTON, D. "The Behavior of the Full-Term Yet Underweight Newborn Infant." *Developmental Medicine and Child Neurology, 18* (1975): 590–602.

ASTBURY, J., ORGILL, A. A., BAJUK, A., AND YU, V. Y. H. "Determinants of Developmental Performance of Very Low Birth-Weight Survivors at One and Two Years of Age." *Developmental Medicine & Child Neurology, 25* (1983): 709–16.

BARNESS, L. W. "Nutrition for the Low-Birth-Weight Infant." *Clinical Perinatology, 2* (1975): 345–52.

BELLER E. K. "Exploratory Studies of Dependency," *Transactions of the New York Academy of Science, 1* (1959), 414–26.

BIRNS, B., AND GOLDEN, M. "Prediction of Intellectual Performance at Three Years from Infant Tests and Personality Measures." *Merrill-Palmer Quarterly, 18* (1972): 53–58.

BJERRE, I. "Physical Growth of 5-Year-Old Children with a Low Birthweight." *Acta Paediatrica Scandinavia* (Stockholm) *64* (1975): 33–43.

BLECK, E. E. AND NAGEL, D. A. *Physically Handicapped Children: A Medical Guide for Teachers.* New York: Grune Stratton, 1975.

BONDS, R. "Growth, Maturation and Performance of Philadelphia Negro and White Elementary School Children. Unpublished doctoral dissertation, University of Pennsylvania, 1969.

BOWLBY, J. *Maternal Care and Mental Health.* Geneva: World Health Organization, 1951.

BRACKBILL, Y. "Obstetrical Medication and Infant Behavior." In J. D. Orofsky (ed.), *The Handbook of Infant Development.* New York: Wiley, 1979.

BREMMER, R. H. (ed.). *Children and Youth in America.* Vol. *II: 1866–1932.* Cambridge, Mass.: Harvard University Press, 1971.

BROWN, J. "Effects of an Integrated Physical Education/Music Program in Changing Early Childhood Perceptual-Motor Performance." *Perceptual and Motor Skills, 53* (1981): 151–54.

BUTLER, R. N. "Cigarette Smoking in Pregnancy: Its Influence on Birthweight and Prenatal Mortality." *British Medical Journal, 2* (1972): 127–30.

CARR, J. *Young Children with Down's Syndrome: Their Developmental Upbringing and Effect on Their Families.* London: Butterworth, 1975.

CLUNIES, R., AND GRAHAM, G. "Accelerating the Development of Down's Syndrome Infants and Young Children." *Journal of Special Education, 13* (1979): 169–77.

CRATTY, B. J. "A Comparison of Fathers and Sons in Physical Ability." *Research Quarterly, 31* (1960): 12–15.

———. *Perceptual-Motor Abilities in Retarded Children and Youth.* Los Angeles County Mental Retardation Services Board, 1968.

———. *Remedial Motor Activity for Children.* Philadelphia: Lea and Febiger, 1975.

———. *Adapted Physical Education for Handicapped Children and Youth.* Denver: Love Publications, 1980.

_____ , MARTIN, M. M., AND MORRISON, M. *Motor Performance, Movement Behavior and the Education of Children*. Springfield, Ill.: Charles C. Thomas, 1970.

CROCKENBERG, S. "Early Mother and Infant Antecedents of Bayley Scale Performance at 21 Months." *Developmental Psychology, 19* (1983): 727–30.

DAVIES, P., AND DAVIS, J. P. "Very Low Birth Weight and Subsequent Head Growth." *Lancet, 2* (1970): 1216–19.

DENNIS, W. "The Effect of Restricted Practice upon the Reaching, Sitting and Standing of Two Infants." *Journal of Genetic Psychology, 47* (1935): 17–32.

_____ . "Does Culture Appreciably Affect Patterns of Infant Behavior?" *Journal of Social Psychology, 12* (1940): 307–17.

_____ . "Causes of Retardation among Institutional Children in Iran." *Journal of Genetic Psychology, 96* (1960): 47–59.

_____ , AND NAJARIAN, P. "Infant Development under Environmental Handicap." *Psychology Monographs, 7* (1957): 71 pp.

DICKS-MIREAUX, M. J. "Mental Development of Infants with Downs Syndrome," *American Journal of Mental Deficiency, 77* (1972), 26–32.

EICHORN, D. H. "Physical Development: Current Foci of Research." In J. D. Osofsky, *Handbook of Infant Development*. New York: Wiley, 1979.

FITZHARDINGE, P. M., AND STEVEN, E. M. "The Small-for-Date Infant. I: Later Growth Patterns." *Pediatrics, 49* (1972a): 671–81.

_____ , AND _____ . "The Small-for-Date Infant. II: Neurological and Intellectual Sequelae." *Pediatrics, 50* (1972b): 50–57.

FRANCIS-WILLIAMS, J., AND DAVIES, P. A. "Very Low Birth Weight and Later Intelligence." *Developmental Medicine and Child Neurology, 16* (1974), 709–28.

FREEDMAN, D. G. *Human Infancy: An Evolutionary Perspective*. Hillsdale, N.J.: Erlbaum, 1974.

GALLER, J. R., RAMSEY, F., SOLIMANO, G., KUCHARSKI, L. T., AND HARRISON, R. "The Influence of Early Malnutrition on Subsequent Behavioral Development. IV: Soft Neurologic Signs." *Pediatric Research, 18* (1984): 826–32.

GERBER, M., AND DEAN, R. F. A. "The State of Development of Newborn African Children." *Lancet, 1* (1957): 1216–19.

GESELL, A., AND AMATRUDE, C. S. *Developmental Diagnosis: Normal and Abnormal Child Development, Clinical Methods and Pediatric Applications*. New York: Hoeber, 1956.

_____ , AND THOMPSON, H. *Infant Behavior: Its Genesis and Growth*. New York: McGraw-Hill, 1934.

GILLBERG, C., RASMUSSEN, P., AND WAHLSTROM, J. "Minor Neurodevelopmental Disorders in Children Born to Older Mothers." *Developmental Medicine and Child Neurology, 24* (1982): 437–47.

GOLDSTEIN, K. M., CAPUTO, D. V., AND TRAUB, H. B. "The Effects of Prenatal and Perinatal Complications on Development at One Year of Age." *Child Development, 47* (1976): 613–21.

GRAY, S. "The Family-Oriented Home Visiting Program." A longitudinal study, Peabody College, 1977.

GUINAGH, B. J., AND GORDON, I. J. *School Performance as a Function early stimulation*. Final Report to Office of Child Development, 1976.

HARBISON, R. D., AND MANTILLA-PLATA, B. "Prenatal Toxicity, Maternal Distribution and Placental transfer of Telralydrocan-malinol." *Journal of Pharmacology and Experimental Therapeutics, 180* (1972): 446–53.

HARRIMAN, A. E., AND LUKOSIUS, P. A. "On Why Wayne Dennis Found Hopi Children Retarded in Age at Onset of Walking." *Perceptual and Motor Skills, 55* (1982): 79–86.

HENDRICK, I. "The Discussion of the 'Instinct to Master.' " *Psychoanalytic Quarterly, 12* (1943): 561–65.

HENNESSY, M. J., AND DIXON, S. D. "The Development of Gait: A Study in African Children Ages One to Five." *Child Development, 55* (1984): 844–53.

HERBER, R., AND GARBER, H. "The Milwaukee Project: A Study of the Use of Family Intervention to Prevent Cultural-Familial Mental Retardation." In B. Z. Friedlander, G. M. Sterrit, and G. E. Kirk (eds), *Exceptional Infant*. New York: Brunner/Mazel, 1975.

HICKS, J. A., AND RALPH, D. W. "The Effects of Practice in Tracing the Porteus Diamond Maze." *Child Development, 2* (1931): 156–58.

HILGARD, J. R. "Learning and Maturation in Preschool Children." *Journal of Genetic Psychology, 41* (1932): 36–56.

HOKE, B. "Promotive Medicine and the Phenomenon of Health." *Archives of Environmental Health, 16* (1968): 269–78.

HOORWEG, J., AND STANFIEL, J. P. "Effects of Protein Energy Malnutrition on Intellectual and Motor Abilities in Later Childhood and Adolescence." *Developmental Medicine, 18* (1976): 330–50.

HOUSTON, K. B. "Review of the Evidence and Qualifications regarding the Effects of Hallucinogenic Drugs on Chromosomes and Embryos." *American Journal of Psychiatry, 126* (1969): 251–54.

HUNTINGTON, D. S. "Supportive Programs for Infants and Parents." J. D. Osofsky (ed.), *Handbook of Infant Development.* New York: Wiley 1979.

HUNTSINGER, P. W. "Differences in Speed between American Negro and White Children in the Performance of the 35-Yard Dash." *Research Quarterly, 30* (1959): 366–68.

Interdepartmental Committee on Nutrition for National Defense. *Manual for Nutrition Surveys,* 2nd ed. Washington, D.C.: U.S. Government Printing Office, 1963.

KALLEN, J. D. (ed.). *Nutrition, Development and Social Behavior.* HEW Publication No NIH 73–242. Washington, D.C.: U.S. Government Printing Office, 1973.

KELLY, H. J., AND REYNOLDS, L. "Appearance and Growth of Ossification Centers and Increases in the Body Dimensions of White and Negro Infants." *American Journal of Retrogenology, 57* (1947): 417–35.

KILBRIDE, P. L. "Sensorimotor Behavior of Baganda and Somia Infants: A Controlled Comparison." *Journal of Cross Cultural Psychology, 11* (1980): 131–49.

KOPP, C. B., AND PARMALEE, A. H. "Prenatal and Perinatal Influences on Infant Behavior." In J. D. Osofsky (ed.), *Handbook of Infant Development.* New York: Wiley, 1979.

KRAUS, H., AND HIRSCHLAND, R. P. "Minimum Muscular Fitness Tests in Children." *Research Quarterly, 25* (1954): 178–85.

LAGERSPETZ, K., NYGARD M., AND STRANDVIK, C. "The Effects of Training in Crawling on the Motor and Mental Level of Infants." *Scandinavia Journal of Psychology, 12* (1971): 192–97.

LEE, A. M. "Child Rearing Practices and Motor Performance of Black and White Children." *Research Quarterly of Exercise and Sport, 51* (1980): 494–500.

LEMOINE, P., HARONSSEAU, H., BORTERYU, J. P., AND MENUET, J. C. "Les enfants de parents alcooliques: Anomalies observees a propoos de 127 cas." [Children of Alcoholic Parents: Anomalies Observed in 127 Cases]. *Ouest Medical, 25* (1968): 476–82.

LEVY, D. M. *Maternal Overprotection.* New York: Columbia University Press, 1943.

LICHT, S. *Towards Prevention of Mental Retardation in the Next Generation.* Fort Wayne, Ind.: Fort Wayne Printing, 1978.

MASSE, G., AND HUNT, E., JR. "Skeletal Maturation of the Hand and Wrist in West African Children." *Human Biology, 35* (1963): 3–10.

MATSUDA, V. Private conversation with director of Physical Fitness Laboratory, Sao Caetano, Sao Paulo, Brazil, 1982.

MCGRAW, M. B. *Growth: A Study of Johnny and Jimmy.* New York: Appleton-Century, 1935.

MEREDITH, H. V. "Somatic Changes during Human Prenatal Life." *Child Development, 46* (1975): 603–10.

MICHAELIS, R., SCHULTE, F. J., AND NOLTE, R. "Motor Behavior of Small for Gestational Age Newborn Infants." *Journal of Pediatrics, 76* (1970): 208–13.

MINERVA, A. N. "Psychomotor Education and General Development of Preschool Children: Experiments with Twin Controls." *Journal of Genetic Psychology, 46* (1935): 433–54.

OUNSTED, M., AND OUNSTED, C. "On Fetal Growth Rate." *Clinics in Developmental Medicine, 46.* London: Heinemann, 1973.

OWEN, G. M., KRAM, K. M., GARRY, P. J., LOWER, J. E., AND LUBIN, A. H. *A Study of Nutritional Status of Pre-School Children in the United States,* 1974, 53, Part II, Supplement 597–646.

PASAMANUCK, B., AND KNOBLACH, H. "Retrospective Studies on the Epidemiology of Reproductive Causality: Old and New." *Merrill Palmer Quarterly, 12* (1966): 7–26.

PIKLER, E. "Data on Gross Motor Development of the Infant." *Child Development and Care, 3* (1972): 297–310.

ROSENTHAL, R., AND JACOBSON, L. *Pygmalion in the Classroom.* New York: Holt, Rinehart and Winston, 1968.

ROSSETT, H. L., AND SANDER, L. W. "Effects of Maternal Drinking on Neonatal Morphology and State. In J. D. Osofsky (ed.), *The Handbook of Infant Development.* New York: Wiley, 1979.

SAINT-ANNE DARGASSIES, S. "Neurological Maturation of the Premature Infant of 28–41 Weeks Gestational Age." In F. Falkner (ed.) *Human Development.* Philadelphia: Saunders, 1966.

SAMUELS, H. R. "The Effect of an Older Sibling on Infant Locomotor Exploration of a New Environment." *Child Development, 51* (1980): 607–10.

SCHAEFER, E. S. *Progress Report: Intellectual Stimulation Culturally Deprived Parents.* National Institutes of Mental Health, 1968.

SCHNABL-DICKEY, E. A. "Relationships between Parents' Child-rearing Attitudes and the Jumping and Throwing Performance of Their Preschool Children." *Research Quarterly, 48* (1978): 382–90.

SCHULTZ, A. G. "Fetal Growth of Man and Other Primates." *Quarterly Review of Biology, 1* (1926): 465–67.

SEARLE, R. W. "The Weight of the Dry, Fat-free Skeleton of American Whites and Negroes." *American Journal of Physical Anthropology, 71* (1959): 37–45.

SOLNIT, A. J., AND PROVENCE, S. "Vulnerability and Risk in Early Childhood." In J. D. Osofsky (ed.), *Handbook of Infant Development.* New York: Wiley, 1979.

SOLOMONS, H. C. "The Malleability of Infant Motor Development: Cautions Based on Studies of Child-rearing Practices in the Yucatan." *Clinical Pediatrics, 17* (1978): 836–40.

SPITZ, R. A. "Hospitalization." *Psychoanalytic Study of the Child, 1* (1945): 53–74.

_____ . "Anxiety in Infancy: A Study of Its Manifestations in the First Year of Life." *International Journal of Psycho-Analysis, 31* (1950): 138–43.

STEINHAUSEN, H. C. "Psychological Evaluation of Treatment in Phenylketnuria: Intellectual, Motor and Social Development," *Neuropaediatrie, 5* (1974), 146–56.

STRAUSS, M. E. "Behavior of Nicotine-Addicted Newborns." *Child Development, 46* (1975): 887–93.

STRESSGUTH, A. P. "Psychological Handicaps in Children with Fetal Alcohol Syndrome: Work in Progress on Alcoholism." *Annals of the New York Academy of Science, 273* (1976): 140–45.

SUPER, C. M. "Environmental Effects on Motor Development: The Case of African Infant Precocity. *Developmental Medicine and Child Neurology, 18* (1976): 561–67.

THELEN, E., FISHER, D. M., RIDLEY-JOHNSON, R., AND GRIFFIN, N.J. "Effects of Body Build and Arousal on Infant Stepping." *Developmental Psychobiology, 15* (1982): 447–54.

TOUWNE, B. C. L., AND PRECHTL, H. F. R. *The Neurological Examination of the Child with Minor Nervous System Dysfunction.* Philadelphia: Lippincott, 1970.

U.S. Department of Health, Education and Welfare. *Ten State Nutrition Survey, 1968–1970.* DHEW Publication (HMS) No 72-8134, 1972, Vols. I–IV.

VORHERR, H. "Placental Insufficiency in Relation to Post-term Pregnancy and Fetal Posmaturity." *American Journal of Obstetrics and Gynecology, 123* (1975): 67–103.

WERNER, E. E. "Infants around the World: Cross-cultural Studies of Psychomotor Development from Birth to Two Years." *Journal of Cross-Cultural Psychology, 3* (1972): 111–34.

WERNER, P. "Education of Selected Movement Patterns of Pre-school Children." *Perceptual and Motor Skills, 39* (1974): 795–98.

WHITE, B. L., AND HELD, R. "Plasticity of Sensorimotor Development in the Human Infant." Paper presented at the American Association for the Advancement of Science, Philadelphia, 1963.

WHITE, R. "Motivation Reconsidered: The Concept of Competence." *Psychological Review, 66* (1959): 297–333.

ZELAZO, P. R. "The Development of Walking: New Findings, Old Assumptions." *Journal of Motor Behavior, 15* (1983): 99–137.

CHAPTER 5

ANDRE-THOMAS, P., AND ST. DARGASSIES, A. *Etudes neurologiques sur de nouveaune et le jeune nourrisson.* Paris: Mason, 1952.

BAYLEY, N. "Behavioral Correlates of Mental Growth—Birth to Thirty-Six Years." *American Psychologist, 23* (1968): 117–23.

FENTRESS, J. C. "Dynamic Boundaries of Patterned Behaviors: Interaction and Self-organization." In P. P. G. Bateson and R. A. Hinde (eds.), *Growing Points in Ethology.* Cambridge, Eng.: Cambridge University Press, 1976.

HOSKINS, T. A., AND SQUIRES, J. E. "Developmental Assessment: A Test for Gross Motor and Reflex Development." *Physical Therapy, 53* (1973): 117–25.

ILLINGWORTH, R. A. *The Development of the Infant and Young Child.* London: Livingston, 1967.

IRWIN, O. C. "Amount of Mobility of 73 Newborn Infants." *Journal of Comparative Psychology, 15* (1932): 415–20.

LOURIE, R. S. "Role of Rhythmic Patterns in Childhood." *American Journal of Psychiatry, 105* (1949): 653–60.

MCGRAW, M. B. *The Neuromuscular Maturation of the Human Infant.* New York: Hafner, 1966.

MEYERS, C. E., AND DINGMAN, H. F. "The Structure of Abilities at Pre-school Ages: Hypothesized Domains." *Psychological Bulletin, 57* (1960): 514–32.

MILANI-COMPARETTI, A., AND GIDONI, E. A. "Pattern Analysis of Motor Development and Its Disorders." *Developmental and Child Neurology, 9* (1965): 631–38.

MILNER, E. *Human Neural and Behavioral Development.* Springfield, Ill.: Charles C. Thomas, 1967.

MINKOWSKY, A. *Regional Development of the Brain in Early Life.* Symposium for International Organizations of Medical Sciences. Philadelphia: Davis, 1973.

MOLNAR, G. "Analysis of Motor Disorders in Retarded Infants and Young Children. *American Journal of Mental Deficiency, 83* (1978): 213–22.

PIEPER, A. *Cerebral Function in Infancy and Childhood.* New York: Consultants Bureau, 1963.

PONTIUS, A. A. "Neuro-Ethics of 'Walking' in the Newborn." *Perceptual and Motor Skills, 37* (1973): 235–45.

RICHARDS, T. W., AND NEWBERRY, H. "Studies in Foetal Behavior." Child Development, 2 (1938): 79–81.

ROBERTON, M. A. "Changing Motor Patterns during Childhood." In J. Thomas (ed.), *Motor Development during Childhood and Adolescence.* Minneapolis: Burgess, 1984.

SCARR, S. "Genetic Factors in Activity Motivation." *Child Development, 37* (1966): 663–73.

SHIRLEY, M. M. *The First Two Years: Postural and Locomotor Development.* Minneapolis: University of Minnesota Press, 1959.

TANNER, J. M. *Education and Physical Growth.* London: University of London Press, 1968.

THELEN, E. "Rhythmic Stereotypes in Normal Human Infants." *Animal Behavior, 27* (1979): 699–715.

————— . "Rhythmical Behavior in Infancy: An Ethological Perspective." *Developmental Psychology, 17* (1981): 237–57.

————— . "Kicking, Rocking and Waving—Contextual Analysis of Rhythmic Stereotypes in Normal Human Infants." *Journal of Animal Behavior, 23* (1981): 3–11.

————— . "Learning to Walk Is Still an 'Old' Problem: A Reply to Zelazo." *Journal of Motor Behavior, 15* (1983): 139–61.

THELEN, E. AND FISHER, D. M. "From Spontaneous to Instrumental Behavior: Kinematic Analysis of Movement Changes during Very Early Learning." *Child Development, 54* (1983): 129–40.

————— , RIDLEY-JOHNSON, R., AND GRIFFIN, N. J. "Effects of Body Build and Arousal on Infant Stepping." *Developmental Psychobiology, 15* (1982): 447–54.

TOUWEN, B. "A Study of the Development of Some Motor Phenomena in Infancy." *Developmental Medicine and Child Neurology, 13* (1971): 435–46.

TWITCHELL, T. E. "The Automatic Grasping Responses of Infants." *Neuropsychology, 3* (1965): 247–59.

————— . "Reflex Mechanisms and the Development of Prehension." In K. Connolly (ed.), *Mechanisms of Skill Development.* New York: Academic Press, 1970.

WALTERS, C. E. "Prediction of Post-Natal Development and Foetal Activity." *Child Development, 33* (1965): 801–8.

ZELAZO, P. R. "The Development of Walking, New Findings, and Old Assumptions." *Journal of Motor Behavior, 15* (1983): 99–137.

————— , ZELAZO, N. A., AND KOLB, S. "Walking in the Newborn." *Science, 176* (1972): 314–15.

CHAPTER 6

BAYLEY, N. A. *The Development of Motor Abilities during the First Three Years.* Monograph, Society for Research on Child Development, 1935, 1–26.

BECK, R. J., ANDRIACCHI, T. P., KUO, K. N., FERMIER, R. W., AND GALANTE, J. O. "Changes in the Gait Patterns of Growing Children." *Journal Bone and Joint Surgery, 63* (1983): 1452–57.

BRUCE, R. "The Effects of Variations in Ball Trajectory upon Catching Performance of Elementary School Children." Unpublished doctoral dissertation, University of Wisconsin, Madison, 1966.

CLARK, J. E., PHILLIPS, S. J. "A Developmental Sequence of the Standing Broad Jump." In J. E. Clark and J. H. Humphrey *Motor Development: Current Selected Research,* Vol I, Princeton N.J.: Princeton Book Co, 1985.

CRATTY, B. J., CORTINAS, D., AND KELLY, J. "The Motor Abilities of Elementary School Children." Unpublished monograph, Perceptual-Motor Learning Laboratory, UCLA, Los Angeles, California, 1973.

_____ , AND MARTIN, M. M. *Perceptual-Motor Efficiency in Children.* Philadelphia: Lea and Febiger, 1970.

DeOREO, K. L. "The Performance and Development of Fundamental Motor Skills in Preschool Children." In M. Wade and R. Martens (eds.). *Psychology of Motor Behavior. Champaign, Ill.: Human Kinetics, 1974.*

_____ , AND WADE, M. "Dynamic and Static Balancing Ability of Preschool Children." *Journal of Motor Behavior, 3* (1971): 325–35.

EAST, W. B., AND HENSLEY, L. D. "The Effects of Selected Socio-Cultural Factors upon the Overhand-Throwing Performance of Prepubescent Children." In J. E. Clark and J. H. Humphrey *Motor Development: Current Selected Research,* Vol I, Princeton N.J.: Princeton Book Co, 1985.

ERBAUGH, S. J. "The Relationship of Stability, Performance and the Physical Growth Characteristics of Pre-school Children." *Research Quarterly for Exercise and Sport, 55* (1984): 8–16.

ESPENSCHADE, A., AND ECKERT, H. M. *Motor Development.* Columbus, Ohio: Charles E. Merrill, 1967.

FORTNEY, V. L. "The Kinematics and Kinetics of the Running Pattern of Two-, Four-, and Six-Year-Old Children." *Research Quarterly for Exercise and Sport, 54* (1983): 126–35.

GOLDSTEIN, D. "The Influence of Training upon the Throwing Patterns of Five-Year-Old Girls." Unpublished study, Perceptual-Motor Learning Laboratory, UCLA, Los Angeles, California, 1983.

HARTMAN, D. M. "The Hurdle Jump as a Measure of Motor Proficiency in Young Children," *Child Development, 23* (1943), 201–11.

HOLBROOK, S. F. "A Study of the Development of Motor Abilities between the Ages of Four and Twelve, Using a Modification of the Oseretzsky Scale." Doctoral Dissertation, No. 5537. Ann Arbor, Michigan: University Microfilms, 1953.

JENKINS, L. M. *A Comparative Study of Motor Achievement of Children Five, Six and Seven Years of Age.* New York: Teachers College, Columbia University, 1930.

KEOGH, J. F. *Motor Performance of Elementary School Children.* Monograph, University of California, Los Angeles, Department of Physical Education, 1968.

LEE, D. N., AND ARONSON, E. "Visual, Proprioceptive Control of Standing in Human Infants." *Perception and Psychophysics, 15* (1974): 529–32.

MAXWELL, G. *Ring of Bright Water.* London: Longmans Green, 1960.

MORRIS, A. M., WILLIAMS, J. M., ATWATER, A. E., AND WILMORE, J. H. "Age and Sex Differences in Motor Performance of 3 through 6 Year Old Children." *Research Quarterly for Exercise and Sport, 53* (1982): 214–21.

NOLLER, K., AND INGRISANO, D. "Cross-Sectional Study of Gross and Fine Motor Development." *Physical Therapy, 64* (1984): 308–16.

NORLIN, R., ODENRICK, P., AND SANDLUND, B. "Development of Gait in the Normal Child." *Journal of Pediatric Orthopedics, 1* (1981): 261–66.

PARIZKOVA, J. *Growth, Fitness and Nutrition in Pre School Children,* Prague (Praha), Charles University: Charles University Press: 1984.

PIKLER, E. "Data on Gross Motor Development of the Infant." *Child Development and Care, 3* (1972): 297–310.

POE, A. "Description of the Movement Characteristics of Two-Year-Old Children Performing the Jump and Reach." *Research Quarterly, 47* (1976): 260–68.

RANDT, R. D. "Ball-Catching Proficiency Among 4, 6, and 8 Year-Old Girls." In J. E. Clark and J. H. Humphrey *Motor Development: Current Selected Research,* Vol I, Princeton N.J.: Princeton Book Co, 1985.

ROSE-JACOBS, R. "Development of the Gait at Slow, Free, and Fast Speeds in 3- and 5-Year-Old Children." *Physical Therapy, 63* (1983): 1251–59.

SAMUELS, H. R. "The Effect of an Older Sibling on Infant Locomotor Exploration of a New Environment." *Child Development, 51* (1980): 607–10.

SARIS, W. H. M., BINKHURST, R. A., CRAMWINCKLE, A. B., WAESBERGHE, F., AND VEEN-HEZEMANS, A. M. "The Relationship between Working Performance, Daily Physical Activity, Fatness, Blood Lipids, and Nutrition in School Children." In K. Berg and B. O. Ericksson (eds.), *Children and Exercise IX*. Baltimore: University Park Press, 1980.

SCHNABL-DICKEY, E. A. "Relationships between Parents' Child Rearing Attitudes and the Jumping and Throwing Performance of Their Preschool Children." *Research Quarterly, 48* (1978): 382–90.

STOTT, D. H. "A General Test of Motor Impairment for Children." *Developmental Medicine and Child Neurology, 8* (1966): 523–31.

ULRICH, B. D. AND ULRICH, D. A. "The Role of Balancing in Performance of Fundamental Motor Skills in 3, 4, and 5, Year-Old Children." In J. E. Clark and J. H. Humphrey *Motor Development: Current Selected Research*, Vol I. Princeton N.J.: Prineton Book Co, 1985.

WELLMAN, B. L. "Motor Achievements of Preschool Children." *Childhood Education, 13* (1937): 311–16.

WILD, M. R. "The Behavior Pattern of Throwing and Some Observations Concerning Its Course of Development in Children." *Research Quarterly, 9* (1938): 20–24.

WILLIAMS, H. *Perceptual and Motor Development*. Englewood Cliffs, N.J.: Prentice-Hall, 1983.

WINTERHALTER, C. "Age and Sex Trends in the Development of Selected Balancing Skills." M.S. Project, University of Toledo, Ohio, 1974.

ZERNICKE, R., GREGOR, R. J., AND CRATTY, B. J. "Balance and Visual Prioception in Children." *Journal of Movement Behavior, 12* (1982): 28–32.

CHAPTER 7

BACHMAN, J. C. "Motor Learning and Performance as Related to Age and Sex in Two Measures of Balance Coordination," *Research Quarterly, 32* (1961): 123–37.

BORDAS, E. "The Effects of Two Methods of Teaching Developmental Movement on Balance of Third and Fourth Grade Children." Unpublished Master's thesis, Springfield College, 1971.

BRACE, D. K. "Studies in the Rate of Learning Gross Bodily Motor Skills." *Research Quarterly, 12* (1941): 181–85.

CAREY, R. A. "A comparison of the Lincoln Revision of the Oseretzsky Tests of Motor Proficiency with Selected Motor Ability Tests on Boys at Elementary Level." Unpublished Doctoral Dissertation, Bloomington: Indiana University, 1954.

CARPENTER, A. "Tests of Motor Educability for the First Three Grades." *Child Development, 11* (1940): 292–99.

————— "Strength Testing in the First Three Grades." *Research Quarterly, 13* (1942): 328–32.

CLARKE, H. *Physical and Motor Tests in the Medford Boy's Growth Study*. Englewood Cliffs, N.J.: Prentice-Hall, 1971.

CLARKE, H. H. "Joint and Body Range of Movement." *Physical Fitness Research Digest, 12* (1975): No 5.

CLARK, J. E., AND PHILLIPS, S. J. "A Developmental Sequence of the Standing Broadjump," in J. E. Clark and J. H. Humphrey, *Motor Development, Current Selected Research*, Vol I, Princeton, N.J.: Princeton Book Co. 1985.

CLARK, J. T. AND WATKINS, D. L. "Static Balance in Young Children," *Child Development, 55* (1984): 133–39.

COTTON, D. J., AND LOWE, S. "Interrelationships among Balance Tests Prior to and after Practice." *Perceptual and Motor Skills, 39* (1974): 629–30.

COWEN, E., AND PRATT, B. "The Hurdle Jump as a Developmental and Diagnostic Test." *Child Development, 5* (1934): 107–21.

CRATTY, B. J., CORTINAS, D., AND KELLY, J. "Perceptual-Motor Abilities of Elementary School Children." Unpublished Monograph. Los Angeles: UCLA, 1973.

—————, AND MARTIN, M. M. *Perceptual-Motor Efficiency in Children*. Philadelphia: Lea and Febiger, 1970.

—————, MORRIS, M., AND JENNET, C. *Movement Behavior, Motor Ability and the Education of Children*. Springfield, Illinois: Charles C. Thomas, 1970.

—————, AND SAMOY, L. "Inter-relationships between Measures of Praxic Behaviors in Children." *Motorik, 7* (1984): 52–58. (In German.)

CUMBEE, F. Z. "A Factorial Analysis of Motor Coordination." *Research Quarterly, 25* (1954): 412–28.

DiNucci, J. M. "Gross Motor Performance: A Comprehensive Analysis of Age and Sex Differences between Boys and Girls Ages 6–9 Years." In J. Broekhoff, *Physical Education, Sports, and the Sciences*. Eugene: Microfilm Publications, 1976.

DOHRMANN, P. "Throwing and Kicking Ability of 8-year-old Boys and Girls." *Research Quarterly, 35* (1964): 464–71.

DUSENBERRY, L. "Study of the Effects of Training in Ball Throwing by Children, Ages 3–7." *Research Quarterly, 23* (1952): 9–14.

FLEISHMAN, E. *The Measurement of Physical Fitness*, Englewood Cliffs, N.J.: Prentice-Hall Inc., 1965.

————, KREMER, E. J. AND SHOUP, G. W. *The Dimensions of Physical Fitness.*" Department of Industrial Administration, and Department of Psychology, New Haven, Conn.: Yale University, 1961.

————, AND RICH, S. "Role of Kinesthetic and Spatial-Visual Factors in Perceptual-motor Learning." *Journal of Experimental Psychology, 66* (1963): 6–11.

GALLAHUE, D. L. *Understanding Motor Development in Children*, New York: John Wiley and Sons, 1982.

GLASSLOW, R. N. AND KRUSE, P. "Motor Performance by Girls Age 6–14 Years." *Research Quarterly, 31* (1960): 425–33.

HALVERSON, L. E., ROBERTON, M. A., LANGENDORFER, S., AND WILLIAMS K. "Longitudinal Changes in Children's Overarm Throw Ball Velocities." *Research Quarterly, 50* (1979) 256–64.

————, ————, AND ———— "Development of Overarm Throw: Movement and Ball Velocity Changes to the 7th Grade." *Research Quarterly of Exercise and Sport, 53* (1982): 198–205.

————, ————, SAFRIT, M. J., AND ROBERTS, T. W. "Effects of Guided Practice on Overhand Throw Ball Velocities of Kindergarten Children." *Research Quarterly, 48* (1977): 311–18.

HODGKINS, J. "Reaction Time and Speed of Movement in Males and Females of Various Ages." *Research Quarterly, 34* (1963): 335–43.

HUPPRICH, F. L., AND SIGERSETH, P. O. "The Specificity of Flexibility in Girls." *Research Quarterly, 21* (1950): 25–31.

JOHNSON, R. D. "Measurements of Achievement in Fundamental Skills of Elementary School Children." *Research Quarterly, 32* (1962): 94–103.

KEOGH, J. F. *Motor Performance of Elementary School Children*, Monograph, University of California, Los Angeles, Physical Education 1965.

———— Physical Performance Test Data for English Boys, Ages 6–9." *Physical Educator, 5* (1966): 65–69.

————, AND SUGDEN, D. *Movement Skill Development*, New York: MacMillan, 1985.

MORRIS, A. M., ET AL. "Age and Sex Differences in Motor Performance of 3 through 6 Year Old Children." *Res. Qrtly. Exer. and Sports, 53* (1982): 214–21.

NOLLER, K., AND INGRISANO, D. "Cross-sectional Study of Gross and Fine Motor Development." *Physical Therapy, 64* (1984): 308–316.

OWINGS, C. L., CHAFFIN, D. B., SNYDER, R. G., AND NORCUTT, R. H. *Strength Characteristics for Product Safety Design*. Report from the Consumer Product Safety Commission, Monograph, University of Michigan, 1975.

PARIZKOVA, J. *Growth, Fitness and Nutrition in Pre-School Children*, Prague, Prague Czechoslovakia: University Press, 1984.

PISSANOS, B. W., MOORE, J. B., AND REEVE, T. G. "Age, Sex and Body Composition as Predictors of Children's Performance on Basic Motor Abilities and Health-related Fitness Items." *Perceptual and Motor Skills, 56* (1983): 71–77.

POE, A. "Description of the Movement Characteristics of Two-year Old Children Performing the Jump and Reach." *Research Quarterly, 47* (1976): 260–68.

RANDT, R. D. "Ball-Catching Proficiency Among 4, 6, and 8 Year-old Girls," in J. E. Clark and J. H. Humphrey, *Motor Development: Current Selected Research* Vol 1, Princeton, N.J.: Princeton Book Co., 1985.

RARICK, G. L. AND DOBBINS, D. A. "Basic Components in the Motor Performance of Children Six to Nine Years of Age." *Medicine and Science in Sports, 17* (1975): 105–10.

SEASHORE, H. G. "The Development of a Beam Walking Test and its Use in Measuring Development of Balance in Children." *Research Quarterly, 18* (1949): 246–59.

SEEFELDT, V., REUSCHLEIN, S., AND VOGAL, P. "Sequenced Motor Skills within the Physical Education Curriculum." Paper presented at the AAHPER National Convention, Houston, Texas, March 1972.

SEILS, L. G. "The Relationships between Measures of Physical Growth and Gross Motor Performance of Primary-grade School Children." *Research Quarterly, 22* (1951): 244–60.

SLAUGHTER, M. H., LOHMAN, T. G., AND MISNER, J. E. "Association of Somatotype and Body Composition to Physical Performance in 7-12 year-old Boys." *Research Quarterly, 48* (1977): 145–49.

————— . "Association of Somatotype and Body Composition to Physical Performance in 7-12 year old Girls." *Journal of Sports Medicine, 20* (1980): 189–97.

STOTT, D. H., MOYES, F. A., AND HENDERSON, S. E. *Test of Motor Impairment,* Guelp, Ontario, Canada: Brook Educational Publishing, 1972.

VANDENBERG, S. G. "Factor Analytic Study of the Lincoln-Oseretzsky Test of Motor Proficiency." *Perceptual and Motor Skills, 17* (1964): 194–98.

WILLIAMS, H. G. *The Perception of Moving Objects by Children,* Unpublished study, Los Angeles: Perceptual-motor Learning Laboratory, UCLA, 1968.

————— . *Perceptual and Motor Development,* Englewood Cliffs, N.J.: Prentice-Hall, 1983.

WILLIAMS, H. G., AND BREIHAN, S. K. "Motor Control Tasks for Young Children." Unpublished manuscript, Univ. of Toledo, 1979.

WYRICK, W. "Effects of Task Height and Practice on Static Balance." *Research Quarterly, 40* (1969): 215–21.

ZIMMERMAN, H. J. "Characteristics, Likenesses and Differences between Skilled and Non-skilled Performance of Standing Broad Jump." *Research Quarterly, 27* (1956): 352–62.

CHAPTER 8

ALLAND, A., JR. *The Artistic Animal: An Inquiry into the Biological Roots of Art.* Garden City, N.Y.: Doubleday, 1977.

————— . *Playing with Form: Children Draw in Six Cultures.* New York: Columbia University Press, 1983.

ARNHEIM, R. *Art and Visual Perception.* Berkeley: University of California Press, 1964.

BERNBAUM, M., GOODNOW, J., AND LEHMAN, E. "Relationships among Perceptual-Motor Tasks: Tracing and Copying." *Journal of Educational Psychology, 66* (1974): 731–35.

BOWER, T. G. R. "The Visual World of Infants." *Scientific American, 215* (1966): 80–97.

————— . *Development in Infancy.* San Francisco: Freeman, 1974.

————— , BROUGHTON, J. M., AND MOORE, M. "1970 Demonstration of Intention in Reaching Behavior of Neonate Humans." *Nature* (1970): 228–34.

BRUNER, J. Heinz Werner Lectures in Developmental Psychology. Worcester, Mass: Clark University, 1968.

BRYANT, W. L. "On the Development of Voluntary Motor Ability." *American Journal of Psychology, 4* (1892): 123–204.

CARON, A. J., CARON, R. F., AND CARLSON, V. R. "Infant Perception of the Invariant Shape of Objects in Slant." *Child Development, 50* (1979): 716–21.

CRATTY, B. J. AND MARTIN, M. M. *Perceptual-Motor Efficiency in Children.* Philadelphia: Lea and Febiger, 1970.

DAY, R. G., AND McKENZIE, B. E. "Perceptual Shape Constancy in Early Infancy. *Perception, 2* (1973): 315–20.

DENCKLA, M. B. "Development of Speed in Repetitive and Successive Finger-Movements in Normal Children." *Developmental Medicine and Child Neurology, 15* (1973): 635–45.

————— . "Development of Motor Coordination in Normal Children." *Developmental Medicine and Child Neurology, 16* (1974): 729–41.

FRANCO, D., AND MUIR, M. "Reaching in Very Young Infants." *Perception, 7* (1978): 385–92.

GARDNER, H. *The Arts and Human Development: A Psychological Study of the Aesthetic Process.* New York: Wiley Interscience, 1973.

GHENT, L., & BERNSTEIN, L. "Influence of the Orientation of the Geometric Figures on their Recognition by Children." *Perceptual and Motor Skills, 12* (1961), 95–101.

GILBRETH, E. F., GILBRETH, L. M., *Applied Motion Study,* New York: Gruen & Stratton, 1917.

GOODENOUGH, F. L., *Measurement of Intelligence by Drawings,* Yonkers, N.Y.: World Book, 1926.

GOODNOW, J. "Children Drawing." In J. Bruner, M. Cole, and B. Lloyd, *The Developing Child Series*. Cambridge, Mass.: Harvard University Press, 1977.

GOODSON, B. D. & GREENFIELD, P. M. "The Search for Structural Principles in Children's Play: A Parallel in Linguistic Development." *Child Development, 46* (1975): 734–46.

GRANT, W. W. "Development Pattern of Two Motor Functions." *Developmental Medicine and Child Neurology, 15* (1973): 171–77.

HALVERSON, H. M. "An Environmental Study of Prehension in Infants by Means of Systematic Cinema Records." *Genetic Psychology Monographs, 10* (1931): 107–86.

HIRSCH, E., AND NIEDERMEYER, F. C. "The Effects of Tracing Prompts and Discrimination Training on Kindergarten Handwriting Performance." *Journal of Educational Research, 67* (1973): 81–83.

HOFSTEN, C. V. "Eye-hand Coordination in Newborns," *Developmental Psychology, 18* (1982), 450–61.

HOLBROOK, S. F. "A Study of the Development of Motor Abilities between Ages 4 and 12, Using a Modification of the Oseretsky Scale." Doctoral dissertation, University of Minnesota, 1945.

ILG, F. L., AND AMES, L. B. *School Readiness: Behavior Tests Used at the Gesell Institute*. New York: Harper & Row, 1965.

KELLOGG, R. *Analyzing Children's Art*. Palo Alto, Calif.: National Press Books, 1969.

KEOGH, J. F. *Analysis of Individual Tasks in the Stott Test of Motor Impairment*. Technical Report 2-68, Department of Physical Education, University of California, Los Angeles, 1968.

KINSBOURNE, M., AND WARRINGTON, E. K. "The Development of Finger Differentiation." *Quarterly Journal of Experimental Psychology, 15* (1963): 132–37.

KUHLMAN, F. *Tests of Mental Development*. Minneapolis: Educational Test Bureau, 1939.

LASKY, R. E. "The Effect of Visual Feedback of the Hand on the Reaching and Retrieval Behavior of Young Infants." *Child Development, 48* (1977): 112–17.

LEFFORD, A., BIRCH, H. G., AND GREEN, G. "The Perceptual and Cognitive Bases for Finger Localization and Selective Finger Movement in Preschool Children." *Child Development. 45* (1974): 335–43.

LEVIN, J. R. "What Have We Learned About Maximizing What Children Learn?" In J. R. Levin and L. L. Allen (eds.), *Cognitive Learning in Children*. New York: Academic Press, 1978.

MOSS, S. C., AND HOGG J. "The Development and Integration of Fine Motor Sequences in 12-18 Month Children: A Test of the Modular Theory of Motor Skill Acquisition." *Genetic Psychology Monographs*. Provincetown, Mass.: The Journal Press, 1983.

NEILSON, J. M. "Gerstmann Syndrome: Finger Agnosia, Agraphia, Confusion of Right and Left, and Acalculia." *AMA Archives of Neurology and Psychiatry, 39* (1938): 536–60.

NOLLER, K., AND INGRISANO, D. "Cross-Sectional Study of Gross and Fine Motor Development." *Physical Therapy, 64* (1984): 308–16.

PARKER, J. L., ROSENFELD, S., AND GILLIAN, T. "Simple Device for Enhancing Feedback in the Acquisition of Visual Motor Skills of Slow Learning Children." *Slow Learning Child, 20* (1973): 164–69.

PECK, M., ASKOV, E., AND FAIRCHILD, S. H. "Another Decade of Research on Handwriting: Progress and Prospect in the 1970s. " *Journal of Educational Research, 74* (1980): 283–98.

PROVINE, R. R., AND WESTERMAN, J. A. "Crossing the Midline: Limits of Early Eye-Hand Behavior." *Child Development, 50* (1979): 437–41.

RAPIN, I., TOURKE, L. M., COSTA, L. D. "Evaluation of the Purdue Peg-board as a Screening Test for Brain Damage." *Developmental Medicine and Child Neurology, 8* (1966): 45–50.

RICHARDS, R., REIMER, D., EAVES, C., AND CRICHTON, L. G. "Name Printing as a Test of Developmental Maturity." *Developmental Medicine and Child Neurology, 17* (1975): 486–92.

RUFF, H. A. "The Development of Perception and the Recognition of Objects." *Child Development, 51* (1980): 981–92.

SCHOFIELD, W. N. "Do Children Find Movements Which Cross the Body Difficult?" *Quarterly Journal of Experimental Psychology, 28* (1976): 571–82.

SCHWARTZ, R. K., AND REILLY, M. A. "Learning Tool Use: Body Scheme Recalibration and the Development of Hand Skill." *Journal of Occupational Therapy, 31* (1981): 13–29.

SHIMRAT, NIUSIA. "Lateral Dominance and Directional Orientation in the Writing of American and Israeli Children." *Dissertation Abstracts, 31* No. 3, 2267-B, 1970.

SOLOKOV, E. N. "Neuronal Models and the Orienting Reflex," in M. A. Brazier, *The Central Nervous System and Behavior*. New York: Macy, 1960.

STENNET, R. G., SYMTHE, P. C., AND HARDY, H. "Developmental Trends in Letter Printing Skills." *Perceptual and Motor Skills, 34* (1972): 182–86.

STOTT, D. H. "A General Test of Motor Impairment for Children." *Developmental Medicine and Child Neurology, 8* (1966): 523–31.

––––––––– , MOYES, F. A., AND HENDERSON, S. E. *Test of Motor Impairment.* Waterloo, Canada: Brook Educational Publishing, 1972.

THELEN, E. "Rhythmical Stereotypes in Normal Human Infants." *Animal Behavior, 27* (1979): 699–715.

TREVARTHEN, C. "The psychobiology of Speech Development." In *Development of Motor, Language, and Cognitive Behavior, Neurosciences Research Program Bulletin, 12* (1979): 570–85.

TWITCHELL, T. E. "Reflex Mechanisms and the Development of Prehension." In K. Connolly (ed.), *Mechanisms of Motor Skill Development.* New York: Academic Press, 1970.

––––––––– . "Development of Motor Coordination in the Presence of Cerebral Lesions." In *Development of Motor Learning and Cognitive Behaviors, Nurosciences Research Program Bulletin, 12* (1979): 565–69.

UZGIRIS, I. C. "Ordinality in the Development of Schemas for Relating to Objects." In J. Hellmuth (ed.), *The Normal Infant.* Seattle: Special Child Publications, 1967.

VANE, J. R. "The Vane Kindergarten Test." *Journal of Clinical Psychology, 24* (1968): 121–34.

VON HOFSTEN, C. "Predictive Reaching for Moving Objects: Human Infants." *Journal of Experimental Child Psychology, 30* (1980): 369–82.

––––––––– , AND LINDHAGEN, K. "Observations on the Development of Reaching for Moving Objects." *Journal of Experimental Child Psychology, 28* (1979): 158–73.

WHITE, B. L., AND HELD, R. "Experience in Early Human Development. Part I: Observations on the Development of Visually-directed Reaching; Part 2: Plasticity of Sensorimotor Development in the Human Hands." In J. Hellmuth (ed.), *The Normal Infant.* Seattle: Special Child Publications, 1967.

WILLIAMS, H. *Perceptual and Motor Development.* Englewood Cliffs, N.J.: Prentice-Hall, 1983.

WOODWORTH, R. S. "The Accuracy of Voluntary Movement." *Psychology Review, 114* monograph supplement 3, 1899.

ZURIF, E. B., AND CARSON, G. "Dyslexia in Relation to Cerebral Dominance, and Temporal Analysis." *Neuropsychologia, 8* (1970): 351–55.

CHAPTER 9

ABERCROMBIE, M. L. J., LINDON, R. L., AND TYSON, M. C. "Associated Movements in Normal and Physically Handicapped Children." *Developmental Medicine and Child Neurology, 6* (1964): 573–83.

ADAMS, M. L. "Effect of Eye Dominance on Baseball Batting." *Research Quarterly, 36* (1965): 3–6.

ANNETT, M. "A Model of Inheritance of Handedness and Cerebral Dominance." *Nature, 205* (1964): 59–60.

––––––––– . "The Distribution of Manual Asymmetry," British Journal of Psychology, 63 (1972): 342–58.

––––––––– . "Handedness in Families." *Annals of Human Genetics, 37* (1973): 93–105.

––––––––– . "Study of Rhythmical Capacity and Performance in Motor Rhythm in Physical Education Majors." *Research Quarterly, 3* (1932): 183–91.

––––––––– , AND TURNER, A. "Laterality and the Growth of Intellectual Abilities." *British Journal of Educational Psychology, 44* (1974): 37–46.

AYRES, J. *Southern California Perceptual-Motor Tests.* Los Angeles: Western Psychological Services, 1969.

BAKAN, P., DIBB, G., AND REED, P. "Handedness and Birth Stress." *Neuropsychologia, 11* (1973): 363–66.

BENTON, A. L., MEYERS, R., AND POLDERG, G. J. "Some Aspects of Handedness." *Psychiatria et Neurologia* (Basel), *144* (1962): 321–37.

BERGES, J., AND LEZINE, I. "The Imitation of Gestures." *Clinics in Developmental Medicine, 18* (1965): 1–122.

BLAU, A. *The Master Hand: A Study of the Origin and Meaning of Right and Left Sidedness and Its Relation to Personality and Language.* Research Monograph No. 5. New York: American Orthopsychiatric Association, 1946.

BOKLAGE, C. E. "The Sinistral Blastocyst: An Embroyologic Perspective on the Development of Brain-Function Asymmetries." In J. Herron (ed.), *Neuropschology of Left-Handedness.* New York: Academic Press, 1980.

BOND, M. H. "Rhythmic Perception and Gross Motor Performance." *Research Quarterly, 30* (1959): 259–65.

BRADSHAW, J. L., AND NETTLETON, N. C. *Human Cerebral Asymmetry. Englewood Cliffs, N.J.: Prentice-Hall, 1983.*

BRUNER, J. *Heinz Werner Lectures in Developmental Psychology.* Worcester, Mass.: Clark University, 1968.

BRYDEN, M. P. *Laterality: Functional Asymmetry in the Intact Brain.* New York: Academic Press, 1982.

————. "Evidence for Sex-Related Differences in Cerebral Organization." In M. A. Wittig and A. C. Peterson (eds.), *Sex-Related Differences in Cognitive Functioning.* New York: Academic Press, 1979.

BUFFERY, A. W. H., AND GRAY, J. A. "Sex Differences in the Development of Spatial and Linguistic Skills." In C. Ounsted and D. C. Taylor, *Gender Differences: Their Ontogeny and Significance.* Edinburgh: Churchill-Livingston, 1972.

CAPLAN, P., AND KINSBOURNE, M. "Baby Drops the Rattle: Asymmetry of Duration of Grasp by Infants. *Child Development, 47* (1976) 532–34.

CHAMBERLAIN, H. D. "The Inheritance of Left-Handedness." *Journal of Heredity, 19* (1928): 557–59.

CONNOLLY, K., AND STRATTON, P. "Developmental Changes in Associated Movements." *Developmental Medicine and Child Neurology, 10* (1968): 49–54.

CONRAD, K. E., CERMAK, S. R., AND DRAKE, C. "Differentiation of Praxis among Children." *American Journal of Occupational Therapy, 37* (1983): 466–73.

COOPER, J. M. *Kinesiology.* St. louis: Mosby, 1982.

CORBALLIS, M. C. *Human Laterality.* New York: Academic Press, 1983.

————, AND MORGAN, M. J. "On the Biological Basis of Human Laterality. I. Evidence for a Maturational Left-Right Gradient." *Behavioral and Brain Sciences, 2* (1978): 261–336.

COREN, S., AND PORAC, C. "Birth Factors and Laterality: The Effect of Birth Order, Parental Age, and Birth Stress on Four Indices of Lateral Preference." *Behavior Genetics, 10* (1980a): 123–38.

———— AND ————. "Family Patterns in Four Dimensions of Lateral Preference." *Behavioral Genetics, 10* (1980): 333–48.

CRATTY, B. J. "Zur ubung manueller fertigkeiten bei schulkindern: Ein pilotstudie. *Motorik 6* (1978): 122–26.

————*Adapted Physical Education for Handicapped Children and Youth.* Denver: Love Publishing, 1981.

————. "A Comparison of Motor Planning in Deaf Children and in the Normal. Unpublished study, 1984.

————, CORNELL, S., AND OMATA, C. "A Comparison of Motor Planning Abilities in Deaf and Hearing Children." Accepted for publication, *American Annals of the Deaf,* 1986.

————, AND GIBSON, S. "Motor Planning and Impulsivity." Publication pending, 1984 *Motorik.*

————, AND SAMOY, L. "A Comparison of Praxic Behaviors in Six-Year-Old Children." *Motorik,* 7 (1984): 112–16.

DEOREO, K. L. "The Performance and Development of Fundamental Motor Skills in Pre-School Children." In M. Wade and R. Martens (eds.), *Psychology of Motor Behavior and Sport.* Champaign, Ill.: Human Kinetics, 1978.

DERENZI, E., FABRIZIA, M. D., MOTTI, M. D., AND NICHELLI, P. "Imitating Gestures: A Quantitative Approach to Ideomotor Apraxia." *Archives of Neurology, 37* (1980): 6–10.

DINNER, B., WAPNER, S., McFARLAND, J., AND WERNER, H. "Rhythmic Activity and the Perception of Time." *American Journal of Psychology, 76* (1963): 287–92.

ELLIOTT, R. "Physiological Activity and Performance: A comparison of Kindergarten Children with Young Adults." *Psychological Monographs, 78* (1964): 1–109.

FOG, E., AND FOG, M. "Cerebral Inhibition Examined by Associated Movements." In M. Bax, R. MacKeith, *Minimal Cerebral Dysfunction.* Clinics in Developmental Medicine, Spastics Society. London: Heinemann, 1963.

GESCHWIND, N., AND LEVITSKY, W. "Human Brain: Left-Right Asymmetries in Temporal Speech Region." *Science, 461* (1968): 186–87.

GESELL, A. *The First Five Years of Life.* New York: Harper and Row, 1946.

————, AND AMES, L. B. "The Development of Handedness." *Journal of Genetic Psychology, 70* (1947): 155–75.

GILBERT, J. A. "Researches on the Mental and Physical Development of School Children." *Studies from the Yale Psychological Laboratory, 13* (1984): 40–100.

GLANVILLE, B. B., BEST, C. T., AND LEVENSON, R. "A Cardiac Measure of Cerebral Asymmetries in Infant Auditory Perception." *Developmental Psychology, 13* (1977): 54–59.

GUBBAY, S. S. "The Management of Developmental Apraxia." *Developmental Medicine and Child Neurology, 20* (1978): 643–46.

HAALAND, K. Y., PORCH, B. E., AND DELANEY, N. D. "Limb Apraxia and Motor Performance." *Brain and Language, 9* (1980): 315–23.

HARRIS, L. J. "Left Handedness: Early Theories, Facts and Fancies." In J. Herron (ed.), *Neuropsychology of Left-Handedness*. New York: Academic Press, 1980.

HAWN, P. R., AND HARRIS, L. J. "Hand Asymmetries in Grasp Duration and Reaching in Two- and Five-Month-Old Infants." Paper presented at the biennial meeting of the Society for Research in Child Development, San Francisco, 1979.

HEILMAN, K. M. "Ideational Apraxia—A Redefinition." *Brain, 96* (1973): 861–64.

————, ROTHI, L. J., AND VALENSTEIN, E. "Two Forms of Ideomotor Apraxia." *Neurology, 32* (1982): 342–46.

HODGKINS, J. "Influence of Age on the Speed of Reaction and Movement in Females." *Journal of Gerontology, 17* (1962): 385–89.

HORINE, L. E. "An Investigation of the Relationship of Laterality Groups to Performance on Selected Motor Ability Tests." *Research Quarterly, 39* (1968): 91–95.

HUFF, J. "Auditory and Visual Perception of Rhythm by Performers Skilled in Selected Motor Activities." *Research Quarterly, 43* (1972): 197–207.

INGRAM, D. "Motor Asymmetries in Young Children." *Neuropsychologia, 13* (1975): 95–102.

IRWIN, L. W. "A Study of the Relationship of Dominance to the Performance of Physical Education Activities." *Research Quarterly, 9* (1938): 98–119.

JACKSON, H. *Selected Writings of John Hughlings Jackson,* J. Taylor (ed.). London: Hodder and Stoughton, 1932.

KELSO, J. A. S., AND TULLER, B. "Toward a Theory of Apractic Syndromes." *Brain and Language, 12* (1981): 224–45.

KEOGH, J. *Developmental Evaluation of Limb Movement Task.* Technical Report 1-68 (USPHS Grant HD 01059), Department of Physical Education, University of California, 1968.

KIMURA, D. "Left Hemisphere Control of Oral and Brachial Movements and Their Relation to Communication." *Phil. Trans. R. Soc.* (London) (1982): 135–49.

————. "The Neural Basis of Language qua Gesture." In H. Whitaker and H. A. Whitaker (eds.), *Studies in Neurolinguistics, Vol. 1.* New York: Academic Press, 1976.

————. "Neuromotor Mechanisms in the Evolution of Human Communication." In H. D. Steklis and M. J. Raleigh (eds.), *Neurobiology of Social Communication in Primates.* New York: Academic Press, 1979.

————, AND ARCHIBALD, Y. "Motor Functions of the Left Hemisphere." *Brain, 97* (1974): 337–50.

KINSBOURNE, M., AND MCMURRAY, J. "The Effect of Cerebral Dominance upon Time Sharing between Speaking and Tapping by Preschool Children." *Child Development, 46* (1975): 240–42.

KOOLS, J. A., AND TWEEDIE, D. "Development of Praxis in Children." *Perceptual and Motor Skills, 40* (1975): 11–19.

LEVY, J., AND NAGYLAKI, T. A. "A Model for the Genetics of Handedness." *Genetics, 72* (1972): 117–28.

LIEDERMAN, J., AND KINSBOURNE, J. "Rightward Motor Bias in Newborn Depends upon Parental Right-Handedness." *Neuropsychologia, 18* (1980): 579–84.

LOO, R., AND SCHNEIDER, R. "An Evaluation of the Briggs-Hebes Modified Version of Annett's Handedness Inventory." *Cortex, 15* (1979): 683–86.

LURIA, A. R. *The Nature of Human Conflicts, or Emotion, Conflict, and Will.* New York: Liveright, 1932.

MANNI, J. L., MARTIN, R., AND SEWELL, T. "Imitation of Gestures Technique: A Preliminary Report on a Preschool Test of Visual-Motor Integration." *Perceptual and Motor Skills, 44* (1977): 1067–72.

MCGLONE, J. "Sex Differences in Human Brain Asymmetry: A Critical Survey." *Behavioral and Brain Sciences, 3* (1980): 215–62.

MELEKIAN, B. "Lateralization in the Human Newborn: Asymmetry of the Stepping Reflex." *Neuropsychologia, 19* (1981): 707–11.

MENDRYK, S. "Reaction Time, Movement Time, and Task Specificity Relationships at 12, 33, and 48 Years of Age." *Research Quarterly, 31* (1960): 156–62.

MICHEL, G. F. "Right-Handedness: A Consequence of Infant Supine Head-Orientation Preference?" *Science, 212* (1981): 685–87.

MOLFESE, D. L., AND FREEMAN, R. B., JR., AND PALERMO, D. S. "The Ontogeny of Brain Lateralization for Speech and Nonspeech Stimuli." *Brain and Language, 2* (1975): 356–68.

MONTESSORI, M. *Marie Montessori's Own Handbook.* New York: Frederick A. Stokes, 1914.

ORFF, C. *Basic Musical Forms for Orff-Schulwerk Classes in the Elementary School.* Mimeograph. Bellflower, Calif.: Bellflower School District, 1969.

PETERS, M., AND DURDING, B. "Handedness as a Continuous Variable." *Canadian Journal of Psychology, 32* (1978): 257–61.

————, AND PETRIE, B. F. "Functional Asymmetries in the Stepping Reflex of Human Neonates." *Canadian Journal of Psychology, 33* (1979): 198–200.

PETRI, B. F., AND PETERS, M. "Handedness: Left-Right Differences in Intensity of Grasp Response and Duration of Rattle Holding in Infants." *Infant Behavior and Development, 3* (1980): 215–21.

PIERSON, W. R. "The Relationship of Movement Time and Reaction Time from Childhood to Senility." *Research Quarterly, 30* (1959): 227–30.

PORAC, C., AND COREN, S. "Individual and Familial Patterns in Four Dimensions of Lateral Preference." *Neuropsychologia, 17* (1979): 543–48.

————, ————, STEIGER, J. H., AND DUNCAN, P. "Human Laterality: A Multidimensional Approach." *Canadian Journal of Psychology, 34* (1980): 91–96.

RAMSAY, D. S. "Beginnings of Bimanual Handedness and Speech in Infants." *Infant Behavior and Development, 3* (1980): 67–77.

————, CAMPOS, J. J., AND FENSON, L. "Onset of Bimanual Handedness in Infants." *Infant Behavior and Development, 2* (1979): 69–77.

RICE, T., PLOMIN, R., AND DeFRIES, J. C. "Development of Hand Preference in the Colorado Adoption Project." *Perceptual and Motor Skills, 58* (1984): 686–89.

RICHMAN, J. S. "Background Music for Repetitive Task Performance of Severely Retarded Individuals." *American Journal of Mental Deficiency, 81* (1976): 251–55.

RIMOLDI, H. J. A. "Personal Tempo." *Journal of Abnormal and Social Psychology, 46* (1951): 283–303.

ROTH, C. "Hand-Eye Dominance as a Factor in Motor Ability." Unpublished doctoral dissertation, New York University, 1942.

ROY, E. A. "Apraxia: A New Look at an Old Syndrome." *Journal of Human Movement Studies, 4* (1978): 191–210.

SATZ, P., ACHENBACH, K., AND FENNELL, E. "Correlations between Assessed Manual Laterality and Predicted Speech Laterality in a Normal Population." *Neuropsychologia, 5* (1967): 295–310.

SEASHORE, R. H. "Studies in Motor Rhythm." *Psychological Monographs, 36* (1926): 142–89.

SEEFELDT, V., REUSCHLEIN, S., AND VOGAL, P. "Sequenced Motor Skills within the Physical Education Curriculum." Paper presented at AAHPER, National Convention, Houston, Texas, March 1972.

SMITH, H. "Implications for Movement Education Experiences Drawn from Perceptual Motor Research." *Journal of Health, Physical Education and Recreation, 4* (1970): 30–33.

SMOLL, F. L. "A Rhythmic Ability Analysis System." *Research Quarterly, 44* (1973): 232–36.

————. "Development of Rhythmic Ability in Response to Selected Tempos." *Perceptual and Motor Skills, 39* (1974): 767–72.

————. "Development of Spatial and Temporal Elements of Rhythmic Ability." *Journal of Motor Behavior, 6* (1974): 53–58.

SPRINGER, S. P., AND DEUTSCH, G. *Left Brain, Right Brain.* San Francisco: Freeman, 1981.

————, AND SEARLEMAN, A. "Left-Handedness in Twins: Implications for the Mechanism Underlying Cerebral Asymmetry of Function." In J. Herron (ed.), *Neuropsychology of Left-Handedness.* New York: Academic Press, 1980.

STEINTHAL, L. *Abriss der spatchweissenschaft.* Berlin, 1871.

SURWILLO, W. W. "Speed of Movement in Relation to Period of the Electro-encephalogram in Normal Children." *Parapsychology, 11* (1974): 491–96.

————. "Human Reaction Time and Period of the EEG in Relation to Development." *Psychophysiology, 8* (1971): 468–82.

THOMAS, J. R., AND MOON, D. H. "Measuring Motor Rhythmic Ability in Children." *Research Quarterly, 47* (1976): 20–32.

—————, AND STRATTON, R. K. "Effect of Divided Attention on Children's Rhythmic Response." *Research Quarterly, 48* (1977): 428–35.

THELEN, E. "Rhythmical Stereotypes in Normal Human Infants." *Animal Behavior, 27* (1979): 699–715.

THOMPSON, A. L., AND MARSH, J. F. Probability Sampling of Manual Asymmetry." *Neuropsychologia, 14* (1976): 217–23.

TOUWEN, B. C. L., AND PRECHTL, H. F. R. *The Neurological Examination of the Child with Minor Nervous Dysfunction.* London: Heinemann, 1970.

TURKEWITZ, G., GORDON, E. W., AND BIRCH, H. G. "Head Turning in the Human Neonate: Spontaneous Patterns." *Journal of Genetic Psychology, 107* (1965): 143–58.

—————, —————, AND —————. "Head Turning in the Human Neonate: Effect of Prandial Condition and Lateral Preference." *Journal of Comparative and Physiological Psychology, 59* (1965): 189–92.

VAN ALSTYNE, D., AND OSBORN, E. "Rhythmic Responses of Negro and White Children 2–6." *Monographs of the Society for Research in Child Development, 2* (1948).

VANDEN-ABELLE, J. "Comments on the Functional Asymmetries of the Lower Extremities." *Cortex, 16* (1980): 325–29.

VOGEL, O. H. "The Relationship of Dominance to Acts of Skill." *Research Quarterly, 6* (1935): 15–18.

WADA, J. A., CLARKE, R., AND HAMM, A. "Cerebral Hemispheric Asymmetry in Humans." *Archives of Neurology, 32* (1975): 239–46.

WATERLAND, J. C., AND HELLENBRANDT, F. A. "Involuntary Patterning Associated with Willed Movement Performed against Progressively Increasing Resistance." *American Journal of Physical Medicine, 43* (1964): 13–30.

WAY, E. E. "An Investigation of the Relationships of Laterality to Success in Certain Physical Activities." Unpublished doctoral dissertion, University of Washington, 1956.

WHITING, H. T. A. *Acquiring Ball Skill: A Psychological Interpretation.* London: Bell, 1969.

WILLIAMS, H. G. "The Perception of Moving Objects by Children." Unpublished study, Perceptual-Motor Learning Laboratory, Department of Kinesiology, University of California, Los Angeles, 1967.

—————, TEMPLE, I. G., LOGSDON, B. J., SCOTT, S., AND CLEMENT, A. "An Investigation of the Perceptual-Motor Development of Young Children." Unpublished monograph, Bowling Green State University, 1971.

WYKE, M. "The Effects of Brain Lesions on the Learning Performance of Bimanual Coordination Tasks." *Cortex, 7* (1971): 59–71.

ZAZZO, R. (ed.). *Manuel pour l'Examination Psychologique de l'Enfant.* Neuchatel de la Chaux, Paris: Neistle, 1960.

ZURIF, E. B., AND BRYDEN, M. P. "Familial Handedness and Left-Right Differences in Auditory and Visual Perception." *Neuropsychologia, 7* (1969): 179–87.

CHAPTER 10

ANSHEL, M. H. "Effect of Age, Sex, and Type of Feedback on Motor Performance and Locus of Control." *Research Quarterly, 50* (1979): 305–17.

BERLYNE, D. E. *Conflict, Arousal, and Curosity.* New York: McGraw-Hill, 1960.

BRUNER, J. S. "Organization of Early Skilled Actions." *Child Development, 44* (1973): 1–11.

CARSON, L. M., AND WEIGAND, R. L. "Motor Schema Formation and Retention in Young Children: A Test of Schmidt's Theory." *Journal of Motor Behavior, 11* (1979): 247–51.

CHI, M. T. "Short-Term Memory Limitations in Children: Capacity or Processing Deficits." *Memory and Cognition, 4* (1976): 559–72.

CHOMSKY, N. "Reading, Writing, and Phonology." In M. Wolf, M. McQuillan, and E. Radwin (eds.), *Thought and Language/Language and Reading.* Cambridge, Mass.: Harvard Educational Review Reprint Series, 1980.

CRATTY, B. J. *Active Learning,* 3rd ed. Englewood Cliffs, N.J.: Prentice-Hall, 1985.

—————, AND SAMOY, L. "Ein verleich praxischer veshalten weisen bei bjahringen kindern" [Relationships of Measures of Motor Planning in Six-Year Olds]. *Motorik, 7* (1984): 52–58.

FANTZ, R. L. "The Origin of Form Perception." *Scientific American, 204* (1961): 66–72.

FLAVELL, J. H. "An Analysis of Cognitive-Development." *Genetic Psychology Monographs, 86* (1972): 279–350.

GACHOUND, J. P., MOUNOUD, P., AND HAUERT, C. A. "Motor Strategies in Lifting Movements: A Comparison of Adult and Child Performance." *Journal of Motor Behavior, 15* (1983): 202-16.

HAITH, M. J. *Rules That Babies Look By: The Organization of Newborn Visual Activity.* Hillsdale, N.J.: Erlbaum, 1980.

HOGAN, J. C., AND HOGAN, R. "Organization of Early Skilled Action: Some Comments." *Child Development, 46* (1975): 233–36.

KELLOGG, R. *Analyzing Children's Art.* Palo Alto, Calif.: National Press Books, 1969.

KELSO, J. A. S., AND NORMAN, P. E. "Motor Schema Formation." *Developmental Psychology, 14* (1977): 153–56.

KERR, R. "Motor Development: A Possible Model." *Motor Skills: Theory into Practice, 6* (1982): 19–28.

LEITHWOOD, K. A., AND FOWLER, W. "Complex Motor Learning in Four-Year-Olds." *Child Development, 42* (1971): 781–92.

MOSS, S. C., AND HOGG, J. "The Development and Integration of Fine Motor Sequences in 12–18-Month-Old Children: A Test of the Modular Theory of Motor Skill Acquisition." *Genetic Psychology Monographs, 107* (1983): 145–87.

NEWELL, K. M., AND KENNEDY, J. A. "Knowledge of Results and Children's Motor Learning." *Developmental Psychology, 14* (1978): 531–36.

PIAGET, J. *The Origins of Intelligence.* New York: International Universities Press, 1952.

THOMAS, J. R. "Acquisition of Motor Skills: Information Processing Differences between Children and Adults." *Research Quarterly, 51* (1980): 158–73.

YARROW, L. J., MCQUISTON, S., MACTURK, R. H., MCCARTHY, M. E., KLEIN, R. P., AND VIETZE, P. M. "Assessment of Mastery Motivation during the First Year of Life: Contemporaneous and Cross-Age Relationships." *Developmental Psychology, 19* (1983): 159–71.

CHAPTER 11

ASLIN, R. N., AND SALAPATEK, R. "Saccadic Localization of Peripheral Targets by the very Young Human Infant." *Perception and Psychophysics, 17* (1975): 293–302.

ASSO, D., AND WYKE, M. "Discrimination of Spatially Confusable Letters by Young Children." *Journal of Experimental Psychology, 11* (1971): 11–20.

AYRES, A. J. "Patterns of Perceptual-Motor Dysfunction in Children: A Factor Analytic Study," Monogram Supplement 3V, *Perceptual and Motor Skills, 18* (1964).

BERLYNE, D. E. *Conflict, Arousal, and Curiosity.* New York: McGraw-Hill, 1960.

BOWER, T. G. R. *Development in Infancy.* San Francisco: Freeman, 1974.

BRONSON, G. W. "The Postnatal Growth of Visual Capacity." *Child Development, 45* (1974): 873–90.

———. *The Scanning Patterns of Human Infants: Implications for Human Learning.* Norwood, N.J.: ABLEX, 1982.

CAMERON, M. I., AND ROBINSON, V. M. J. "Effects of Cognitive Training on Academic and on Task Behavior of Hyperactive Children." *Journal of Abnormal Psychology, 8* (1980): 403–19.

CARRIERE, L., AND BELLEC, J. "Components of the Coincident-Anticipation Behavior of Children Aged from 6–11 Years." *Perceptual and Motor Skills, 52* (1981): 547–56.

COHEN, L. B., AND SALAPATEK, P. *Infant Perception: From Sensation to Cognition.* New York: Academic Press, 1977. Vols. I and II.

COHEN, R., SCHLESER, R., AND MEYERS, R. "Self-instructions: Effects of Cognitive Level and Active Rehearsal." *Journal of Experimental and Child Psychology, 34* (1982): 65–76.

COLARUSSO, R. P., AND HAMILL, D. D. *Motor-Free Visual Perception Test.* Novato, Calif.: Academic Therapy Publications, 1972.

CONEL, J. L. *The Postnatal Development of the Human Cerebral Cortex, Vols. 2–5.* Cambridge, Mass.: Harvard University Press, 1941–1959.

CRATTY, B. J. *Adapted Physical Education for Handicapped Children, and Youth.* Denver: Love Publications, 1980.

———. *Active Learning,* 3rd ed. Englewood Cliffs, N.J.: Prentice-Hall, 1985.

———, APITZSCH, E., AND BERGEL, R. *Dynamic Visual Acuity: A Developmental Study.* Los Angeles: University of California, Perceptual Motor Learning Laboratory, 1973.

————— , AND MARTIN, M. M. *Perceptual Motor Efficiency in Children.* Philadelphia: Lea and Febiger, 1975.

CRUIKSHANK, R. M. "The Development of Visual Size Constancy in Early Infancy." *Journal of Genetic Psychology, 58* (1941): 327–51.

Davidson, H. P. "A Study of Reversals in Young Children." *Journal of Genetic Psychology, 44* (1934): 452–65.

————— . "A Study of the Confusing Letters B, D, P, Q." *Journal of Genetic Psychology, 47* (1935): 4658–68.

DEACH, D. "Genetic Development of Motor Skills of Children, 2–6 Years of Age." Unpublished doctoral dissertation, University of Michigan, 1951.

DiFRANCO, D., MUIR, D. W., AND DODWELL, P. C. "Reaching in Very Young Infants." *Perception, 7* (1978): 385–92.

DUKE-ELDER, S., AND COOK, C. *Systems of Ophthalmology, Vol. III.* St. Louis: Mosby, 1963.

ELKIND, D., KOEGLER, R. R., AND KOEGLER, E. G. "Studies in Perceptual Development. II: Whole-Part Development." *Child Development, 35* (1964): 81–90.

FANTZ, R. L. "The Origin of Form Perception." *Scientific American, 204* (1961): 66–72.

————— . "Pattern Discrimination and Selective Attention Determinants of Perceptual Development from Birth." In A. H. Kidd and J. L. Rivoire (eds.), *Perceptual Development in Children.* New York: International Universities Press, 1966.

FROSTIG, M. *Developmental Test of Visual Perception.* Palo Alto: Conslting Psychologists Press, 1963.

HAITH, M. M. "Visual Competence in Early Infancy." In R. Held, H. Leibowitz, and H. L. Teuber (eds.), *Handbook of Sensory Physiology.* Berlin: Springer-Verlag, 1978.

————— . *Rules That Babies Look By: The Organization of Newborn Visual Activity.* Hillsdale, N.J.: Erlbaum, 1980.

HELLWEG, D. A. "An Analysis of Perceptual and Performance Characteristics of the Catching Skill in 6 and 7 Year Old Children." Ph.D. dissertation, University of Wisconsin, Madison, 1972.

HERSHENSON, M. "Visual Discrimination in the Human Newborn." *Journal of Comparative Physiological Psychology, 58* (1964): 270–76.

HOADLEY, D. "A Study of the Catching Ability of Children in Grades 1–4." M.S. thesis, University of Iowa, Iowa City, 1941.

JEFFREY, W. E. "Discrimination of Oblique Lines by Children." *Journal of Comparative Physiological Psychology, 62* (1966): 154–56.

JOHNSON, B., AND BECK, L. F. "The Development of Space Perception. I. Stereoscopic Vision in Pre-School Children." *Journal of Genetic Psychology, 58* (1941): 247–54.

KAGAN, J. "The Growth of the 'Face' Schema: Theoretical Significance and Methodological Issues." In J. Hellmuth (ed.), *The Exceptional Infant.* Vol. I: The Normal Infant. New York: Brunner/Mazel, 1967.

KARMEL, B. Z., AND MAISEL, E. B. "A Neuronal Activity Model for Infant Visual Attention." In L. B. Cohen and P. Salapatek (eds.) *Infant Perception: From Sensation to Cognition: Basic Visual Processes, Vol I,* New York: Academic Press, 1975.

KAVALE, K. "One Jumped Off the Balance Beam: Meta-analysis of Perceptual-Motor Training." *Journal of Learning Disabilities, 16* (1983): 165–72.

KENDALL, P. C., AND FINCH, A. J., JR. "Developing Nonimpulsive Behavior in Children: Cognitive-Behavioral Strategies for Self-Control." In P. C. Kendall and S. D. Hollon (eds.), *Cognitive-Behavioral Interventions: Theory, Research, and Procedures.* New York: Academic Press, 1979.

KEPHART, N. C. *The Slow Learner in the Classroom.* Columbus, Ohio: Charles E. Merrill, 1964.

LAST, P. *Eugene Wolff's Anatomy of the Eye and Orbit.* London: Lewis, 1968.

LING, B. C. "Form Discrimination as a Learning Cue in Infants." *Comparative Psychological Monographs, 2* (1941): 1–49.

MAUER, D. "Infant Visual Perception: Methods of Study." In L. B. Cohen and R. Salapatek (eds.), *Infant Perception, From Sensation to Cognition: Basic Visual Processes,* Vol. I. New York: Academic Press, 1975.

McDANIEL, E. D. *Motion Picture Tests to Measure Perceptual Abilities in Children, Vols. 1–2.* Lafayette Ind.: Purdue Research Foundation, 1972.

MEICHENBAUM, D. H., AND GOODMAN, J. "Training Impulsive Children to Talk to Themselves: A Means of Developing Self-Control." *Journal of Abnormal Psychology, 77* (1971): 115–26.

MEYERS, P. E., AND HAMMILL, D. *Methods for Learning Disabilities,* 3rd ed. New York: Wiley, 1982.

PARMALEE, A. H., AND SIGMAN, D. "Development of Visual Behavior and Neurological Organization in Pre-Term and Full-Term Infants." In A. D. Pick (ed.), *Minnesota Symposia on Child Psychology*, Vol. 10. Minneapolis: University of Minnesota, 1976.

PEIPER, A. *Cerebral Function in Infancy and Childhood.* New York: International Behavioral Science Series, Consultants Bureau, 1963.

RANDT, R. D., "Ball-Catching Proficiency Among 4, 6, and 8, Year Old Girls." In J. E. Clark and J. H. Humphrey, *Motor Development: Current Selected Research, Vol I.* Princeton, N.J.: Princeton Book Co, 1985, pp. 35–43.

RUDEL, R. G., AND TEUBER, H. L. "Discrimination of Direction of Line in Children." *Journal of Comparative Physiological Psychology, 56* (1963): 892–97.

SALTZ, E. "Let's Pretend: The Role of Motoric Imagery in Memory for Sentences and Words." *Journal of Experimental Child Psychology, 34* (1982): 77–92.

——————, AND DONNENWERTH-NOLAN, S. "Does Motoric Imagery Facilitate Memory for Sentences? A Selective Interference Test." *Journal of Verbal Learning and Verbal Behavior, 20* (1981): 322–32.

SMITH, O. W., AND SMITH, P. C. "Developmental Studies of Spatial Judgements by Children and Adults." *Perceptual and Motor Skills,* Monograph Supplement, 22 (1966): 3–73.

SOKOLOV, E. N. *Perception and the Conditioned Reflex.* New York: Macmillan, 1963.

STADULIS, R. "Coincidence Anticipation Behavior of Children." Ph.D. dissertation, Teachers College, Columbia University, New York, 1971.

—————— "Coincidence-Anticipation Behavior of Children." In J. E. Clark and J. H. Humphrey, *Motor Development: Current Selected Research, Vol I.* Princeton, N.J.: Princeton Book Co, 1985, pp. 1–17.

TELLER, D. Y. A. "A Visual Psychophysicist Turns to Infants." Paper presented to the Society for Research in Child Development, Philadelphia, March 1973.

THORNBURG, K. R., AND FISHER, V. L. "Discrimination of 2-D, Letters by Children after Play with 2 or 3 Dimensional Letter Forms." *Perceptual and Motor Skills, 30* (1970): 979–86.

TORRES, J. A. "The Relationships between Figure-Ground Perceptual Ability and Ball Catching Ability in 10- and 13-Year-Old Boys and Girls." M.S. thesis, Purdue University, Lafayette, Indiana, 1966.

VICTOR, E. A. "A Cinematographical Analysis of Catching Behavior of a Selected Group of 7- and 9-Year-Old Boys. Ph.D. dissertation, University of Wisconsin, Madison, 1961.

VON HOFSTEN, C. "Predictive Reaching for Moving Objects by Human Infants." *Journal of Experimental Child Psychology, 30* (1980): 369–82.

——————, AND LINDHAGEN, K. "Observations on the Development of Reaching for Moving Objects." *Journal of Experimental and Child Psychology, 28* (1979): 158–73.

VURPILLOT, E. *The Visual World of the Child.* New York: International Universities Press, 1976.

WALK, R. D. "The Development of Depth Perception in Animals and in Human Infants." In H. W. Stevenson (ed.), *Concept of Development.* Monograph of Society for Research in Child Development, 1966, serial no. 107.

——————, AND GIBSON, E. J. A. "A Comparative and Analytic Study of Visual Depth Perception." *Psychological Monographs, 75* (1961).

WALTERS, C. P., AND WALK, R. D. "Visual Placing by Human Infants." *Journal of Experimental Child Psychology, 18* (1974): 34–40.

WATSON, J. S. "Perception of Object Orientation in Infants." *Merrill Palmer Quarterly, 12* (1966): 72–94.

WHITE, B. "Development of Perception during the First Six Months." Paper read at the American Association for the Advancement of Science, 1963.

WHITE, C. T., WHITE, C. L., FAWCETT, W., AND SOCKS, J. "Color Evoked Potentials in the Newborn." Paper presented at the meeting of the Society for Research in Child Development, New Orleans, March 1977.

WILLIAMS, H. G. "The Perception of Moving Objects by Children." Unpublished monograph, Perceptual-Motor Learning Laboratory, UCLA, 1968.

YAKOVLEV, P., AND LECOURS, A. "The Mylogenetic Cycles of Regional Maturation of the Brain." In A. Minkowski (ed.), *Regional Development of the Brain in Early Life.* Oxford, Eng.: Blackwell, 1967.

ZINCHENKO, V. P., VAN CHIZI-TSIN, V., AND TARAKANOV, V. V. "The Formation and Development of Perceptual Activity." *Soviet Psychology/Psychiatry, 1* (1963): 3–12.

CHAPTER 12

ASTRAND, P. *Experimental Studies of Physical Working Capacity in Relation to Sex and Age.* Copenhagen: Ejnir Munksgaard, 1952.

_____ . "Commentary—International Symposium on Physical Activity and Cardiovascular Health." *Canadian Medical Association Journal, 96* (1967): 760–65.

ASTRAND, P. O., ET AL. "Girl Swimmers." *Acta Paediatrica, 147* (1963): 1–75.

ASTRAND, P. O., AND RODAHI, K. *Textbook of Work Physiology.* New York: McGraw-Hill, 1977.

BAILEY, D. A. "Sport and the Child: Physiological Considerations." In R. A. Magill, M. J. Ash, and F. L. Smoll, (eds.) *Children in Sport: A Contemporary Anthology.* Champaign, Ill.: Human Kinetics, 1978. pp. 103–12.

BAR–OR, O., AND SWIREN, L. D. "Physiological Effects of Increased Frequency of Physical Education Classes and Endurance Conditioning on 9 to 10 Year Old Boys and Girls:" In Bar–Or (ed.) *Pediatric Work Physiology: Proceedings of the Fourth International Symposium.* Tel Aviv: Technodaf, 1972.

BRANDFONBRENER, M., LANDOWNE, M., AND SHOCK, H. W. "Changes in Cardiac Output with Age." *Circulation, 12* (1955): 557–66.

BROZEK, J. "The Measurement of Body Composition." In J. Brozek, (ed.) *Human Body Composition.* Oxford, Eng.: Pergamon Press, 1960, pp. 1–29.

EDINGTON, D. W., AND EDGERTON, V. R. *The Biology of Physical Activity.* Boston: Houghton Mifflin, 1976.

ERIKSSON, B. O. "Physical Training, Oxygen Supply and Muscle Metabolism in 11–13 Year Old Boys." *Acta Physiologica Scandinavica Suppl, 384* (1972), 2–48.

_____ , KARLSSON, J., AND SALTIN, B. "Cardiac Output and Arterial Blood Gases During Exercise in Pubertal Boys." *Journal of Applied Physiology, 31* (1971): 348–52.

_____ , AND SALTIN, B. "Muscle Metabolism During Exercise in Boys Aged 11–16 Years Compared to Adults." *Acta Paediatrica Belgica, 28* (1974): 257–65 (Supplement).

FERRIS, B. G., JR., WHITTENBERGER, J. L., AND GALLAGHER, J. R. "Maximum Breathing Capacity and Vital Capacity of Male Children and Adolescents." *Pediatrics, 9* (1952): 659–70.

FREEDSON, P. S., GILLIAM, T. B., SADY, S. P., AND KATCH, V. L. "Transient VO_2 Characteristics in Children at the Onset of Steady-Rate Exercise." *Research Quarterly for Exercise and Sport, 52* (1981): 167–73.

FRISCH, R. E., AND MCARTHUR, H. W. "Menstrual Cycles: Fatness as a Determinant of Minimum-weight for Height Necessary for their Maintenance or Onset." *Science, 185* (1974): 949–55.

GATCH, W., AND BYRD, R. "Endurance Training and Cardiovascular Function in 9 and 10 Year Old Boys." *Archives of Physical Medicine and Rehabilitation, 60* (1979): 574–77.

GILLIAM, T. B., SADY, S., THORLAND, W. G., AND WELTMAN, A. L. "Comparison of Peak Performance Measures in Children Ages 6 to 8, 9 to 10, and 11 to 13 years." *Research Quarterly, 48* (1977): 695–701.

HARRE, D. *Principles of Sports Training.* Berlin: Sportverlag, 1982.

ILIFF, A., AND LEE, V. A. "Pulse Rate, Respiratory Rate and Body Temperature of Children between Two Months and Eighteen Years of Age." *Child Development, 23* (1952): 237–45.

JENSS, R. M., AND SHOCK, N. W. "A Mathematical Expression for Oxygen Consumption following Violent Exercise." *Am. J. Hygiene, 24* (1936): 83–93.

LYDIRAD, A., AND GILMORE, G. *Run to the Top,* 2nd ed. Auckland: Minerva Ltd, 1967.

MAUTNER, H., LUISADA, A., AND WEISZ, L. "Physiological Tachycardia in the Young." *Arch Pediat. 58* (1941): 562–69.

MAYER, J. "Nutritional Relationships to Exercise and Obesity." *Nutr. Abstr Rev. 25* (1955): 597–871.

MCARDLE, W. D., KATCH, F. I., AND KATCH, V. L. *Exercise Physiology, Energy Nutrition, and Human Performance.* Philadelphia: Lea and Febiger, 1981.

OGDEN, E., AND SHOCK, N. W. "Circulatory Changes During Recovery from Intense Exertion." *Proc. Soc. Exp. Biol. Med, 33* (1935): 5–8.

PARIZKOVA, J. "Age Trends in Fat in Normal and Obese Children." *J. Applied Physiology, 16* (1961): 172–74.

_____ . "Body Composition and Exercise During Growth and Development." In G. L. Rarick (ed.) *Physical Activity: Human Growth and Development.* New York: Academic Press, 1973.

_____ *Body Fat and Physical Fitness.* The Hague: Martinus Nijhoff, 1977.

_____ *Growth, Fitness and Nutrition in Pre-School Children.* Charles University, Prague (Praha): Charles University Press, 1984.

POWERS, S. K. "Children and Exercise." In J. Thomas (ed.) *Motor Development During Childhood and Adolescence.* Minneapolis, Minn: Burgess Publishing Co., 1984.

RICHEY, H. G. "The Blood Pressure in Boys and Girls before and after Puberty, Its Relation to Growth and to Maturity." *American J. Dis. Child, 42* (1931): 1281–1330.

ROBINSON, S. "Experimental Studies of Physical Fitness in Relation to Age." *Arbeitsphysiologie, 10* (1938): 251–323.

SHOCK, N. W. "Physiological Responses of Adolescents to Exercise." *Texas Rep. Biol. Medicine, 4* (1946): 289–310.

————— "Physiological Growth." In F. Falkmer (ed.) *Human Development.* Philadelphia, Pa.: W. B. Saunders, Co., 1966.

SHOCK, N. W., AND SOLEY, M. H. "Average Values for Basal Respiratory Functions in Adolescents and Adults." *J. Nutrit., 18* (1939): 143–53.

SPRYRANOVA, S. "Development of the Relationship between Aerobic Capacity and the Circulatory and Respiratory Reaction to Moderate Activity in Boys 11–13 Years of Age." *Physiol. Bohenoslov, 15* (1966) 253–64.

SWEENEY, H. "When Interest Dies." In *The Young Runner.* Mountain View, California: World Publications, 1973.

TANNER, J. M., AND WHITEHOUSE, R. H. "Standards for Subcutaneous Fat in British Children." *Brit. Med. J., 1* (1962): 446–50.

THORLAND, W. G., AND GILLIAM, T. B. "Comparison of Serum Lipids between Habitually High and Low Active Pre-adolescent Males." *Medicine and Science in Sport Exercise, 13* (1981): 316–21.

VACCARO, P., AND CLARKE, D. H. "Cardiorespiratory Alterations in 9 to 11 Year Old Children following a Season of Competitive Swimming." *Medicine and Science in Sports, 10* (1978): 204–7.

CHAPTER 13

AINSWORTH, M. D. S., BELL, S. M., AND STAYTON, J. D. "Individual Differences in Strange-Situation Behavior of One-Year-Olds." In H. R. Schaffer (ed.), *The Origins of Human Social Relations.* London: Academic, 1972.

ALDERMAN, R. B., AND WOOD, N. L. "An Analysis of Incentive Motivation in Young Canadian Athletes." *Canadian J. of Applied Sport Sci., 1* (1976): 169–76.

ALLEN, S. "The Effects of Verbal Reinforcement on Children's Performance as a Function of Type of Task." *J. Exp. Child. Psych., 13* (1965): 57–73.

ANASTASIOW, N. J. "Success in School and Boys' Sex Role Patterns." *Child Development, 33* (1965): 1053–66.

AZRIN, N. J., AND LINDSLEY, O. R. "The Reinforcement of Cooperation between Children." *J. Abnorm. Soc. Psych., 52* (1956): 100–102.

BELL, R. Q. "A Congenital Contribution to Emotional Response in Early Infancy and the Preschool Periods." In R. Porter and M. O'Conner (eds.), *Parent-Infant Interaction.* CIBA Foundation Symposium 33, New York: Associated Science, 1975.

BENDER, L., AND RAPPAPORT, J. "Animals Drawings of Children." *Am. J. of Orthopsych., 14* (1944): 521–27.

BRAZELTON, T. B. "Neonatal Behavioral Assessment Scale." *Clinics in Devlpmtl. Med., 50.* Philadelphia: Spastics International Medical Corp., Lippincott, 1973.

BRIDGES, K. M. B. "Occupational Interest of Three-Year-Old Children." *Ped. Sen. J. Genet. Psych., 34* (1928): 413–23.

————— . *The Social and Emotional Development of the Pre-School Child.* London: Kegan Paul, 1931.

BRONSON, W. C., AND PANKEY, W. B. "The Evolution of Early Individual Differences in Orientation toward Peers." In L. A. Strouf, *The Organization of Early Development and of Continuity in Adaptation.* New Orleans: Society for Research in Child Development, March 1977.

BÜHLER, C. "Die Ersten Socialen Verhaltungsweisen des Kindes." In "Sociologische und Psychologische Studien Ueber das Erste Lebensjahr." *Quell. u. Stud. Z. Jugendk, 5* (1927): 1–102.

CHALLMAN, R. "Factors Influencing Friendships among Pre-School Children." *Child. Dev., 3* (1932): 146–58.

CLARKE-STEWART, K. A. "The Father's Impact on Mother and Child." Paper presented at the biennial meeting of the Society for Research in Child Development, New Orleans, 1977.

COCKRELL, D. L. "A Study of the Play of Children of Pre-School Age by an Unobserved Observer." *Genet. Psych. Monog., 17* (1935): 372–469.

COX, F. N. "Some Effects of Test Anxiety and Presence or Absence of Other Persons on Boys' Performance on a Repetitive Motor Task." *J. Exp. Child. Psych., 3* (1965): 100–112.

CRATTY, B. J. *Social Dimensions of Physical Activity,* Englewood Cliffs, N.J.: Prentice-Hall, 1967, chap. 6.

CRUM, J. F., AND ECKERT, H. M. "Play Patterns of Primary School Children." In J. E. Clark and J. H. Humphrey, *Motor Development: Current Selected Research,* Vol. 1. Princeton, N.J.: Princeton Book Co., 1985, p. 99.

DAVITZ, J. R. "Social Perception and Sociometric Choice of Children." *J. Abnorm. Soc. Psych., 50* (1955): 173–76.

DESTEFANO, C. T. "Environmental Determinants of Peer Social Activity in 18-Month-Old-Males." Unpublished Ph.D. dissertation, Boston University, 1976.

ECKERMAN, C. O., WHATLEY, J., AND KUTZ, S. "Growth of Social Play with Peers during the Second Year of Life." *Develop. Psych., 11* (1975): 42–49.

FRIES, M., AND WOLFF, P. "Some Hypotheses on the Role of the Congenital Activity Type in Personality in Development." *Psychoanalytic Study of the Child,* 8 (1953): 48–62.

GERSON, R. "Intrinsic Motivation: Implications for Children's Athletics." *Motor Skills: Theory into Practice, 2* (1978): 111–19.

GEWIRTZ, H. B., AND GEWIRTZ, J. L. "Visiting and Caretaking Patterns for Kibbutz Infants: Age and Sex Trends." *Am. J. of Orthopsychiatry, 38* (1968): 427–43.

GOODENOUGH, F. L. "Measuring Behavior Traits by Means of Repeated Short Samples." *J. Juv. Res., 12* (1928): 230–35.

————————. "Inter-Relationships in the Behavior of Young Children." *Child. Dev., 1* (1930): 29–48.

GREENBERG, P. J. "Competition in Children: An Experimental Study." *Amer. J. Psych., 44* (1932): 221–48.

HALVERSON, C. F., AND WALDROP, M. F. "The Relations between Pre-School Activity and Aspects of Intellectual and Social Behavior at Age 7½." *Dev. Psych., 12* (1976): 107–12.

HARDY, M. C. "Social Recognition at the Elementary School Age." *J. Soc. Psych., 8* (1937): 365–84.

HARTRUP, W. "Some Correlates of Parental Imitation in Young Children." *Child Dev., 33* (1962): 85.

HEATHERS, G. "Emotional Dependence and Independence in Nursery School Plays." *J. Genetic Psych., 87* (1955): 37–57.

HEISE, B. *Effects of Instruction in Cooperation on the Attitudes and Conduct of Children.* Ann Arbor: University of Michigan Press, 1942.

HURLOCK, E. B. "Experimental Investigations of Childhood Play." *Psych. Bull., 31* (1934): 47–66.

JONES, H. E. *Motor Performance and Growth.* Berkeley: University of California Press, 1949.

JONES, M. C. "Adolescent Friendships." *Amer. Psych., 3* (1948): 352.

————————, AND BAYLEY, N. "Physical Maturing among Boys as Related to Behavior." *J. Educ. Psych., 41* (1950): 129–48.

KAGAN, J., AND MOSS, H. A. *Birth to Maturity: A Study in Psychological Development.* New York: Wiley, 1962.

KEILEY, R., AND STEPHENS, M. W. "Comparison of Different Patterns of Social Reinforcement in Children's Operant Learning." *J. Comp. Physiol. Psych., 57* (1964): 294–96.

KEMPE, H. Paper presented at the Perinatal Medicine Meeting, Snowmass, Colorado, 1976.

KORNER, A. F. "Visual Alertness in Neonates: Individual Differences and Their Correlations." *Perceptual and Motor Skills, 31* (1970): 499–509.

KOTELCHUCK, M. "The Nature of the Child's Tie to His Father." Unpublished Ph.D. dissertation, Harvard University, 1972.

————————. "The Infant's Relationship to the Father: Experimental Evidence." In M. E. Lamb (ed.), *The Role of the Father in Child Development.* New York: Wiley, 1976.

LAMB, M. E. "The Development of Mother-Infant, and Father-Infant Atachments in the Second Year of Life." *Develop. Psych., 13* (1977): 639–49.

LATANE, B., AND ARROWWOOD, A. J. "Emotional Arousal and Task Performance," *J. Appl. Psych., 47* (1963): 324–27.

LEHMAN, H. C., AND WITTY, P. A. *The Psychology of Play Activities.* New York: Barnes, 1927.

LEWIS, M., AND LEE-PAINTER, S. "An Interactional Approach to the Mother-Infant Dyad." In M. Lewis and L. A. Rosenblum (eds.), *The Effect of the Infant on Its Caregiver.* New York: Wiley, 1974.

_____ , WALL, M., AND ARONFREED, I. "Developmental Change in the Relative Values of Social and Non-Social Reinforcements." *J. Exp. Psych., 66* (1963): 133–37.

LICHTENBERGER, W. *Mitmenschliches, Verhalten eines Zwillingspaares in seinen ersten Lebensjahren.* Munchen: Ernest Reinhardt, 1965.

LUSK, D., AND LEWIS, M. "Mother-Infant Interaction among the Wolof Senegal." *Hum. Devel., 15* (1972): 58–69.

MAHLER, M., PINE, F., AND BERGMAN, A. *The Psychological Birth of the Human Infant.* New York: Basic Books, 1975.

MISSIURO, W. "The Development of Reflex Activity in Children." In E. Jokl and E. Simon (eds.), *International Research in Sport and Physical Education.* Springfield, Ill.: Charles C. Thomas, 1964.

MOSS, H. A. "Sex, Age, and State as Determinants of Mother-Infant Interaction." *Merrill Palmer Qtrly., 13* (1967): 19–36.

MUELLER, E., AND BRENNER, J. "The Growth of Social Interaction in a Toddler Playgroup: The Role of Peer Experience." *Child Devel., 48* (1977): 854–61.

_____ , AND DESTEFANO, C. "Sources of Toddlers' Peer Interaction in a Playground Setting." Unpublished paper, Boston University, 1973.

MUKERJI, N. P. "An Investigation of Ability to Work in Groups and in Isolation." *Br. J. Psych., 30* (1940): 352–56.

MURPHY, L. B., AND MURPHY, G. "The Influence of Social Situations upon the Behavior of Children." In C. Murchison (ed.), *Handbook of Social Psychology.* Worcester, Mass.: Clark University Press, 1935.

MUSTE, M. J., AND SHARPE, D. F. "Some Influential Factors in Determination of Aggressive Behavior in Preschool Children." *Child Devel., 18* (1947): 11–28.

NELSON, D. O. "Leadership in Sports." *Res. Quart., 37* (1966): 268–75.

NOER, D., AND WHITTAKER, J. "Effects of Masculine-Feminine Ego Involvement on the Acquisition of a Mirror-Tracing Skill." *J. Psych., 56* (1963): 15–16.

PARKE, R. D., AND O'LEARY, S. "Father-Mother-Infant Interaction in the Newborn Period: Some Feelings, Some Observations and Some Unresolved Issues." In K. Riegel and J. Meacham (eds.), *The Developing Individual in a Changing World.* Vol. 2: *Social and Environmental Issues.* The Hague: Mouton, 1975.

_____ , AND SAWIN, D. B. "The Father's Role in Infancy: A Re-evaluation." *The Family Coordinator, 25* (1976): 365–71.

_____ , AND _____ . "The Family in Early Infancy: Social, Interactional and Attitudinal Analyses." Paper presented to the Society for Research in Child Development, New Orleans, March, 1977.

PARTEN, M. B. "Social Play among Preschool Children." *J. Abnorm. Soc. Psych., 28* (1933): 136–47.

PATTERSON, G. R., AND ANDERSON, D. "Peers as Social Reinforcers." *Child Dev., 35* (1964): 951–60.

PAYNE, D. E., AND MUSSEN, P. H. "Parent-Child Relations and Father Identification among Adolescent Boys." *J. Abnorm. Soc. Psych., 52* (1956): 358–62.

PHILIP, A. J. "Strangers and Friends as Competitors and Cooperators." *J. Genet. Psych., 57* (1940): 249–58.

PINTNEY, R., FORLANDS, F., AND FREEDMAN, H. "Personality and Attitudinal Similarity among Classmates." *J. Appl. Psych., 21* (1937): 48–65.

QUILITCH, H. R., AND RISLEY, T. "The Effects of Play Materials on Social Play." *J. App. Beh. Anal., 6* (1973): 575–78.

RARICK, G. L., AND MCKEE, L. "A Study of Twenty Third-Grade Children Exhibiting Extreme Levels of Achievements on Tests of Motor Proficiency." *Res. Quart., 20* (1950): 142–50.

REANEY, M. J. "The Correlation between General Intelligence and Play Abilities as Shown in Organized Group Games." *Br. J. Psych., 7* (1914): 227–52.

REDICAN, W. K. "Adult Male-Infant Interactions in Nonhuman Primates." In M. Lamb (ed.), *The Role of the Father in Child Development.* New York: Wiley, 1976.

RENDINA, I., AND DICKERSCHEID, J. D. "Father Involvement with First-Born Infants." *Family Coordinator, 25* (1976): 373–79.

ROSENBERG, B. G., AND SUTTON-SMITH, B. "The Measurement of Masculinity and Femininity in Children: An Extension and Revalidation." *J. Genet. Psych., 96* (1960): 165–70.

RUBIN, J. Z., PROVENZANO, F. J., AND LURIA, Z. "The Eye of the Beholder: Parents' Views on Sex of Newborns." *Amer. J. Orthopsych., 43* (1974): 720–31.

RUBENSTEIN, J., AND HOWES, C. "The Effects of Peers on Toddler Interaction with Mother and Toys." *Child Devel., 47* (1976): 597–605.

SADUSKY, A. S. "Collective Behavior of Children of a Pre-School Age." *J. Soc. Psych., 1* (1930): 367–78.

SCHAEFER, E. S. "Converging Conceptual Models for Maternal Behavior and for Child Behavior." In J. C. Glidewell (ed.), *Parental Attitudes and Child Behavior*. Springfield, Ill.: Charles C. Thomas, 1961.

————, AND BELL, R. Q. "Patterns of Attitudes Toward Child Rearing and the Family." *J. Abnorm. Soc. Psych., 54* (1957): 39–95.

SCHAFFER, H. R., AND EMERSON, P. E. "Patterns of Response to Physical Contact in Early Human Development." *J. Child Psych. Psychiatry, 5* (1964): 1–13.

SEARS, R. R., MACCOBY, E. C., AND LEVIN, H. *Patterns of Child Rearing*. Evanston, Ill.: Row, Peterson, 1957.

SPITZ, R. A., AND WOLF, K. M. "The Smiling Response: A Contribution to the Ontogenesis of Social Relations." *J. Genet. Psych. Monogr., 34* (1946): 57–156.

STEVENSON, H. W. "Social Reinforcement with Children as a Function of CA, Sex of E, and Sex of S." *J. Abnorm. Soc. Psych., 63* (1961): 147–54.

STONEMAN, Z., BRODY, G. H., AND MACKINNON, C. "Naturalistic Observations of Children's Activities and Roles While Playing with Their Siblings and Friends." *Child Devel., 55* (1984): 617–27.

VANDELL, D. L. "Toddler Sons' Social Interaction with Mothers, Fathers, and Peers." Unpublished Ph.D. dissertation, Boston University, 1976.

VINCZE, M. "The Social Contacts of Infants and Young Children Reared Together." *Early Child Devel. Care, 1* (1971): 99–109.

WOLFF, P. H. "Mother-Infant Relations at Birth." In J. G. Howels (ed.), *Modern Perspectives in International Child Psychiatry*. New York: Brunner/Mazel, 1971.

YARROW, L. J., RUBENSTEIN, J. L., PEDERSEN, F. A., AND JANKOWSKI, J. J. "Dimensions of Early Stimulation and Their Differential Effects on Infant Development." *Merrill-Palmer Qtrly., 18* (1972): 205–18.

ZIGLER, E., AND KANZER, P. "The Effectiveness of Two Classes of Reinforcers on the Performance of Middle and Lower Class children." *J. Personal., 30* (1962): 155–63.

CHAPTER 14

ALS, H., TRONICK, E., LESTER, B. M., AND BRAZELTON, T. B. "Specific Neonatal Measures: The Brazelton Neonatal Behavioral Assessment Scale." In J. D. Osofsky (ed.), *Handbook of Infant Development*. New York: Wiley, 1979.

APGAR, V. "A Proposal for a New Method of Evaluation of the Newborn Infant." *Current Researches in Anesthesia and Analgesia, 32* (1953): 260–67.

————, AND JAMES, L. S. "Further Observations on the Newborn Scoring System." *Amer. J. Dis. Child., 104* (1962): 419–28.

BAILER, I., DOLL, L., AND WINSBERG, B. G. *Modified Lincoln-Oseretsky Motor Development Scale*. New York: New York State Department of Mental Health and Hygiene, 1973.

BAKOW, H., SAMEROFF, A., KELLY, P., AND ZAX, M. "Relation between Newborn and Mother: Child Interactions at Four Months." Paper presented at the biennial meeting of the Society for Research in Child Development, Philadelphia, 1973.

BEITEL, P. A., AND MEAD, B. J. "Bruinicks-Oseretsky Test of Motor Proficiency: A Viable Measure for 3–5 Year Old Children." *Perc. Mtr. Skls., 51* (1980): 919–23.

BENDER, A. L. *A Visual-Motor Gestalt Test*. New York: American Orthopsychiatric Association, 1938.

BERGES, J., AND LEZINE, L. *The Imitation of Gestures*, A. H. Parmalee, trans. London: W. Heinemann, 1965.

BRAZELTON, T. B. "Neonatal Behavioral Assessment Scale (Clinics in Developmental Medicine, No. 50)." *Spastics International Medical Corporation*. Philadelphia, Pa.: Lippincott, 1973.

BRIGANCE, A. *Inventory of Early Development*, 2nd ed. North Billerica, Ma.: Curriculum Associates, 1977.

BRUININKS, R. H. *Bruininks-Oseretsky Test of Motor Proficiency*. Circle Pines, Minn.: American Guidance Service, 1978.

CATTELL, P. *The Measurement of Intelligence of Infants and Young Children.* New York: New York Psychological Corporation, 1940.

CHARLOP, M., AND ATWELL, C. W. "The Charlop-Atwell Scale of Motor Coordination: A Quick and Easy Assessment of Young Children." *Perc. Mtr. Skls., 51* (1980): 1291–1308.

COLARUSSO, R. P., AND HAMMILL, D. D. *Motor-Free Visual Perceptual Test.* Novato, Ca.: Academic Therapy Publications, 1972.

CONNOLLY, K., AND STRATTON, P. "Developmental Changes in Associated Movements." *Devel. Med. Child Neurol., 10* (1968): 49–56.

CORMAN, H. H., AND ESCALONA, S. K. "Stages of Sensiromotor Development: A Replication Study." *Merrill-Palmer Qrtly., 15* (1965): 351–61.

CRATTY, B. J. "Qualitative Aspects of Movement." In B. J. Cratty, *Remedial Motor Activity for Children.* Philadelphia, Pa.: Lea and Febiger, 1975.

————. *Adapted Physical Education for Handicapped Children and Youth.* Denver, Co.: Love Publications, 1980.

————, AND GIBSON, S. "Impulsivity and Motor Planning in School Children." Publication pending, *Motorick,* 1985.

————, AND SAMOY, L. "Inter-relationships of Motor Planning Measures." Publication pending, *Motorik,* 1984.

DRAGE, J. S., KENNEDY, C., BERENDES, H., SCHWARZ, B. K., AND WEISS, W. "The Apgar Score as an Index of Infant Morbidity." *Devel. Med. Child Neuro., 8* (1966): 141–48.

EDWARDS, N. "The Relationship between Physical Condition Immediately After Birth and Mental and Motor Performance at Age Four." *Genet. Psych. Monog., 78* (1968): 278–89.

FLEISHMAN, E. *The Measurement of Physical Fitness.* Englewood Cliffs, N.J.: Prentice-Hall, 1965.

FRANKENBURG, W. K., AND DODDS, J. B. "The Denver Developmental Screening Test." *J. Pediat., 71* (1967): 181–91.

FREEDMAN, D. G., AND FREEDMAN, H. "Behavioral Differences between Chinese-American and European-American Newborns." *Nature, 224* (1969): 122–35.

FRIES, M. "Psychomatic Relationships between Mother and Infant." *Psychomatic Med., 6* (1944): 159–65.

GALLAGHER, J. D. "Making Sense of Motor Development: Interfacing Research with Lesson Planning." In J. R. Thomas (ed.), *Motor Development During Childhood and Adolescence.* Minneapolis, Minn.: Burgess Publishing Co., 1984.

GAUSSEN, T. "Developmental Milestones or Conceptual Millstones? Some Practical and Theoretical Limitations in Infant Assessment Procedures." *Childcare, Health, and Development, 10* (1984): 99–115.

GESELL, A. *The Mental Growth of the Pre-School Child.* New York: MacMillan, 1925.

HARRIS, G. *Childrens' Drawings as Measures of Intellectual Maturity.* New York: Harcourt, Brace and World, 1963.

HARTER, S., AND PIKE, R. *The Pictorial Scale of Perceived Competence and Aceptance for Young Children.* Unpublished monograph, University of Denver, 1981.

HOFSTAETTER, P. R. "The Changing Composition of 'Intelligence': A Study in T-Technique." *J. Genet. Psych., 85* (1954): 159–64.

HOSKINS, T. A., AND SQUIRES, J. E. "Developmental Assessment: A Test for Gross Motor and Reflex Development." *Phys. Thpy., 53* (1973): 117–25.

HUGHES, J. E. *Manual for the Hughes Basic Motor Assessment.* Golden, Co.: University of Colorado, 1979.

HUNT, J. V. "Mental and Motor Development of Preterm Infants during the First Year." Paper presented at the biennial meeting of the Society for Research in Child Development, 1975.

KEOGH, B. K., AND SMITH, C. E. "Visuo-Motor Ability for School Prediction: A Seven Year Study." *Percept. and Motor Skills, 32* (1967): 152–55.

KNOBLOCH, H., AND PASAMANICK, B. "The Developmental Screening Inventory." In H. Knoblock and M. Pasamanick (eds.), *Gesell and Amatruda's Developmental Diagnosis,* 3rd ed. New York: Harper and Row, 1974.

KOONTZ, C. C. *Koontz Child Developmental Program.* Los Angeles: Western Psychological Services, 1974.

KOPPITZ, E. M. *The Bender Gestalt Test for Young Children. Vol II: Research and Application 1963–1973.* New York: Grune and Stratton, 1975.

LOOVIS, E. M., AND ERSING, W. F. *Ohio Motor Assessment.* Cleveland Heights, Ohio, 1979.

MILANI-COMPARETTI, A., AND GIDONI, E. A. "Pattern Analysis of Motor Development and Its Disorders." *Devel. Med. Child Neurol., 9* (1967): 625–35.

NICHOLS, P. L., AND BROMAN, S. H. "Familial Resemblance in Infant Mental Development." *Devel. Psych., 10* (1974): 124–30.

OSERETZKY, N. A. "A Metric Scale for Studying the Motor Capacity of Children in Russia." *J. Clin. Psych., 12* (1948): 37–47.

PARMELEE, A. H., JR. "Newborn Neurological Examination." Unpublished manuscript, August, 1974.

PIERS, E. V., AND HARRIS, D. B. "Age and Other Correles of Self-Concept in Children." *J. Educ. Psych., 55* (1964): 19–95.

POWELL, L. F. "The Effect of Extra Stimulation and Maternal Involvement upon the Development of Low Birth Weight Infants and upon Maternal Behaviors." *Child Development, 45* (1974), 106–111.

PRECHTL, H., AND BEINTEMA, D. *The Neurological Health of the Full Term Newborn Infant.* Clinics in Developmental Medicine, No. 12, London, Spastics Society: Heinemann, 1964.

ROSENBLITH, J. F. "The Modified Graham Behavior Test for Neonates. Test Re-Test Reliability, Normative Data, and Hypothesis for Future Work." *Biologia Neonatorum, 3* (1961): 174–85.

——————— . "Prognostic Value of Behavioral Assessment of Neonates." *Biologia Neonatorum, 6* (1964): 76–103.

SCAMMON, R. E. "First Seriatim Study of Human Growth." *Amer. J. Phys. Anthro., 10* (1927): 329–33.

SERUNIAN, S. A., AND BROMAN, S. H. "Relationship of Apgar Scores and Bayley Mental and Motor Scores." *Child Devel., 46* (1975): 696–700.

SHIPE, D., VANDENBERG, S., AND WILLIAMS, R. D. B. "Neonatal Apgar Ratings as Related to Intelligence and Behavior in Pre-School Children." *Child Devel., 39* (1968): 861–66.

SLOAN, W. "The Lincoln-Oseretsky Motor Development Scale." *Genet. Psych. Monog., 51* (1955): 183–252.

STOTT, D. H. "A General Test of Motor Impairment for Children." *Devel. Med. Child Neurol., 8* (1966): 523–31.

——————— , MOYES, F. A., AND HENDERSON, S. E. *Test of Motor Impairment.* Guelph, Ontario, Canada: Brook Educational Pub. Co., 1972.

THAMS, P. F. "A Factor Analysis of the Lincoln-Oseretsky Motor Development Scale." Unpublished Doctoral dissertation, University of Michigan, 1955.

TOUWEN, B. C. L., AND PRECHTL, H. F. R. *The Neurological Examination of the Child with Minor Nervous Dysfunction.* London: Clinics in Developmental Medicine, Heinemann, 1970.

UZGIRIS, I. C., AND HUNT, J. M. *Toward Ordinal Scales of Psychological Development in Infancy.* Champaign, Ill.: University of Illinois Press, 1975.

WILSON, R. S. "Twins: Mental Development in Pre-School Years." *Devel. Psych., 10* (1974): 580–88.

YANG, R. K. "Early Infant Assessment: An Overview." In J. D. Osofsky (ed.), *Handbook of Infant Development.* New York: Wiley, 1979.

Index